Understanding Acupuncture

About the authors

Dr Stephen Birch has practiced acupuncture since graduating from acupuncture school in 1982. He studied acupuncture extensively in Japan with Yoshio Manaka and senior Toyohari instructors. He has a PhD from the Centre for Complementary Health Studies at Exeter University, Exeter UK, focusing on acupuncture research methods. He has coauthored six books on acupuncture (one with Manaka) has taught acupuncture in both undergraduate and postgraduate level training programs, and has become an internationally renowned instructor in acupuncture. He has also lectured at a number of medical schools and medical conferences in the US. In addition he has been involved in academic and research debates in the field. He helped found the Society for Acupuncture Research, was project director of a clinical trial of acupuncture at Yale University for two years, was involved with acupuncture research at Harvard Medical school, and a consultant to other studies. He participated in both the US Food and Drug Administration's review and eventual approval of acupuncture, and the recent US National Institutes of Health consensus development conference on acupuncture which led to a greater recognition of the value of acupuncture. He currently practices in Holland with his wife where he also continues to pursue his diverse interests in the field of acupuncture.

In 1973, after studying massage, medicinal cooking and acupuncture, **Bob Felt** founded Redwing Book Company, the first US bookseller to concentrate on complementary medicine. In 1981, with his partner Martha Fielding, he founded Paradigm Publications, a publishing company specializing in advance texts and language resources for the study and practice of traditional East Asian medicines. He has edited several of the fields seminal texts, served as the first publically-elected director of the New England School of Acupuncture, and is a member of the Mercy College and CAOMJ advisory boards.

The authors are participants in the Council of Oriental Medical Publishers and support their effort to inform readers of how works in Chinese medicine are prepared. *Understanding Acupuncture* is an original work prepared from the sources referenced. Unless otherwise noted, translated terms follow: N. Wiseman and Y. Feng; *A Practical Dictionary of Traditional Chinese Medicine, Paradigm Publications, Brookline, MA, 1998.*

For Churchill Livingstone

Publishing Manager: Inta Ozols
Design Direction: Judith Wright

Understanding Acupuncture

Stephen J. Birch PhD BA LicAc
Society for Acupuncture Research, Toyohari Association

Robert L. Felt
Paradigm Publications
Brookline, MA, USA

Foreword by
C. David Lytle PhD
Research Biophysicist, Division of Life Sciences,
Food and Drug Administration, Rockville MD, USA

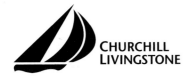

CHURCHILL
LIVINGSTONE

EDINBURGH LONDON NEW YORK PHILADELPHIA SYDNEY TORONTO 1999

CHURCHILL LIVINGSTONE
An imprint of Harcourt Brace and Company Limited

First published 1999

ISBN 0 443 061793

British Library Cataloguing in Publication Data
A catalogue record for this book is available from the
British Library.

Library of Congress Cataloging in Publication Data
A catalog record for this book is available from the Library
of Congress.

Note
Medical knowledge is constantly changing. As new
information becomes available, changes in treatment,
procedures, equipment and the use of drugs become
necessary. The authors and the publishers have, as far as
it is possible, taken care to ensure that the information
given in this text is accurate and up to date. However,
readers are strongly advised to confirm that the information,
especially with regard to drug usage, complies with latest
legislation and standards of practice.

Neither the Publishers nor the authors will be liable for any
loss or damage of any nature occasioned to or suffered by
any person acting or refraining from acting as a result of
reliance on the material contained in this publication.

The
publisher's
policy is to use
**paper manufactured
from sustainable forests**

Printed in China

Contents

Foreword

Understanding Acupuncture is a book whose time has come. In fact, the information, perspective and objective analyses were sorely needed a few years ago when the US Food and Drug Administration and the National Institutes of Health's Office of Alternative Medicine were wrestling with 'what to do about acupuncture.' It is especially important now that acupuncture is starting to break out of the alternative medicine mold and become a serious candidate for complementary medicine.

For the first time in English, we have an up-to-date scholarly treatise on the various forms of acupuncture practiced around the world. The evolution of each different form is traced against the social, economic, medical and scientific settings of that time and place. *Understanding Acupuncture* commences with treatments described in classic Chinese texts and arrives at the current situation in the West, relating the 'theoretical' basis of acupuncture to the tenets of modern medicine and science.

The practice of acupuncture can sound rather mystical. *Understanding Acupuncture* removes the mysticism while retaining the esthetic and practical value of the Qi paradigm. The book is readable, with the many aspects of acupuncture necessary for a thorough and balanced understanding illustrated clearly by carefully chosen examples. It is not a how-to book. Its purpose is to promote understanding by stressing careful scholarship and objective analysis. A particularly educational feature is the side-by-side presentation of the different systems of diagnosis and treatment to illuminate the diverse approaches to acupuncture practice. Boxes, that explain important issues without breaking the flow of the main text, are interspersed throughout. Several models developed to explain acupuncture are presented, from the neurophysiological model to Yoshio Manaka's X-signal model. The reasons for the high

level of acceptance by the Western biomedical world of the neurophysiological model for analgesia are elucidated, along with reservations that show just how limited such a model is.

Perhaps one of the most important issues addressed is how biases and assumptions in research can lead to misinterpretations and misrepresentations, misleading all but the most discerning and knowledgeable. An unfortunate result has been the delayed acceptance of acupuncture by the medical and scientific communities in the West. *Understanding Acupuncture* provides an objective examination of some key studies to illuminate many of the pitfalls waiting to dupe the naive and uninformed. An unbiased comprehension of these issues will continue to be important in the foreseeable future.

Understanding Acupuncture should be required reading for several groups. Most importantly, it should serve as a primary source for regulators and policy makers, including those who must discriminate among who should be regulated and in what manner. This book addresses several issues critical to the regulatory process. One of the most frustrating issues recently has involved discerning which scientific or clinical studies should be given attention, since most published studies have not met the standards of rigor normally demanded by the scientific and clinical communities. The authors have chosen key illustrative examples to educate the reader, drawing reasonable interpretations that policy makers should find helpful.

Inquiring acupuncture students, their instructors and other, practicing acupuncturists should know how the particular acupuncture scheme they are employing fits into the overall picture. *Understanding Acupuncture* will help them be better able to interact with their peers from other acupuncture traditions and, more importantly, with future patients who in turn arrive having had different levels and sources of acupuncture experience. This book will provide physicians, dentists and other members of the allopathic medical community with information to help them understand the utility of acupuncture and interact with patients who use acupuncture as a complementary or alternative health care modality. Indeed, this book would serve well as the acupuncture textbook for a medical school course on alternative/complementary medicine.

Clinical and laboratory investigators need to understand the current models of acupuncture mechanisms, but not be misled into unduly limiting paradigms. *Understanding Acupuncture* gives guidance on how to ask the right research questions and how to or how not to design and interpret experiments on acupuncture efficacy or mechanisms. Researchers also will benefit from detailed explanations on what constitutes adequate treatment (e.g., number and stimulation of needles, number and timing of treatments, individuality of treatment, etc) and what constitutes appropriate treatment controls.

The authors clearly have an impressive breadth and depth of perspective on the various forms of acupuncture practice and how those forms mesh with the medical and scientific worldviews. Few indeed are those with such depth and breadth of knowledge and experience, and fewer still are those who can enlighten others. Both authors know the acupuncture literature and have authored or edited English texts and participated in the evolution of

acupuncture's acceptance in the United States. These latter activities have included dealing with bureaucrats with little, or no, initial understanding of acupuncture. The senior author is an experienced acupuncturist who was a major contributor of material submitted to the FDA, including the manner of presentation and analysis. Perhaps that experience motivated the substantial scholarly effort represented by *Understanding Acupuncture*.

There is a refreshing candor throughout the text. The importance of accurate translations and critical scholarship is stressed. The explanations and descriptions are presented with clarity and thoughtful organization, pointing out the strengths and weaknesses of one issue after another. Many assumptions about acupuncture are challenged, many answers are documented. This will hopefully raise and broaden the comprehension of proponents and opponents alike to the truths and limitations of the various issues in acupuncture and their supporting data.

Understanding Acupuncture belongs on the bookshelf of everyone interested in acupuncture, whatever their reason for interest. The broad, deep, objective perspective will earn it the position of 'first reference' when questions arise. Even my first quick skim through the chapters convinced me of its value. You will agree, and then place it in your place of 'first reference' on acupuncture.

Rockville, MD USA 1999   C. David Lytle

Preface

This is an acupuncture textbook. That may seem an odd claim for a book that offers history, research, and science but no needling instructions. Yet, acupuncture, like many familiar Western arts and sciences, is intellectually hierarchal. Learning acupuncture has never been solely a matter of learning technical details. History shows that some acupuncturists have always been technicians trained only to follow the established procedures of a family tradition, teacher, or school. Others have been medical artists whose refined sensory and physical skills were honed by a social, moral, or religious philosophy. Some have been eminent teachers and innovators, who extended acupuncture through scholarship and experimentation. Fewer have been of such rare brilliance that their inspirations and realizations are the landmarks of acupuncture's history and substance of its practice.

In Asian societies the practise of traditional acupuncture is not unlike many modern Western careers. For example, some electricians are trained to follow instructions known as 'codes.' They know how to install electrical equipment that will pass commercial and governmental inspections. But those code books contain no history, no science, no references; none of the information by which to judge the intellectual or scientific foundations of the devices they install. On the other hand, the electrical engineers who design those devices learn not only the historical development of the principles, but also the science necessary to create new systems. They are guided not by codes but by qualitative and quantitative standards, some of which derive from allied fields. They are taught not to follow rules but to understand and apply measures and standards. Those standards are developed by physicists who refine their ideas by subjecting them to experimental trials. Following this extended analogy, this is a

textbook for those who must judge for themselves the utility of information provided by academic, clinical, commercial, and scientific sources.

When traders arrive on a foreign shore they bargain for what most brightly shines of their own values. It is thus reasonable that the idea of acupuncture that has reached the broadest Western audiences reflects the values of those who first discovered it. Some information, particularly that carried by scholarly and scientific vehicles, has received little attention, not only because it is not always applicable to the acquisition of clinical skill, but also because commercial sources are more quickly and easily available. This too is expected, because acupuncture's economic application is the most powerful stimulus for its survival and transmission. However, there is more.

Whether it is for students evaluating a career in acupuncture, acupuncturists who must judge the services and products they are offered, teachers who hope to develop better courses, or the rapidly expanding corps of physicians whose patients need to know if acupuncture can help, technical knowledge alone is not enough. Acupuncture must be understood as a human intellectual pursuit in order to best choose a course of study, to make referrals, to judge efficacy, or to advise a complex health care system.

This is not a theoretical need. Because more and more people associated with the practice or delivery of medicine feel, along with a majority of their patients, that there is a useful role for acupuncture in modern medical systems, acupuncture must now adapt not only to the needs of new patient populations but also to the demands of Western culture. This is nothing new. Acupuncture's 2000 year history is a story not only of gradual dissemination to virtually every country on Earth, but also of adaptation to the needs of many different cultures in many different eras. Thus we have concentrated on the presentation of principles. By examining ideas common to most views and systems, we are best prepared to understand and apply the technical details. However, if only because there is no consensus among systems and cultures, we have considered many views while preparing this book. We have taken a survey approach, reporting facts, thoughts, and opinions gathered from experts and practitioners.

Among the things that are clear from this survey is that, without understanding the broad outlines of Chinese medical history, it is easy, and perhaps even inevitable to misunderstand acupuncture. The themes and techniques of acupuncture begin in history and can only be clearly understood in relation to the needs of those who created·them. A tradition can only be understood through its history. Indeed, even the most basic technical features of acupuncture — needle selection, insertion technique, and stimulation — vary with time, culture, and school of thought. It is also true that acupuncture has been widely practiced in many countries besides China, in some for more than a millennium. Without recognizing the contribution of these societies, acupuncture's story is incomplete. It is also necessary to understand something about other traditional medicines, for example, traditional pharmaceutics and massage, to understand acupuncture's place among China's traditional medical arts.

Acupuncture's breadth must also be understood. Acupuncture is as broad as it is ancient. It includes techniques beyond the use of needles. Historically, not only was there a selection of needles, nine to be exact, but several of those needles were never used to puncture. Acupuncture also was, and is, routinely used with moxibustion, a heat therapy. Its therapeutic repertoire has also included a bloodletting very different from that of medieval Europe, a suction stimulation now called 'cupping,' massage and physical manipulation in several forms, as well as disciplines like *qi gong* that apply movement arts to medicine.

Practitioners in different times and different cultures have thought many different things when they used the Chinese term that today we call 'acupuncture'. It is still a word that is difficult to define, precisely because it is sometimes used in a very narrow sense, and sometimes more broadly, with meanings that include many commonly (but not universally) associated techniques. In this book we use the term 'acupuncture' in its narrow sense; that is, as the therapeutic use of needles by those

specifically trained to do so. We describe moxibustion as a separate tradition.

Today, acupuncturists use a range of tools and techniques, from disposable needles to electric stimulators and lasers. Each defines what they do as acupuncture. Speaking precisely, however, *zhen* in Chinese refers to the use of needles. Although individual practitioners have combined needling with other techniques, there has never been any absolute link between one treatment method and another. Although the time required to master the skills has tended to keep clinician's practices fairly narrow, the choice to combine different therapies has always been a mix of personal preference, the training available, social needs, and economic advantages.

In sum, there is no quick and easy description of acupuncture; there is no one and only answer we can ask you to believe at the expense of all others. There is no one and only explanatory analogy that diminishes all others. There is no unique access to clinical success. There is only a fascinating story of human genius applied to the universal human quest for a long, happy, and healthy life.

It is hard to tell that story without superlative, even mythic terms. Words such as 'ancient' and 'cosmological' are so often mixed with a space-age vocabulary of 'energetics,' that acupuncture has acquired the reputation of something fantastic. It often sounds as if writers were claiming to have found a fully functional electrical stimulator among the wood ash and flint tools of an ancient cave. However, acupuncture's roots are not fantastic but indistinct. It begins in mythology and archeology, reaches the domains of philology, anthropology, and history as early as the −3rd century, and arrives in modern times entwined with sufficient complexity to challenge linguistics, biology, psychology, political science, economics, and sociology. In fact, making any statement about any of Asia's indigenous medicines requires the knowledge of experts in several arts and sciences.

Yet, even for experts the facts are elusive. China has not only burned books but has re-written them almost routinely. Thus scholars must search for unknown authors' meanings in texts that have been re-edited, re-written, re-attributed, re-interpreted, and censored. As the wisdom of one age lost favor, tradition and history, logic and philosophy, and science and medicine were rewritten. Neither were Asian cultures pure or isolated. Over caravan trails and through oft-told tales, shared myths, Asian religions and cultural institutions have migrated among populations for nearly three millennia. Thus their cultures reflect one another, often as imperfect mirrors distorted by longevous memories of invasions, wars, and ethnic hatreds.

Neither is reporting on acupuncture in the modern era free of problems. In China nothing escaped the turmoil of the 20th century. Even the so-called objective sciences suffered in China's political upheavals. For example, China's once considerable progress in genetics was surrendered to a politically correct but fallacious Soviet theory. Then, during a devastating cultural revolution, peasants became laboratory directors and senior scientists were sent to distant villages for 'rural re-education,' a euphemism for social isolation and psychological, and even physical, torture. Purges, plagues, and the starvation brought about by vastly mismanaged resources may have killed as many as 20 million Chinese in the post-liberation (1949) period. During this time, elements of acupuncture changed dramatically, as it was conscripted to serve not only China's vast health-care needs but also its political imperatives.

Within the lives of China's current political leaders acupuncture has been described as a vile feudal superstition that should be entirely purged from communist society. It has been seen as a primitive, pre-Marxist dialectic and as a treasury of techniques that might be useful if integrated with modern medicine. Then, as acupuncture and Chinese traditional pharmacotherapies were enfused with modern medicine to produce the synthesis known as Traditional Chinese Medicine (TCM), acupuncture became a secondary component of the now-proposed 'World Medicine,' a policy-derived goal where traditional and modern practices are to be integrated and imparted to other nations. However, the theoretical co-equality of integrated medicine has been comfortable for neither biomedical nor traditional practitioners, and preserving the integrity of traditional medicine against the encroachment of its Western rival continues to be a strong impetus for its adaptation and development.

Today, TCM is officially one of three theoretically co-equal branches of medicine in the People's Republic of China. In this policy, known as 'The Three Roads,' traditional practices such as acupuncture, herbal medicine, qi gong, and the martial arts are permitted to seek their own ground in a competitive coalition with biomedicine and the TCM supported by the state. In fact, China's struggle to bring its native medicine into harmony with modern biomedicine has been a consistent theme throughout the 20th century. In the face of truly vast public-health problems, innovations such as the barefoot doctors, and massive people's campaigns against epidemic disease, have made the integration of traditional techniques with Western science a matter of acute attention in the West. While once highly visible techniques such as so-called 'acupuncture anesthesia' are now known as less worthwhile than when first brought to Western attention, and the budgets for their development have become accordingly less generous, the integration of traditional techniques into the Western medical infrastructure continues to fascinate writers.

In fact, this is so much the case that some of acupuncture's outstanding accomplishments in China and the rest of East Asia have received almost no attention. In an era when managed care is the central focus of Western medical economics, China's experience using traditional medicine in a vast, cost-driven public health-care system is of considerable potential value to the West. Although Japan, Korea, and Taiwan are less often investigated than is China, acupuncture nonetheless plays a role in the modern managed medical institutions in these countries. Although acupuncture has earned a stable and not insignificant role, often in regard to conditions for which Western patients seek acupuncture treatment, this has gone nearly unnoticed in the West. Today, for example, the courses and tests used to qualify acupuncturists in the USA are mostly drawn from TCM sources.

Although Western views of acupuncture have been less politically driven than in China, they are nonetheless just as strongly colored by cultural needs and desires. Some Western writers see in China's medicine an antidote to what they believe to be a dangerously technological and impersonal medicine. Others see acupuncture as the product of a golden age, believing not only that it was fully formed in antiquity, but also that it suffers no deficit except a loss of purity. Quoting Chinese texts that long ago discussed lost, ancient wisdom, these writers proffer images of pure sages who lived long lives uncorrupted by pain or disease. While righteousness and wellness are so inextricably linked in Chinese thought that even bubonic plagues in the 20th century were attributed to the misbehavior of the victims, such views better mirror our own culture's religious images of 'before the fall' than they reflect the evidence of archaeology or history.

In Western thought a long-lived idea is no more or less true than one just now conceived; if anything, we are biased in favor of the new, of progress. However, perhaps stimulated by our dimming infatuation with technology, age does give ideas a patina of truth. Because acupuncture's patina is amazing by any culture's standards, its longevity often lures Western authors into projecting modern ideas backward into antiquity. This happens even to the most cautious and well intentioned. When George Soulie de Morant, the father of acupuncture in the West, arrived in China in 1901, Chinese archaeology and history were still tightly bound by tradition. Thus he returned to the West with a story that began in the −3rd millennium. Although he accurately represented his sources, he delivered unlikely dates that have been quoted and re-quoted. Even today, dates of −2800 or earlier are commonly ascribed to Chinese books written in the first century.

Today, Chinese medical history is often treated like a rich but unpleasant uncle whom we call when in need but otherwise ignore. Although tradition, which can only be understood through history, is often offered as proof of acupuncture's clinical validity, history plays almost no role in the education of Western acupuncturists. Authors who link modern acupuncture technically to the ancient past are so rarely challenged that there is a popular impression that peasants in ancient China were treated exactly like patients in modern London or Beijing. This image obliterates not only the actual social order of feudal China, but also the adaptive genius of acupuncture. It also burdens modern acupuncture with a reputation for religiosity. Because acupuncture is by any measure ancient, and by anyone's standard one of the most longevous products of human genius, its history cannot be so profoundly abbreviated. It did not rise fully grown like a Mediterranean Venus but rather earned its keep in thousands of dusty marketplaces by continual change and adaptation — an accomplishment that needs no fantastic antiquity to earn our conscientious attention.

In China, age is still honored to a greater degree than the West. Furthermore, Western ideas of scholarship have never been universal. Even today Chinese writers are rarely edited or conform to the scholarly conventions of the West. It has been common for Chinese authors to ascribe their writings to some ancient writer, borrowing credibility for their ideas. The *Huang Di Nei Jing* of −100 to −200 was ascribed to Huang Di, the Yellow Emperor of −2800. The *Nan Jing*, written near the first century, was ascribed to the famous clinician Bian Que of the −5th century. This practice continues throughout the history of acupuncture in China, indeed, into the 20th century. Thus historical accounts need to be screened carefully in order to do justice to the story.

How to proceed

In avoiding the presentation of an entirely personal or fanciful version of acupuncture, it is not only important to follow the journalist's regimen of 'who, what, when, and where,' but also to describe what parts of the story we have chosen not to tell. The subject is so large that its is easy to misrepresent. Therefore, we have followed a set of principles we have taken from the consensus of experts.

In studying any subject as vast as acupuncture, there is considerable room for disagreement. Sinologists have already filled that room with competing ideas of Chinese intellectual history. However, there are principles about which there is no significant disagreement, and it is these that we have tried to honor. For example, sinologists agree that acupuncture, like all Chinese traditional medicines, must be understood in its cultural context. In addition, experts agree that Chinese traditional medicine is not a smooth and invariant monolith, but an aged sculpture of great complexity. Some features have been worn smooth and indistinct by time, while others are being constantly re-sculpted. Thus, sinologists understand that we must examine the specifics of acupuncture's practice in each particular era. And, for example, although scholars may disagree about the precise extent of Confucian influence, there is no disagreement that the major Asian religions must be studied. We have thus reported the major cultural influences.

Sinologists also agree that the history of acupuncture cannot be divorced from the history of Chinese culture. If we are to understand acupuncture, we must also understand the social, economic, and political activities of each era. Thus, in the historical summary that begins this book we have reported the major intellectual, social, political, and economic events that affected Chinese culture. Because Chinese history is usually reported in eras named for a hereditary ruling family, what are called 'dynasties,' our report is ordered chronologically by the generally accepted modern dates for each. However, this is only a useful way to write a chapter, not a truth. Acupuncture probably developed in a far less orderly way, but too much of acupuncture's development remains unknown for even experts to make definitive statements.

Another area of broad agreement among experts regards the heterogeneity of Chinese traditional medicine. Chinese traditional medicine is roughly equivalent to Western medicine in the extent of its written history. Its library includes more than ten-thousand texts, by thousands of writers. It is a history with hundreds of critical events and thousands of schools of thought and practice, many of which have never been explored by Western clinicians or scholars. It is simplistic, but not unfair, to summarize this complexity as if there were three general categories of Chinese traditional medicine. The first is the uncapitalized 'Chinese traditional medicine' — the heterogeneous medicine of China's long recorded history. The second is the 'traditional East Asian medicines' (TEAM) that evolved as other Asian societies imported medical practices and ideas from China. The third is the capitalized Traditional Chinese Medicine (TCM). This is the synthesis of internal medicine and biomedicine currently taught in Chinese medical schools to which modern Chinese acupuncture has conformed. TCM is what is best known in the West. As such, we afford it a greater emphasis than its relatively few years of existence would allow in an academic history.

The newer TCM is, of course, a subset of the others. All three categories are complexes of related ideas, some of which have been dominant at times, dormant at others. Furthermore, these ideas are linked, intertwined and inseparable to the point that undue concentration on any aspect can de-emphasize much of what is important. In fact, the subject is so vast that any concentration can be misleading. Fortunately, the work of Professor Paul Unschuld has provided us with a central theme with which to guide your tour of acupuncture past and present.

Through his study of the surviving artifacts and primary documents — the foundation texts of Chinese medicine and acupuncture — Professor Unschuld has described the logical process by which information was gathered, processed, and used to arrive at medical conclusions. This he termed the 'medicine of systematic correspondence.' This is what we have taken as an organizing theme. Its principal feature, the recognition of observable patterns in nature as the basis for medical categorization and decision-making, is not only the development we will follow from the beginning of Chinese history into the future, but also the essence of each aspect of acupuncture we explore.

The medicine of systematic correspondence

Although we will later describe the medicine of systematic correspondence in greater detail, for now, begin by thinking of it as the discovery that humans interact with their environment in patterns that can be realized through observation using the trained but naked human senses. Although China never developed the science of statistics, the observation of pattern plays a role parallel to that of statistics in the West. Both disciplines assume that repeatability substantiates ideas. Pattern in Chinese traditional medicines describes the most probable outcome of a particular set of clinical observations, just as statistics are used to predict trends. Pattern is not absolute, just as statistics are not absolute, both represent what is probable.

Although Chinese clinical researchers still do not use statistical analysis to any great extent, the patterns used in acupuncture were observed over very long times. Although the mathematical safeguards of statistics allow many misperceived relationships to be discovered, they also tend to limit research to problems that can be assessed by statisticians. The so-called 'test of time' has allowed Chinese traditional medicine to accrete scientifically untested assumptions, but it has also provided the ability to recognize patterns that were unseen or untestable in the West. For example, among the patterns of acupuncture are conditions that, with the appropriate training can be seen, felt, and even intuited.

This reliance on the naked senses and human perceptions has had a profound influence on all of Chinese traditional medicine but is critical to acupuncture, which is essentially a hands-on skill. To understand this more intuitively, imagine that you have a time machine fitted with language translators of the utmost sophistication. Imagine that you are able to return to China in antiquity, find the finest physicians, the greatest physician-scholars, chosen by whatever standards you wish. Follow them through their days and you will certainly find that theirs was a bedside medicine. Unlike the clinical orientation of today's acupuncturists, these ancients and their apprentices worked at their patients' bedsides, providing acute care, and following the progression of disease through patient observation. Although there were social reasons for the development of a beside medicine, the critical point is that practitioners' senses were their most important tools.

No matter how sophisticated your time machine, whether you looked in the imperial palace or a peasant hut, you would not find a thermometer or a blood-pressure cuff. Acupuncture would be already ancient before these, the most basic measurement tools of biomedicine, would arrive. Clinicians thought about the heat perceived at the body's surface ('heat effusion') rather than the measure of the temperature within ('fever'). Thus, there is very little in acupuncture that was quantified in the way of the West. In the medicine of systematic correspondence the microcosm is not the world of measurable bacteria, viruses, genes or the energies of subatomic process; it is the sensorial world of humanity, our thoughts, our feelings, our bodily experiences, the sensations of our lives. The universe was not the infinity our modern instruments describe — vast galaxies separated by measured expanses of invisible, cold, dark matter — but the subtle seasons of human life revealed by steady observation. Not only were heaven, human, and earth closer than our modern view proposes, they were intimately linked. Thus patterns in the medicine of systematic correspondence are at times related to calendric cycles (natural phenomena), but are always reported according to their sensory qualities. The same is true of disease identifications. For example, what modern TCM physicians routinely label 'acute conjuctivitis,' their traditional Chinese counterparts called 'wind fire eye,' for its cause, sensation, and color. What we call 'organs,' Chinese doctors thought of as 'depots and palaces,' images that reflected their view of order in life and society.

These naked sense observations and trained perceptions can be seen forming into a coherent system in three landmark documents: the Ma Wang-dui scripts of the late –3rd or early –2nd second century, the *Huang Di Nei Jing* texts of the –1st century, and the *Nan Jing* of the 1st century. These documents trace over approximately 400 years the development of the major conceptual features of the medicine of systematic correspondence. These features include the development of the *qi* concept, the functional description of bodily process, and the theory of *qi* circulation on which modern acupuncture depends — what we call the 'qi paradigm.'

'*Qi*' and 'paradigm' are both powerful words. Because *qi* is so often translated as 'energy' and paradigm is usually thought of in its Khunian but not its linguistic sense, both words have come to note a thinker's place in a presumed East-versus-West, tradition-versus-science conflict. This is sometimes explained as a shift of 'paradigms.' Thus, for example, questioning the equation of *qi* to energy, or proposing that acupuncture shares means and methods with biomedicine, is sometimes considered a challenge to acupuncture itself. Some writers have even proposed that modern medical thinkers and traditional theorists inhabit such different paradigms that they cannot share methods of research, or even participate in a productive medical pluralism.

This is a pessimism we do not share. Traditional and conventional medicines share many ideas and observations. Although *qi* is not a shared concept, the observations upon which it is based are often familiar. When considered individually there are some traditional ideas of *qi* that can be fairly described and researched as energy. There are also traditional ideas of *qi* that are entirely lost when submerged in this connotively powerful Western idea. Thus, to understand acupuncture we must stand aside from positions in today's debates and examine it on its own terms.

Acupuncture is paradigmatic, not because it conflicts with Western ideas, but because it is a set of concepts linked, stored, and transmitted through the linguistic relations that reflect the experience of Asian peoples. It is true that when traditional acupuncturists labeled an individual's state as a 'lung *yin* vacuity' they were not referencing laboratory tests. However, they were logically using features of their language to access the treatment knowledge it stored, in this case by following the top-down logic of vacuity–*yin*–lung to determine acupoints known to positively affect the signs they observed. Thus, although there are instances where Western ideas of what can be true, and how truth must be tested, do affect how proponents and skeptics think about acupuncture, particularly in East Asia where the faith in Western science has had considerable cultural impact, the paradigmatic characteristic with which this text is most concerned, is acupuncture's coherence with the cultural constructs from which it was derived.

Thus using the term 'qi paradigm' is a way to emphasize that acupuncture is more than any one of its aspects. It is a reminder that the whole must be explored. This text is meant as a beginning to that exploration. Practically, however, we have arranged the text recognizing that the materials presented are of greater or lesser interest to readers whose primary interests are in different disciplines.

A readers' guide

The first section of this book, 'What Acupuncture is,' focuses on acupuncture's history up to the 20th century, and the traditional and modern models used to explain its function. This is the ideal starting point for any investigation. However, those who require immediate access to information regarding acupuncture's efficacy can begin with the second section, 'How Acupuncture is Practised,' using the first section as a reference when required. The second section concerns the theoretical and practical issues of efficacy, diagnostic processes and methods, therapeutic techniques, and clinical examples.

Section 1 What acupuncture is

In Chapter 1 you will find a history of acupuncture from its earliest references to the present. This history focuses on the Ma Wang-dui scripts, the *Nei Jing*, and the *Nan Jing* as the foundation for the development of acupuncture in China. With its diversity, contradictions, and mythologic qualities, it is impossible to understand many of acupuncture's theories and techniques without understanding their history. The sense of a theory or practice in acupuncture is often best described by its relationship to the social environment.

In Chapter 2 acupuncture's acculturation to the present is described in roughly chronological and nation-by-nation sequences. There you will see the scope of acupuncture's adaptability and its current status in representative countries where it is practiced throughout the world. The emphasis in this chapter is on how modern societies are using acupuncture. Whereas the information in Chapter 1 could be drawn from sources that have been subject to academic scrutiny, there are few peer-reviewed sources of historical, clinical, or economic data for the last half of the 20th century. Thus much of the information is from our interviews with the persons involved. Where it was possible to do so, we have based our estimates and assumptions on non-academic sources that may be verified independently; for example, counts of advertisements and article subjects in professional periodicals, and commercial sales and mailing lists.

In Chapter 3 these historical trends are summarized in the basic traditional models of acupuncture, in particular the theory of *qi* and the medicine of systematic correspondence. Because for most of its service to humanity acupuncture has been a skill taught by apprenticeship, different schools of thought have arisen. In each of these traditions some correspondence sets have been considered more valuable than others, and some skills have been more highly refined. Thus, in this chapter we have concentrated on correspondences and patterns common to most, with particular emphasis on those that are refined in representative traditions. Here we have relied largely on secondary literature that is commonly available in English-speaking countries, with an emphasis on texts that are documented as to primary language source and translation method.

In Chapter 4 we explore the major contemporary explanations of acupuncture. Both Chinese and Western scientists have investigated various ideas of how acupuncture accomplishes change in the human body. This is an important chapter even for those who are not immediately concerned with research, because it is in the scientific study of acupuncture where East must truly meet West. Until there is an acceptable rationale for acupuncture the longevity of its current Western acculturation remains in doubt. This chapter concentrates on the subjects that have been most widely researched. However, speculative concepts for which there is some evidence are also discussed.

Section 2 How acupuncture is practiced

In Chapter 5 the matter of efficacy is addressed in a broad sense by looking at the entirety of the treatment model, including how researchers understand who seeks acupuncture and the different ways in which questions of efficacy are asked and answered. The discussion includes a list of conditions for which there is reasonable evidence for referrals or further investigation. Although you may access this chapter directly if your only interest is the medical utility or economics, acupuncture research issues can only be focused fully in the light of Section 1.

In Chapter 6 we examine the diversity of practice in acupuncture by describing several currently active systems of evaluation, diagnosis, and, where applicable, prognosis. The emphasis in this chapter is the commonality of practical treatment options within the diversity of methods. Again, this and the following chapter will give you a broad idea of what acupuncturists actually do in clinic; the diversity in acupuncture must be seen fully as an outgrowth of its long history.

Chapter 7 is based on actual cases drawn from published sources and the clinical records of our colleagues who afforded us the time to edit accurate but succinct case stories. We also used questionnaires and interviews with several working practitioners who follow particular systems of practice to insure that we did not unfairly represent anyone's clinical approach. Although the survey is not scientifically valid, its results closely match the experience of relevant commercial sources.

Finally, we attempt to speculate regarding the outcome of current trends and to draw conclusions from the latest decisions and consensus statements from American and European governmental and regulatory agencies.

IJmuiden, The Netherlands, 1998   S.B.
Brookline, MA, USA, 1998   R.F.

Acknowledgements

The writers' most sincere acknowledgements are their references. Those are the people who made our own work possible. It is they who are ultimately responsible for the successes of *Understanding Acupuncture;* we are responsible for its failures.

Without Paul Unschuld's steady and persistent investigation of the primary sources of Chinese medicine, the first two chapters could not have been written. Many of the major themes we present begin with Dr Unschuld's insights. Nigel Wiseman's research is equally seminal. His dedication to Chinese sources and to the Chinese view of Chinese medicine provides us all with insight and information not found in the literature of personal perspective and Western interpretation.

Yoshio Manaka's generosity in sharing his work, his network of colleagues, his intelligence, wit, and inspiration were also very important in writing this book. We would like to thank Ido No Nippon Sha, in particular Mr Soichiro Tobe, for sending us important historical documents, books, and papers.

We are also grateful to those who took time from their own busy schedules to comment on particular chapters in their formative stages. Richard Hammerschlag's contribution cannot be overstated. Without his careful critique, readers would have been more often confused. Paul Unschuld, Nigel Wiseman, Arthur Margolin, David Lytle, Marnae Ergil, Harriet Mann, and Rod Sperry all contributed in a similar manner. We thank all who generously provided cases, completed questionnaires, answered calls, sat through interviews, answered e-mail, and attended discussions. We hope the book lives up to your expectations and is worthy of your contributions.

Pat Culliton, Mike Smith, Bill Prensky, Charles Chace, Hannah Bradford, Zoe Brenner, Jing-feng Cai, Dan Kenner, Dan Bensky, Joseph Helms, Miki Shima, June Brazil, Roberta Chow, Mark Friedman, Peter Eckman, Kouei Kuwahara, Michael Helmeh, Paul Zmiewski, Marnae Ergil, Kevin Ergil, and Craig Mitchell each materially contributed.

Others who contributed through their support of our work include Bob Jamison, Kodo Fukushima, Akihiro Takai, and Kiichiro Tsutani. Inta Ozols critically reviewed the work in progress and substantively improved it. We would like to thank numerous unnamed patients, students, peers, authors, and clients who contributed their experiences. We thank Sam Bercholz for the push it took to get the project started, and Jesse Jacobs for the technical skill to bring the project to a close. Finally, we would not have been able even to begin *Understanding Acupuncture* without the unfailing support of Junko Ida and Martha Fielding. Both were generous concerning our time away from our families, despite the energy with which sons Nigel and Dylan dashed around their feet. Junko assisted with translations and some of the scholarship. Without the time provided by Martha Fielding and Redwing Book Company's tolerance of Bob's inattention, the book would never have been finished.

What acupuncture is

1

History

The mythologic past

Modern Chinese archeology came of age in the social and political environment that followed the revolution of 1949, what the Chinese call 'Liberation.' It was a time of supreme skepticism, not only concerning traditional medicine, but also all that was traditional to China. The conclusions reached in this period countered what had been an often fanciful chronology of events that exaggerated the antiquity of Chinese discoveries. Previously, even careful Western writers had accepted the −3rd millennium as the earliest date for the practice of acupuncture. In fact, the Chinese people had been taught for generations that their culture had existed intact for 5000 years.[1] However, the archaeological record tells a different story.

The beginning of Chinese medicine is traditionally dated to the period −23 000 to −2000. This is a long blank period in the record of human habitation in China. There is evidence of a non-Mongolian race migrating from north to south following the last ice age, but then modern archaeology reveals nothing until a late stone age mongolian culture appears around −2000. This blank period is known as the 'neolithic hiatus' and is established by geologic evidence that the climate of northern China was so arid that it could not support a population. Suddenly though, a change occurs around −2000: there is plentiful evidence of villages, even large towns hunting, husbandry, and agriculture.[2]

In short, after a long blank period, a late stone-age culture appropriate to human development of the time appears. However, the first real evidence of culture, beyond pottery and tools, begins with the Shang society of approximately –1523. Recognizing that we are passing over the mythology of the vast period between these dates, some of which evidences a continuum of mythologic themes with India and the Middle East, we can divide our historic exploration into periods that begin with the Shang (Table 1.1).

Shang, –1523 to –1027: the classic bronze age in China

The culture of the Shang was agrarian, based on small towns and villages. There was a hereditary nobility and a king, but the majority of people lived as stone-age peasants. From the Shang through to the middle Zhou, the –8th century, Chinese civilization corresponded to that of India in these regards. What is outstanding about this period is how little is

Table 1.1

China	Japan
–1523 to –1027: Shang, *the classic Chinese bronze age.* Demonological beliefs and ancestral propitiation indicate that a medicine distinct from religion has yet to develop	– 4500 to – 250: primitive **Jomon** culture emerges
–1027 to –772: early Zhou, *a period of classical feudalism.* Agricultural advances permit the raising of larger armies and workforces led by hereditary, absolute rulers. Wu shamen lead a ritual-based religious system in which medicine is rooted in magical and demonological beliefs	
–772 to –480: middle Zhou, *a period of declining feudalism.* Recorded history begins, Confucianism arises in the midst of 'farm and fight' principalities. Medicine, although dominated by magical correspondences and demonology, begins to develop as a distinct activity	
–480 to –221: late Zhou, *the period of Warring States.* Chinese culture descends into a chaos of warring principalities. Daoism arises and the five phases emerge as medicine begins to develop as an institution	–300 to 300: **Yayoi** culture establishes rice agriculture
–221 to –206: Qin, *the period of book burning.* Autocratic rule creates an empire that establishes and consolidates social and cultural institutions by creating a governmental bureaucracy	
–206 to 220: Han, *the period of systematization.* In a flowering of Chinese culture, the medicine of systematic correspondence dominates acupuncture through seminal texts such as the *Nei Jing* and *Nan Jing.* Although the *Shang Han Lun* is also written in this era, its incorporation of naturally occurring drugs into the medicine of systematic correspondence fails to find followers	–150: small tribal towns have developed into federations
220 to 589: Six Dynasties, *a period of disunity.* Buddhist influences are active in China. The medicine of systematic correspondence becomes more formal and a technical literature develops	330: **Yamato** government established
590 to 617; Sui, *a period of reunification.* Chinese culture, including an acupuncture that has refined its clinical details, spreads throughout Asia	552 to 710: **Asuka** period. Import of Chinese culture begins. The Japanese begin a conservative and detailed absorption of Chinese ideas

Table 1.1 *(cont'd)*

China	Japan
618 to 906: Tang, *a period of culmination.* While Chinese medical ideas are diffused and absorbed throughout Asia, Chinese developments are dominated by the search for alchemical immortality during a period of immense wealth and cultural fecundity	710 to 794: **Nara** period. Expansion of contact with China. The first Imperial Medical College opens
907 to 960: Five Dynasties, *a period of disunity.* A period of governmental inadequacy	794 to 1185: **Heian** period. Curtailment of contact with China encourages native Japanese developments
960 to 1264: Song, *the period of neo-Confucianism.* The medicine of systematic correspondence predominates. Traditional medicine as drug therapy is incorporated into the qi paradigm	1185 to 1333: **Kamakura** period. Introduction of Zen Buddhism, first Shogunate established
1264 to 1368: Yuan, *the period of Mongol control.* European influences begin to take hold. First independent medical college established	1333 to 1568: **Muromachi**. A time of increasing restlessness. The first appearance of Europeans
1368 to 1643: Ming, *a period of restoration.* Democratization of the Confucian bureaucracy leads to an information explosion, greater heterogeneity, individualism. The extremely influential *Zhen Jiu Da Cheng* and *Ben Cao Gang Mu* are written	1568 to 1600: **Momoyama**, the unification of Japan. The first resistance to Europeanization appears. A resurgence of Japanese innovations in acupuncture begins to flourish
1644 to 1911: Qing, *the end of the empire.* The decline of traditional medicine becomes severe as the Chinese people lose faith in their traditions. Acupuncture largely lost. The *Yi Xue Yuan Liu Lun* is written	1600 to 1853: **Edo-Tokugawa**. Isolationism, but the importation of Western science and medicine continues
	1853 to 1868: transition to modern Japan. Rapid import and assimilation of Western culture
	1868 to 1912: **Meiji Restoration**. Intense and universal modernization and industrialization leave acupuncture reduced and politically marginalized

actually known. Not only is most of the information archaeological rather than historical, the objects must be interpreted from a mythic tradition that has been extensively doctored.[3] In mythologist Joseph Campbell's words:

...all of the myths (or rather, as we now have them, moralizing anecdotes) of the Chinese golden age have to be recognized as the productions rather of a Confucian forest of pencils than any 'good earth' or 'forest primeval.' And, if gems or jades are to be found among them for the actual mythology of Yangshao, Lungshan [Longshan], Shang, or even Chou [Zhou] (anything earlier, that is to say, than Shih Huang Ti's [Shi Huang Di's] burning of the books, 213 B.C.), we have to realize that they have been lifted from the primitive, and remounted carefully in a late, highly sophisticated setting, like

an old Egyptian scarab mounted as a ring for some fine lady's hand.[4]

In short, we are dealing with a history that has been rewritten to suit a later age, something we will meet again and again in acupuncture's story. However, and to whatever extent the tales have been remounted, the Shang period begins with an intact and clearly earlier mythology. These myths describe the Chinese founders of civilization. Three of these five rulers of ancient China were revered as the founders of Chinese medicine, as they were through the following Zhou dynasty, and they are as myths to the present day: Fu Xi, Shen Nong, and Huang Di (Fig. 1.1).

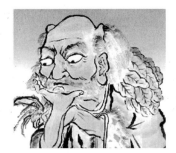

Figure 1.1 Detail of Shen Nong, by Yoshio Manako. (Watercolour on parchment, courtesy of R. Felt.)

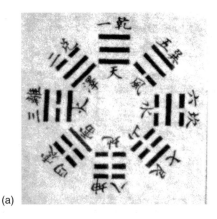

(a)

Fu Xi was the inventor of picture symbols, who taught humankind the rules of marriage and the arts of fishing, husbandry, cooking, and music. To philosophy, and by extension medicine, he contributed the *ba gua*, or eight trigrams, on which the *Yi Jing* is based.

Shen Nong is said to have discovered the curing virtues of plants, to have established markets for the exchange of commodities, and to have extended the eight trigrams Fu Xi formed into the 64 hexagrams of the *Yi Jing*. He is the reputed author of the *Shen Nong Ben Cao*, an early materia medica of Chinese traditional medicine. However, even Shen Nong is eclipsed in importance by Huang Di, the so-called 'Yellow Emperor.'

Huang Di is said to have written with his minister Qi Bo the *Nei Jing*, or 'Canon of Internal Medicine.' He is also said to have taught humankind to manufacture with wood, ceramics, and metal, and to have ordered the building of the first boats and wheeled vehicles. From his 25 sons came 12 of the feudal families ruling during the Zhou.

The archaeological record provides a picture of a spiritual order quite different than that of benign ruler–doctors presiding over a golden age. Between 1928 and 1937 the royal graves of the Shang were excavated by J. G. Anderson at the ancient Shang capital of Anyang.[5] These tombs were not unlike the tombs of Egypt. The royal warrior is buried in the deepest part, covered by the artifacts and weapons he used in life, as well as animals and humans sacrificed to his death. China's participation in human sacrifice at the death of a king evidences, as it

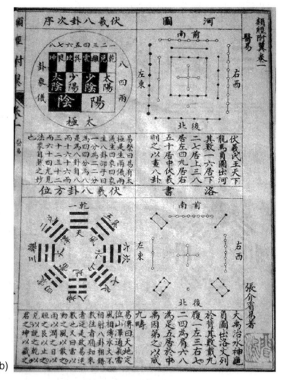

(b)

Figure 1.2 Detail of *Yi Jing* patterns. (Courtesy of R. Felt.)

did in the cultures of Egypt, Crete, and India, that the king was believed to be more than a secular ruler. Kings served as a link between humanity and the supernatural in an ancestral, demonological belief system that would survive in various forms until the modern era. These ideas in their most ancient forms were alive for a considerable period in China. As late as –420 the philosopher Mo Zi would complain that:

...in the case of an Emperor, sometimes several hundred and never less than twenty or thirty of his servants are slain to follow him; for a general or a principal minister sometimes twenty or thirty people are slain, and never less than four or five.[6]

In Shang China the dead were believed to influence the living but to depend on the living for their provisions. 'Di,' as the supreme or divine ancestor was known, provided good harvests and assistance in battle. Yet, only the king's ancestors were able to influence Di. Thus the king was also the chief diviner and used 'oracle bones' to communicate with his ancestors and seek the cooperation of Di. Cattle bones, and later turtle shells, were drilled and heated. This caused cracks and these cracks were interpreted by the king or a diviner.[7] Medical questions are among the more prominent requests.

However, medicine was not a system distinct from religion. Treatment was essentially propitiation and medicine had no distinct conceptual foundation. Because the hostility of a neglected ancestor could result in crop failure, a battlefield loss, or the offending descendant becoming ill, all these calamities were similarly treated. Thus, like combat and the harvest, medicine was a life-and-death matter that belonged to religion. Shang China had developed no distinct theory

of nature that attributed control of the harvest, illness, or personal outcomes to anything other than the supernatural. However, there were exceptions, and among these were elements of what would become medicine in succeeding generations. Natural causes of disease were recognized, and questions as to whether it was 'snow' or an 'evil wind' that caused an illness are inscribed on oracle bones.[8]

Physicians or medical training did not exist as separate social institutions and it was the Wu-shaman, a class of diviners and magicians, who were called on to pacify 'evil wind' (Fig. 1.3). It can be supposed from the earlier myth of Shen Nong that there was a practical herbal lore, but even that remains undocumented. However, despite the tradition established by claims in the *Nei Jing* that stone was the original material of acupuncture needles, there is no actual evidence that acupuncture was practiced during the Shang. What is probably the oldest mention of needles, although acupuncture is not noted, is in the *Shan Hai Jing* (*The Classic of Mountains and Rivers*). These scripts contain materials that range in age from the –8th to the –4th century, although the text was probably produced in the –5th century.[9] Thus, as regards the medicine of systematic correspondence, the medicine of *qi* that we now call 'Chinese traditional medicine,' the Shang provides only the crudest beginnings (Fig. 1.4).

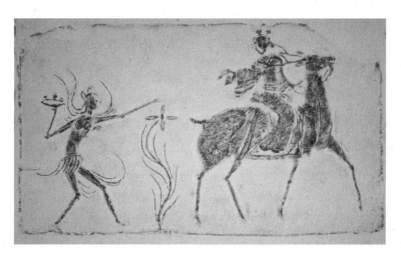

Figure 1.3 Wu Shaman, Han era, Rubbing from stone tablet. (Courtesy of Paradigm Publications.)

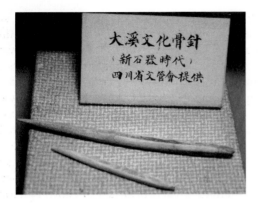

Figure 1.4 Bone needles. (Courtesy of Paradigm Publications.)

Early Zhou, −1027 to −772: classical feudalism in China

The Zhou dynasty, like many to succeed it, established itself by conquest. Once the Zhou family had consolidated their power over the loosely supervised territories of the Shang frontier with the aid of dissident Shang nobles, they conquered the central Shang. Their conquest had its roots not only in the failure of the Shang monarchy to guard its territories adequately, but also in the Zhou's superior agricultural productivity. This productivity came from the use of communally managed irrigation systems. This innovation permitted agricultural surpluses and lessened the number of laborers required to feed the population. Thus the Zhou rulers were free to conscript larger armies from the peasantry. The Zhou form of government physically was much like European feudalism. Their new capital in Shensi was surrounded by the fiefdoms of royal relatives; beyond these lay the fiefs of the surviving Shang ruling clan. The fief holders provided labor for the ruler's lands and soldiers for his armies, but otherwise occupied themselves with their own interests.[10]

As is evidenced by the fact that Shang nobles survived the Zhou victory, the link between nobility and the supernatural was still an effective force in Zhou China. This 'chivalry' is based on the perception of an ancestral link to a common deity. The Zhou first adopted the Wu, or shaman leaders of the Shang, continuing the belief that they were possessed of magical powers. They were believed responsible for the provision of rain, quieting violent storms and purging poisonous creatures and evil influences. The higher ranking Wu, who were possibly members of the royal family, were responsible for sacrifices to Di, the supreme ancestor. However, during the Zhou period, Di of the Shang was gradually replaced by the celestial deity Tian. As Tian became the most important subject of propitiation, the Wu's supposed access to Di became less and less important. Thus, with their access to the supernatural devalued, the Wu gradually returned to the lower classes. A new class of priests, the Zhu, took their place in the feudal hierarchy.[11]

As with the Shang, there is no evidence of acupuncture, although needles made of perishable materials are a possibility.[12] The *Shi Jing* (*Book of Odes*) of the −7th century refers to gathering mugwort (*Artemisiae Argyi Folium*) the plant from which the material for moxibustion is made, but not to its use. In fact, the predominant feature of the period is the rise of the idea that demons were a harmful influence on humankind.[13]

Middle Zhou, −772 to −480: the decline of feudalism

The early Zhou feudal arrangement was disrupted in −771. The foreign powers with whom the Zhou king had allied to win a bloody succession war refused to surrender the territory they had conquered. This forced the establishment of a new Zhou capital further east in Le-yi, from which the period takes the name given it by Chinese historians, 'The Eastern Zhou.' Thus began a period of shifting alliances and power struggles among ruling families that diminished their authority. Although the initial fragmentation of the Zhou territory into many small political units was partially reversed by alliances that produced fewer but larger political entities, their struggles for power resulted in an end of feudal society in the later Zhou, a period appropriately known as 'The Warring States.'[14]

History in the modern sense begins in the Zhou around −722. However, in the middle and late Zhou it is a history of considerable human ruthlessness. In the last years of the Zhou dynasty this trend reached the extreme, with the establishment of a 'farm and fight' state. We can fairly assume that the arts did not flourish under the patronage of this government. However, medicine did begin to have an existence separate from ancestral propitiation and demonology. It was beginning to earn a place distinct from religion in the social order. There were, for example, four kinds of doctor listed in the Zhou archives: physicians, surgeons, dieticians, and veterinary surgeons. The text of Zhou rituals *Zhou Li Tian Guan* says:

The chief doctor superintends all matters relating to medicine and collects drugs for medicinal purposes. He directs the doctors to take charge of the different departments so that those who are sick or wounded may go to see them. At the end of the year their work is examined and the salary of each fixed according to the results shown. If all cases get well, it is excellent; if there is one failure in ten cases, it is second; if two out of ten, third; three out of ten, fourth; and if four out of ten, it is bad.[15]

Although it is wise to keep in mind that any document from this period was probably subject to later editing, the middle Zhou period provides the oldest traces from which references to acupuncture may be supposed. At least, the development, production, and fashioning of metals begins in these times. In −540 there is also the first evidence of what will become the theory of six environmental evils. This appears in a story about the physician Yi-He's attendance on the prince of Jin. In the form of the time, *yin* and *yang* are represented as hot and cold. These are joined by wind, rain, darkness, and brightness as the influences that can cause disease — concepts that reappear later in medical literature. When a modern Chinese acupuncturist speaks of 'cold damp wind,' he or she is referring to a secularized and modernized version of the concept of evil influences that begins in this period.

The most seminal influence to arise in the middle Zhou was Confucianism. Gong Qiu, born in −551, was the son of a lower-order noble house. Legend has it that Gong Qiu, known in the West by the latinization of his name — Confucius — rose to become a prime minister. However, in this tale, he became disenchanted with the ruler's depravity, and resigned his post to wander in the company of his disciples. Together they sought a state that would apply his philosophy. Of course, it is important to remember that there is little, if anything, about the life and writings of Confucius that is certain. What is important, however, is that the philosophical structure known as Confucianism became one of the 'three pillars,' i.e. the three central influences of Chinese thought: Confucianism, Daoism (Taoism), and Buddhism.

Confucianism proposes that what causes social unrest is the difference between the actual conduct of society's members, including the ruler and ruling class, and what that conduct should be for society to function properly.[16] Whether or not any of the *Analects* or other texts ascribed to Confucius contain his actual words, the consequence of the rise of Confucianism in Chinese culture was the establishment of a solid connection between responsible human behavior and desirable outcomes:

If a person utilizes his body and his nature, his insight, understanding, and mature consideration in the manner prescribed by custom, order and success will ensue; otherwise, the result is unpredictability and upheaval, idleness and unruliness. If the consumption of food and drink, clothing, lodging at home and outside the home, as well as movement and rest are carried out in the manner prescribed by custom, one will achieve harmony and order; otherwise, one is subject to attack and betrayal, and illness will occur.[17]

In a way, Confucianism re-established the by now ancient moral order wherein a king and his ministers were thought to use their link to the supernatural to provide for the general good. However, instead of assigning that capacity to a king's unique ability to contact the divine Di or Tian, Confucius ascribed it to a neutral moral way. In effect, the king's divinity became a ruler's responsibility. Ritual that had once been justified by the king's access to his direct ancestors came to reflect a moral social order. Custom and universal order merged.

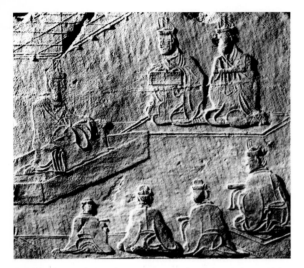

Figure 1.5 Lecturing. (Rubbing from stone tablet, courtesy of Paradigm Publications.)

This recycling of customary behaviors and social institutions through absorption into a new view is another Chinese trait that recurs throughout history. Thus it was natural that the Confucian link between human behavior and social outcomes found parallel expression in the development of medicine, and that the language of medicine would acquire meaning from the older ideas for which the characters had originally stood. One of the root assumptions of the medicine of systematic correspondence is that the trends and tendencies of human life are subject to intelligent human intervention and appropriate individual behavior. Those who believe that illness comes from a supernatural agent's displeasure do not look to the natural world that surrounds them, or to their own behavior, for either cause or cure. Although the transition from demonic causation and magic intervention to the theory of *qi* was neither immediate nor solely Confucian in origin, the medicine of *qi* could not have existed without a relationship between human well-being and human action. Confucianism provided that link.[18]

This was also true in details of what influenced Chinese medicine. Confucian philosophy emphasized moderation in eating and drinking; the *Analects* purported that 'diseases enter by the mouth,' and advised 'eat nothing that is not properly cooked,' and 'meat and wine bought at street stands should not be taken.' Although these proscriptions are quite reasonably seen as recognition that tainted food could cause disease, moderation was deeply rooted in the philosophical propositions of Confucianism — if a man is irregular in his sleep, intemperate in his eating, and immoderate in his work, sickness will kill him. Here too there is an element of concept recycling: what once would have been cured by shamanic offerings to ancestors or demons, is to be cured by a behavioral change with a particular moral tone.

Late Zhou, −480 to −221: the Warring States

The era of the Warring States was precisely that — the final dissolution of Chinese feudalism into vicious bloody contests between principalities large and small. In warfare all traces of 'feudal chivalry' were forgotten as fights to the finish became the rule. Kings were no longer seen as literal or figurative relatives in a supernatural hierarchy; they had become just another piece to be removed from the game. The period is the culmination of a philosophy in which it was the peasants' place to 'farm and fight.' However, as unpleasant as life in this time may have been, its chaos sets the stage for the consolidation of China into an empire. By making it possible for the first Qin monarch to eliminate his rivals and consolidate his power, it set Chinese culture on course to one of its most memorable periods.

In the dissolution of the Warring States period, more of the socio-political seeds of the medicine of systematic correspondence took root. Just as the chaos of the declining Zhou dynasty was fertile soil for the political and cultural developments that would become the essentials of Chinese culture, in particular Confucianism and Daoism, it was the ground substance of the qi paradigm.

At this time, there were two main trends in medicine: magical correspondence and systematic correspondence. In both these views the order of nature was believed to relate the seen and unseen. Because things correspond, affecting one affects the other.[19] However, neither magical nor systematic correspondences require the elimination of the other. Unlike Western intellectual history, where a new model succeeds by eliminating a previously dominant model, Chinese thinkers tended to absorb existing ideas, thus permitting the application of whatever model worked best in a particular situation.[20] Thus the older *yin-yang* concept and the newer five-phase doctrine introduced by Zou Yan during this period both incorporated aspects of the older magico-demonic tradition. In fact, the language of Chinese traditional medicine still retains terms that reflect both demonic medicine and the strife of feudalism's demise. The body may be attacked so it has 'defense,' or 'guards,' (*wei*) and 'army camps' (*ying*). The five-phase relationship between organ systems includes one where the stronger 'restrains' or 'subdues' (*ke*) the weaker.[21]

Thus, when Daoism, the second of China's Three Pillars, arose during the period of the Warring States, it eliminated neither Confucianism nor the earlier religious traditions. Daoism is now a term used to group different and sometimes contradictory philosophies that share the conception of Dao as a law of nature beyond humankind's comprehension. Confucianism also refers to 'Dao,' but in that context it is more an idea of how humans can correctly coexist in society. The Daoists were less concerned with humanity and more impressed by nature. They sought to know how humans could best conform to nature, not how they should act toward one another. Daoism and Confucianism are in fact often philosophically contradictory. Where, for example, Confucianism sees the establishment of hierarchical order as a blessing to humankind, Daoism sees the same structure as a disorder-inducing intervention in nature. From this ideal derived *wu wei*, the well-known Daoist concept of non-intervention.[22]

Lao Zi is the legendary author of the best-known Daoist text, the *Dao De Jing*. According to the legends, he got his name, 'The Old Boy,' because he spent 72 years in his mother's womb. Lao Zi stressed the concept of *wu wei*, passive non-action, to realize the Dao. Zhuang Zi, a later contemporary, stressed that the Dao can be realized through our actions (as opposed to inaction). Lao Zi and Zhuang Zi are the best known Daoists, as their works developed the mystic and philosophical system; however, there was also an active Daoist occultism that included the demonological practices that were ever-present in early China. There are very early records of ceremonies to ward off pestilence, and Confucius himself is said to have participated in such ceremonies. Shi Huang-di of the Qin frequently consulted magicians, and sought the elixir of life, itself one of the longest-lived concepts in Chinese culture, and one with Daoist roots. Wu Di, the Han emperor, also supported such beliefs.[23] Daoism was also the ground from which deep breathing and the search for the elixir of life (immortality drugs) developed. Its precepts affected the form and substance of the *Nei Jing*, the concept of *qi*, and the techniques of medicine and health that would characterize Chinese traditional medicine from this time forward.[24]

Qin, −221 to −206: the burning books

Beginning in −249 with the home state of Confucius, where Confucian precepts had been most generally accepted, the Qin state proceeded to conquer all the states and principalities of China. Being thus the first to unify China, the Qin ruler not only declared himself emperor, but also replaced the feudal elite with his own officials, appropriating their lands in the process.[25] In what is perhaps the act typifying his rule, King Zhen, as the newly imperial Shi Huang-di, ordered the burning of all literature except that on medicine, drugs, oracles, agriculture, and forestry, subjects he considered to have some practical value. Shi Huang-di also began the earliest version of the so-called 'Great Wall of China,' in Joseph Campbell's words of unbridled disdain, 'to protect the Empire from further inroads by barbarians such as himself.'[26] However, unrest was unceasing as two groups contested Shi Huang-di's powers.

This period sees a transformation resulting from the policies of the Qin state. The Qin ruler was guided by a Legalist philosophy that directed its attention to the acquisition of wealth and power. In legalism, power and good, wealth and right were equated. The old ancestor-centered chivalry of the feudal period was irrevocably replaced by the finality of winner-take-all.

Thus the short rule of Shi Huang-di passed, leaving behind forced-labor projects, the ashes of pre-Han philosophical works, and the cultural effects of the first and last Chinese Legalist government. However, among those effects were those that laid the foundations for the prosperity and creativity of the Han. For example, Shi Huang-di simply ordered 120 000 families to move to his new capital, thus ending with a word China's long tradition of small, self-reliant towns. The interdependent, currency-driven population centers thus established became the future of the empire and the base for the Han's cultural flowering. His government standardized weights and measures, set the value of coinage, standardized writing, and imposed the construction of a transportation system on subjects who either complied or died.[27] In this inadvertent way Shi Huang-di's ruthless drive to wealth and power left a socioeconomic legacy that would later empower one of the most revered periods in Chinese history. It also established a bureaucracy that would be the basis of China's government until the modern era.

Han, −206 to 220: the period of systematization

Gao-zu, founder of the Han dynasty, apparently never forgot his humble origin, and his monarchy was one of responsible leadership. He moderated the harshness of Qin rule, lowered taxes, and loosened government control, while retaining its organization. His supporters were rewarded with fiefdoms. Gao-zu decentralized power, broadened the social and political elite, and humanized policy. However, his reign was cut short when he died in his forties. The 15 years of unrest that followed Gao-zu's death in −195, and his widow's assumption of power, ended with the establishment of the Han dynasty. The Han developed into a period of peace and stability through the reigns of the emperors Wen to Wu (−180 to −87).[28] By the end of the reign of Wu the political system that would serve China for the next 1900 years would be in place, and the qi paradigm had become the future course for acupuncture, as well as all medicine in China, until the arrival of Western medicine.[29]

It is no wonder that writers cannot resist mythologizing the Han. The Chinese have many times pointed to this era as a period of supreme cultural achievement worthy of emulation. During this period, Chinese culture, including medicine, changed with a swiftness rarely found in Chinese history. The harsh policies of the Qin weeded out the institutions and social powers that might have opposed change, clearing the cultural soil for the germination and flowering of innovation, exploration, and invention. Not only were cultural barriers eliminated, Chinese society and economy were physically accessible as never before. Roads and canals connected once largely autonomous cities, and all classes of society benefited from an ever-increasing wealth from trade and ordered economic interdependence. At the very least, the court and the wealthy were able to obtain foreign goods.[30] Feudal lords no longer controlled social and religious life, and an educated class survived independent of their wealth or favor.

Han China was no longer isolated, and the Chinese reached outward in all directions. The famous silk road opened in the −1st century during the reign of Wu-di, and contact with Western Asia commenced. Wu-di also is said to have commissioned a mission to the 'Huns' as part of an effort to reach an aristocrat who had migrated West after a defeat in war.[31] Within China itself the Han opened an exchange of ideas with the nomads of the north and north-west and colonized the far south. Medicine may also have been fertilized by foreign ideas, but this can be neither proven nor discounted.[32]

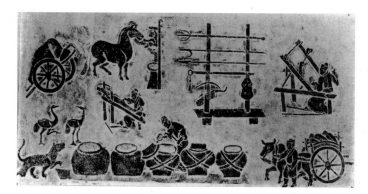

Figure 1.6 Han tools. (Rubbing from stone tablet, courtesy of Paradigm Publications.)

From the viewpoint of medicine generally, and acupuncture in particular, the Han was the period during which the medicine of systematic correspondence comes of age. The Ma Wang-dui scripts of the late –3rd or early –2nd century, the *Huang Di Nei Jing* texts of the minus second to first century, and the *Nan Jing* of the first century provide an historical window on this process. These documents trace over approximately 400 years the development of the major conceptual features of the medicine of systematic correspondence. The theories of anatomy, physiology, pathology, and treatment that formed China's indigenous medicine to the present day matured during the Han.[33]

It is not clear how all the aspects of the medicine of systematic correspondence arose, and our chronological presentation should not imply that it was a steady and orderly progress. For example, while Zou Yan (–350 to –270) is credited with the origination of the five-phase concept, both the Greek conception of four elements and the Indian series of five are products of approximately –600 and are reasonable ancestors for Chinese five-phase ideas.[34] However, it is clear that at the beginning of the Han the qi paradigm had not been fully elaborated. Thus, although it is certain that the five-phase ideas most popular today in the UK can be traced to the Han, the logic by which modern treatments are formed had yet to evolve and mature.

During this formative period, the idea of wind, which had been considered the principal cause of illness in the most ancient times, evolved. From a willed spirit entity it became an environmental phenomenon, just as Chinese civilization was transforming from a mythologically justified aristocracy to a secular nation. In the process of that transition, *qi*, subtle influences, was identified as the ground substance of all that is. Next, the human body came to be seen as relationships between functional units. Where in the West we describe organs as biological factories linked in an internal metabolic economy, China's medical thinkers conceived poetic images that explained biological functions in social and political terms. The organs were divided into *zang* ('depots' in the language of the time) and *fu* ('palaces'), reflecting their role in a complex system of functional interactions.

The images and terms used to describe this system were borrowed from the social and natural environments and often reflect the political state at the time of their conception. Chinese writers found in their social and philosophical vocabulary processes that they thought were analogous to what goes on in the human body. When, finally, through the great accomplishment of the *Nan Jing* author, the human organism came to be seen as linked in an endless circulation of *qi*, these *jing* would be named for the watercourses that were the high technology of the day, 'conduits' or 'channels.' This discovery would result in most of the principles and some of the practices that survive in acupuncture today.

The archaeological record

Acupuncture arose in an essentially classically feudal state governed by an elite whose power was absolute. It is from their burial sites that we have learned much about early Chinese medicine. In −168 the Lord of Dai, then aged around 30, was buried along with manuscripts written on silk. These, the Ma Wang-dui archaeological discoveries, include 14 texts, two of which are landmarks in the early history of Chinese medicine. They document virtually all the ancient indigenous treatments: demonology, magic, minor surgery, and pharmacology, as well as nascent concepts of systematic correspondence.[35] Because the writing resembles Qin bronze inscriptions it is possible that these manuscripts were old before the young prince was born. The burial also contains a copy of the *Yi Jing* written on silk that presents an order of the hexagrams that may be earlier than the classical order. Certainly, these scripts are older than the *Nei Jing*.

Ma Wang-dui

In the later Han work of Fu Jian (c 165 to 185), the transition from stone to iron needles was attributed to the early Han.[36] Yet, evidence to this effect has not been found. Although Joseph Needham's interpretation of a passage in the *Shi Ji*, a text of −90, has been quoted as the earliest mention of acupuncture: 'No (needle) can penetrate to it, no drug can reach it. There is nothing to be done,'[37] later research does not support his assumption. The text actually reads:

To attack it is impossible. [If one attempted] to advance to it, [he would] not reach it. [The reason is:] drugs cannot proceed to it. [Hence,] nothing can be done about it.[38]

Thus, although there is no clear beginning for acupuncture, the Ma Wang-dui texts and the first appearance of the *Nei Jing* in the late −2nd or early −1st century are reasonable boundaries.

It is clear that the medical theory presented in the Ma Wang-dui scripts is unfinished, showing Chinese traditional medicine early in the process of becoming distinct from religion.

It contains descriptions of acupuncture channels, but only 11. Six rise from the feet to various points above the waist. Five descend from the hands to the chest or head. Diseases are related to one of these unconnected vessels, each of which is associated with an individual set of symptoms. Although the vessels are said to be filled with *qi*, and subject to repletion, vacuity, and undesirable movement — concepts that the system permanently retained — no specific treatment points are identified, and therapy is limited to burning herbs on the afflicted channel. There is no indication of *qi* circulation. There is little evidence of the five phases, and no theory of disease.[39]

In fact, it is the absence of acupuncture in the Ma Wang-dui texts that is remarkable. Although spells and rituals, exercise, sexual practices, drugs, massage, cupping, bathing, and fumigation are discussed — sometimes based on systematic correspondence and sometimes based on demonology — acupuncture is not mentioned and specific acupoints are not described.[40] Thus it is reasonable to assume that the Han began with medicine in a transitional state. The raw conceptual materials of the qi paradigm were present, but its elaboration and interrelation through the logic of systematic correspondence had yet to be achieved.

Evidently, China in the −2nd century was following a course similar to that of Greece 3 centuries earlier. The principles of pathology, anatomy, and physiology were being established as distinct human disciplines, as medicine. As Paul Unschuld expresses it:

The distinct feature of emerging Greek and Chinese philosophy in the last half of the last millennium B.C. is the attempt to explain the phenomena of the perceptible world as natural occurrences, without referring to mysterious forces such as gods or ancestors.[41]

This image of the early Han is confirmed by other historical evidence. Shortly after the Prince of Dai's burial around −176, Cang Gong would report the first clinical histories known in Chinese traditional medicine. However, this was a practice that would not find followers for another 1500 years. Although the early pharmacopoeia do not contain references to moxibustion, *jiu jing* or 'moxibustion manuals' were available by Han times and the *Meng Zi* book contains one of the earliest references to the medical use of moxa.[42] Indeed, based on this and other evidence preserved by the work of physician Shun Yu-yi, Joseph Needham expresses the general scholarly conclusion that:

...there can be no further room for skepticism concerning the virtual consummation of the system's general outlines by the end of minus second century, and this must surely mean, as already suggested, that the beginnings of it must be older than several centuries.[43]

Although the Han is a focal point for the development of the qi paradigm, the demonological and magical traditions remained very much alive. Amulets and talismans, for example, were also features of Han medicine. These were not decrepit ideas surviving only in the medical periphery. By the early Han, the cruder ceremonials of the Zhou period had become more subtle means of warding off demons and enlisting the help of spirits to cure illness. In the herbal text *Wu Shi Er Bing Fang* from the Ma Wang-dui grave, for example, 27 of the prescriptions are based on spells.[44] In the later Han reign of Shun Di, 125 to 145, Zhang Daoling would introduce the first entire book of charms for curing illnesses.[45] In fact, magical and demonological instructions are found in both the Ma Wang-dui and *Nei Jing* texts.

Huang Di Nei Jing

If the Ma Wang-dui texts are the earliest of the important Han documents, it is the *Huang Di Nei Jing* (*The Yellow Emperor's Canon of Internal Medicine*) that is best known and most revered now in the West, as it has been for 1900 years in Asia. This work is composed as a supposed dialogue between the Yellow Emperor, Huang Di, and his minister, Qi Bo. There are two sections, each composed of multiple books: the *Su Wen* or 'Fundamental Questions' and the *Ling Shu* or 'Spiritual Axis/Pivot.' In the former the conversation elucidates points of medical theory. The latter is essentially an acupuncture

manual. Traditionally dated from −2698 to −2598, the period also ascribed to the Yellow Emperor, scholars today agree that the *Nei Jing* was probably completed in the −2nd to −1st century.[46]

The text's contribution and place in history is clear. It can stand for nothing less than the genesis of medicine in China, even if there were more important texts and events that we will never know. It symbolizes the point when the essential ideas of disease and treatment reached maturity. Disease was no longer just one of the many catastrophes for which humankind sought supernatural aid. Medicine had become a human endeavor distinct from religion. The text not only assembles in a single source the most fundamental aspects of the medicine of systematic correspondence, but also begins a focus on differential treatment of individual symptoms that continues to the present. Like raw gems, the ideas have rough edges and have yet to be polished and elegantly set. Yet, the 162 articles of the *Nei Jing* show not only the absorption and extension of *yin-yang* theory and the incorporation of the relatively newer concept of five phases,[47] but also a focus on individual symptoms as somatic rather than supernatural events.

As important as these accomplishments are, the *Huang Di Nei Jing* is neither rigorously structured nor systematic. It is best conceived as a first, most ancient attempt to assemble a medical art from the many schools of medical thought that had survived to the Han. Thus the *Nei Jing* allows us to look at the foundations of Chinese traditional medicine as regards anatomy, physiology, and the root theories of pathology and treatment. It is a window onto the medicine of systematic correspondence as it matured; a transitional stage where acupuncture had become a principal therapy and the concepts of systematic correspondence had assumed the prominent role. However, neither the techniques nor their conceptual roots had reached final elaboration.

Although by the time of the *Nei Jing*, probably through dissections, Chinese medical writers were aware of the internal structure of the human body, it is descriptions of the non-material acupuncture channels that are principal among its facts. These channels present no physical evidence that could have been recognized by physicians of this period, although there is one reference to observing them through dissection of corpses. Thus they probably represent a logical relationship inferred from naked-sense observations. Some speculate that the idea of channels came from observing people who were sensitive to acupoint or channel stimulation or palpation, or even the dermatological phenomena that sometimes appear along these lines.[48]

However accomplished, by this time medical thinkers had identified all the currently defined 12 regular channels as well as 135 bilateral acupoints. The two midline channels, the conception or controller and governing vessels, were also known, along with another 25 acupoints. In total, counting bilateral points twice, some 295 points of the 670 presented in current modern Chinese texts were known, just less than half.[49] These channels carry a *qi* that is described in part as a product of the body and in part as a product of the environment. The bodily *qi* are spoken of as inherently healthy, although they can be internally disrupted, producing illness. An important concept is even named 'right *qi*' to indicate this quality. External *qi* on the other hand are 'evils' that induce illness as they permeate the channels to reach the viscera and bowels.

The body's physical, internal anatomy was seen as composed of 11 organs. The five *zang* were the heart, liver, spleen, lungs, and kidney. The six *fu* were the gallbladder, stomach, large intestine, small intestine, bladder, and the *san jiao* or 'triple burner,' a nonphysical entity linked to a variety of systemic chores such as control of the body's fluids. However, these organs were seen to relate to one another not as mere primitive analogs of the biochemical factories that modern medicine describes, but as features of a functional economy that was logically parallel to the social order of the newly founded empire. And, as such, the concepts can present considerable difficulty for modern readers.

In the *Nei Jing* the condition of the viscera and bowels is ascertained by palpation at points all over the body. The principal forms of treatment are bloodletting, the insertion of needles, or the burning of herbs at specific locations on all 12 of the channels. It is here that we find the beginnings of the practices found in virtually every modern style. It is certain, for example, that the bloodletting methods used today can be traced to the *Nei Jing*, and it is the *Ling Shu* that details many of the technical aspects of acupuncture.

Depending on who is telling the story, the *Nei Jing* theories, which are retained today in modified forms, are either praised as 'holistically functional' or damned as 'mostly imaginary.' However, both these descriptions tell us more about the 20th century than the Han. *Nei Jing* physiology, like its anatomy and pathology, is rooted in the observations that were possible at the time. It is indeed holistic from a modern viewpoint. However, the rigid boundaries of modern Western science that the philosophy of holism means to overcome were not only many centuries in the future, even in the West, but also unimaginable to those who read the *Nei Jing*. Thus it is more useful to think of these constructs as part of a Chinese philosophy of correspondence rather than as expressions of a modern Western response to specialization and fragmentation.

Chinese ideas of anatomy and human function can likewise be called imaginary only from the perspective of the 20th century. The body's functions in the *Nei Jing* are not only some of those that can be observed by modern medicine (the relation of nutrition to health), but also those observed in humans living in their environment (the relationship of cold and damp to illness). Thus, what the *Nei Jing* accomplishes is a theory of how the observable elements of the human body function in life. These ideas were expressed through images grounded in the theories of *yin-yang* and the five phases.

These interwoven and sophisticated analogies describe human functions through systematic relationships at all levels of human experience.

For example, the spleen and stomach are related to the earth of the five phases. Earth is 'yellow,' a shade in which the Chinese include what Westerners would call 'tan.' It is said to match the soil of the region. Earth relates to 'long summer' (the harvest season in Chinese thought) and ripe crops and fruits (the produce of the harvest). It is a common experience in agrarian societies that when people have a good diet they are healthy. When the earth is fecund, food is plentiful and the nation thrives. If digestion is effective, the body is healthy. If digestion fails, humans wither and die. If earth has rain, it flourishes; if not, the people starve. By analogy then the spleen, as is said in the *Inner Canon*, 'holds the office of the granaries.' The spleen is to the person as the department of agriculture is to the people — things go well if the minister's job is well done.[50] The spleen is like soil; if its balance within the environment is correct, the body will thrive.

Likewise, pathology in the *Nei Jing* fits these same analogies. Just as farmers' fields that are undrained produce only rotting vegetation, a damp spleen cannot properly nourish the body.[51] Although the *Nei Jing* continues the prominence of wind as a source of illness, it also begins the formalization of the idea that disease has both internal and external causes, and that natural phenomena can lead to illness. In accord with the same analogies, dampness, dryness, heat, and cold can damage the body. So too can the specific effects related to an organ; anger, for example, can injure the liver. If the kidneys, the root of life, are ill, there will be fear, because fear is the emotion of threatened survival.

However, as curious as this approach may be to Westerners who are culturally imbued with the principles of biomedicine, we should not forget that the medical theory of the *Nei Jing* also shares much with Western thought. For example, some diseases are described so precisely that modern scholars believe they can accurately identify malaria, diabetes, nephritis, gastric ulcer, bronchitis, and various pathologies of the spine.[52] Chapter 41 of the *Su Wen* describes the differentiation and treatment of more than 20 manifestations of low-back pain,

which arguably can be mapped to modern pathologies. Furthermore, treatment in the *Nei Jing* is allopathic (treatment by opposites), like modern medicine. But, where biomedicine attacks a particular germ with a specific drug, the *Nei Jing* considers only functional and environmental qualities. The physician is instructed to heat what is cold, or cool what is hot, to supplement what is insufficient, or to drain that which is replete. There are also striking linguistic similarities. What we call 'stroke' was identified as 'wind strike.' The Latin roots of 'malaria' mean 'bad air.' The Chinese term reflects exactly the same assumption.

Finally, particularly in light of the decline of Chinese public health that occurred in the early 20th century, it is important to note that Han medicine understood the importance of balance within the environment. In fact, the reputation of the ancient sources for emphasis on prevention represents the very practical understanding that the environment was a source of illness. In the Han there were sanitary inspectors who were to fumigate buildings, remove dead bodies, and control pollution. Clean drinking water was an important goal, communal cleaning a public responsibility. Public lavatories were maintained and human excrement was transported to the countryside by barge.[53]

In sum, there is less to be gained from dwelling on the differences between *Nei Jing* postulates and Western thought than from focusing on its accomplishment of laying down China's foundation medical theories. It is a principal feature of these theories that the analogies describing disease provide the basis for treatment. A damp spleen must be treated just as rotting vegetation must be cleared from a flooded field so that the soil can dry as the water mists upward in the sun. Again, the Chinese terms fit the picture — waste must be 'broken' and 'drained,' water must be 'diffused' upward or 'percolated' downward, the spleen must be 'dried,' and its *qi* 'boosted.' In addition, the *Nei Jing* represents the distinction of acupuncture as a theoretically justified medicine. Although other forms of treatment are mentioned, acupuncture is the orthodox treatment and the *Ling Shu*, the second volume of the *Nei Jing*, is devoted almost exclusively to it.[54]

It is difficult to understand the mind-set of thinkers whose thoughts were formed in a context far removed from our own. On the one hand, to think of these complex analogies as merely flawed theories of causation is overly chauvinistic. For example, the idea that the kidney produces urine is quite probably attributable to actual observation of the anatomical structures, as is the relation to reproduction. These principles are not unfairly categorized as early gross anatomy. However, to then say that the idea of *jing*, the reproductive essence that is linked to the kidney, is merely a misperception of the reproductive role of sperm and egg, is to suppose that the early medical writers were not conscious of their own reasoning. First, an earlier meaning of the character (*shen*) used for 'kidney' referred to the testicles, without which men are not fertile. Second, Chinese thought about the kidney is philosophically related to the idea of water. Water is the giver of all life without which everything dies. Its association with reproduction is not primitive anatomy, but an expression of natural patterns.

It is wise, nonetheless, to keep our ideas about these ancient analogies in their own era. It is very unlikely that ancient medical thinkers put forward the idea of *jing* as a way to describe a mysterious generative matter–energy at work in a quantum world beneath what can be observed. Although this is another idea that has proven irresistible to modern writers, it assigns to ancient medical thinkers a god-like anticipation of modern events. Such an energy was not only beyond the range of naked-sense observation, but also completely outside the cultural context of the *Nei Jing*. In fact, it is ideas of magical correspondence that are the more probable rationale. More importantly, however, *qi*, the Chinese idea of what lay beneath and beyond the world of the physical senses, needs no speculative reinterpretation in modern terms. Although it is far fuzzier than modern scientific concepts, and perhaps forever untranslatable into popular Western words, it is not a prim-

itive expression waiting for interpretation into Western ideas of energy or matter. It is a perfectly useful concept that expresses the recognition that human health, and all things, depend on harmony in their environment.

In sum, the *Nei Jing* texts represent a transitional stage at which acupuncture had reached the state of a principal therapy and the concepts of systematic correspondence had assumed a prominent role. However, neither the techniques nor their conceptual roots were entirely mature at this point. This would be the accomplishment of the unknown author of the *Nan Jing*.

Nan Jing

The *Nan Jing* or *Classic of Difficult Issues* takes its name from its composition of 81 articles named '*nan*.' Today, most scholars assign it a date between the 1st and 2nd centuries.[55] The contents have been arranged in different ways and there is a variety of theories about its authorship.[56] It is also the text most commented upon by authors in later periods. Thus, while there have been many opinions expressed, the text is now generally considered the mature development of the medicine of systematic correspondence, because it integrates for the first time all aspects of health care into the *yin–yang* and five-phase doctrines.

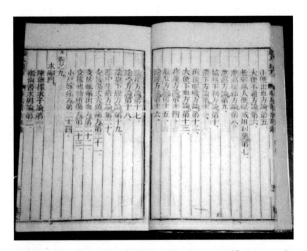

Figure 1.7   *Nan Jing*: 'Eighth Difficult Issue.' (Courtesy of Paradigm Publications.)

Although Chinese traditional pharmacotherapies would not be integrated into the qi paradigm until the 12th century,[58] the *Nan Jing* marks the point at which the heterogeneity of the *Nei Jing* had been resolved. The gems had now been culled, cut, and polished and, even if the settings not entirely finished, the extent and value of the treasure was clear. Although many of the terms from the *Nei Jing* remain, they are used in different ways. Demonology and magic are entirely absent.[59] Like the *Nei Jing*, acupuncture is the principal form of treatment; in fact, it is the only form of treatment. But a breakthrough has occurred. The choice of acupoints is now based on a systematization rooted in the idea of *qi* circulation.

By the time of the *Nan Jing*, the 12 principal interconnected channels had expanded to 14 with the addition of two midline channels on the front and back of the body. The channel system was further developed and a greater number of acupoints identified. The channels were still thought to carry *qi*; *qi* was still seen as arising in both the body and the environment, but the idea of circulation predominated. Practice was systematized by the idea of circulating *qi*. The system of *jing*, 'conduits' or 'channels,' had achieved the form it would retain until today, although the pathways were simplified in the modern development of TCM. Among the heirs of this innovation are many principles and practices that survive in acupuncture today.[60]

Perhaps the best example of a longevous *Nan Jing* contribution to acupuncture is the idea of the 'movement in the vessels,' what is called 'the pulses' in English-language acupuncture books. In the *Nei Jing* the condition of someone's *qi* was assessed by palpation of points all over their body. In the *Nan Jing* the wrists were identified as sites where the movement in the vessels could be assessed by identifying one of many qualitatively distinct patterns. These qualities diagnose not just the immediate area, but the entire body. *Qi* has become a circulating, whole-body phenomenon and it is the *Nan Jing* author who forwarded the idea that the 'hand great *yin* channel' (the channel associated with the lung) was the primary meeting point of all the body's channels. Thus the condition of the body's channels, viscera, and bowels is shown by the quality of the movement in the vessels felt at the radial artery near both wrists.[61]

In practice, practitioners place their third and fourth fingers to either side of the radial styloid process (the bump found on the outside of the inner surface of the wrist, slightly toward the elbow), spaced relative to the size of the patient. Once positioned, the practitioner assesses the rate, thickness, length, smoothness of flow, and rhythm in three positions on each wrist. A pulse that can be felt only with pressure is termed 'sinking.' A pulse that can be felt only with light pressure at the surface is called 'floating,' and one that can be felt further outward than usual is labeled 'long.' These qualities combine, and the combinations reflect particular patterns. These patterns are not diagnoses of uniquely named diseases but qualitative statements that mesh neatly with the analogies of the qi paradigm and thus the capabilities of acupoints. For example, it is said today that a pulse that is sinking and weak to the point that it can hardly be felt without pressing to the bone indicates cold and pain.[62]

Today, a more generalized pulse diagnosis is taught in modern Chinese medical schools. Yet, the classical *Nan Jing* tradition survives, particularly in Japan where acupuncture training retains more of the apprentice tradition. For example, many of the blind acupuncturists, who make up 40% of Japan's acupuncturists, regulate their treatment by repeatedly checking a patient's pulse. Because pulse-taking is an apprentice skill that is passed from one generation to another by rigorous training supervised by a master, a process that requires apprentices to practice with, and patients to practice upon, pulse diagnosis tends to have a less important role in other nations where classroom teaching is dominant.

Nan Jing pulse examination requires recognition of the relative strength and quality of the pulsation at three different depths of palpation at each of three pulse positions on each wrist.

The qualities of the pulse wave found at each of these 18 locations indicate the condition of the channels, the *zang* and *fu*. Thus the possible diagnoses are numerous and specific. Once the acupuncturist has pictured the relationships indicated by the pulse qualities, *yin-yang* and five-phase logic are used to choose acupoints for treatment. In this model acupoints are not chosen so much to treat a disease, or even to ameliorate a particular symptom, but more to adjust the *qi* to an ideal state. In the language of treatment, *qi* is 'rectified, boosted, supplemented' or 'drained' according to the indications of the pulse. In some modern adaptations of this approach, especially in Japan, the pulse is also used as an immediate feedback mechanism by which the success of treatment is judged. Each step of the treatment, each acupoint stimulated, will be followed by re-examination of the pulses. In some traditions, treatment cannot finish until the desired changes in the pulses have been observed.[63]

Of course, a theory and a technique that allow greater specificity are of little use without a treatment of similar precision. This too is achieved in the *Nan Jing*. Where in the *Nei Jing* acupoints were needled relative to a very localistic idea of the channel affected (e.g. those close to the pain), the *Nan Jing* proposed choosing one of several acupoints on each channel as determined by *yin-yang* and five-phase theory. Instead of merely needling the site or channel affected, the acupuncturist was to choose an acupoint that might, for example, increase *qi* 'downstream' in the flow, thus harmonizing the system. Again, acupoints are chosen in accord with the principles of the qi paradigm. For example, one might select points according to a rule known as 'mother–child.' In this case, rather than treating an affected channel, acupuncturists stimulate points that increase the flow of *qi* from the 'mother channel,' the one preceding the affected channel in one of the five-phase cycles.

It is the *Nan Jing* that founds modern practice models that depend upon five-phase logic. In less explicit form, these five-phase relationships, for example, the relationship between a phase and color, are also found in modern TCM acupoint treatments and in the selection of medicinal substances. Keep in mind, however, that the more localistic *Nei Jing* approach also survives today, as does the use of what are known as *ashi* ('it's there') points. Although these techniques do not depend on the theory of *qi* circulation, they are no less traditional. Acupuncturists whose principal therapeutic model derives from the *Nan Jing* nonetheless apply ideas and techniques from the *Nei Jing*. This is another example of how traditional Chinese medicine preserves effective practices without prejudice against one or another theoretical or philosophical root.

In sum, at all levels of medicine, in both theory and practice, the unknown *Nan Jing* author systematized an image of the human organism. This system is linked internally by influences that behave according to the principles of *yin-yang* and five phases, thus providing a vast range of therapeutic options — what Japanese master acupuncturist Yoshio Manaka would 1800 years later describe as the 'software' of the human body. These options can be selected via a diagnostic method, pulse-taking, that permits an assessment of everything required to form a mental picture of any patient's condition. That assessment is the product not only of the natural images derived from earlier texts, but also of specific channels and organ states related to one another by the repeating cycles of *qi*. The human is also seen to be linked to the surrounding environment, again by *qi*, and again in the images of the qi paradigm.

From the *Nan Jing* onward, medicine not only freed itself from its roots in religion and divination, but also was supplied with an image of humankind linked to nature in an infinite and eternal flow of *qi*.

The Later Han

The *Nan Jing* is not the only accomplishment of the later Han, nor was its unknown author the only genius of the era. This is also the period of the first attempt to incorporate herbal pharmacotherapy into the medicine of systematic correspondence. In 198, Zhang Zhong-jing wrote the *Shang Han Lun* (*A Discourse on Cold-induced Disorders*), today recognized as central to Chinese medical thought on natural drug therapy. Ironically, Zhang Zhong-jing, who is now called 'the greatest physician China has produced' or 'the Chinese Hippocrates,' would have relatively little influence on China's traditional medicine for nearly a thousand years.[64]

Although the *Shang Han Lun* and Zhang Zhong-jing's second seminal work, *Jin Gui Yu Han Yao Lue* (*Survey of the Most Important Elements from the Golden Chest and Jade Container*) would remain intact for centuries between the Han and Song, they would inspire less than 10 Chinese authors to follow their lead.[65] Indeed, the works seem to have more powerfully influenced Japanese traditional medicine. This theoretical and therapeutic approach would have such a profound effect on Japanese medicine that it still retains a significant place in modern Japan, particularly in Japanese traditional pharmaceutics. Only later in the Song-Jin-Yuan period would virtually all the important Chinese authors adopt the principles expressed in these texts.

The *Shang Han Lun* details the progression of epidemic disease in six levels, and describes specific treatments for each stage. The treatments are multiple medicinal substances decocted together according to *yin-yang* principles.[66] Each was to be modified according to the manifestations observed at the patient's bedside. The text has a few brief references to needling, including the use of the *wenjiu* (warming) needle method, and thus is probably the source of modern moxa-heated needle techniques.[67] Zhang Zhong-jing eventually had a profound and lasting effect on the practice and development of Chinese pharmaceutics, but had much less influence on the practice of acupuncture. References to his ideas in acupuncture appear only in the Ming dynasty, over 1000 years later, and these do not seem to have been in common use.

Zhang Zhong-jing's contemporary, Hua To, born in approximately 190, is famous for his use of surgical and anesthetic procedures, his diagnostic skills, and his creation of the 'animal frolics,' a set of exercises for promoting health.

Six Dynasties, 220 to 589: the period of disunity

The Later Han dynasty gradually disintegrated from lack of consistent administration, a succession of under-age rulers, none of whom were over 15 years old, and the political miseries of revolts and self-seeking generals. By 220 the central government was no longer functional. A succession of dynasties came and went. China was fractured, with much of its territory under foreign control, until 589 when the country was finally reunified.[68]

Another seminal influence on Chinese culture during this period was the advancement of China's third pillar, Buddhism. Buddhism had possibly entered China during the 1st century.[69] Emperor Ming Di of the Han (58 to 76) is said to have dreamt that a brilliant God entered his palace. This dream was interpreted to mean that Buddha required worship in China. Ming Di thus sent ambassadors to India who, after an extended journey, returned with Buddhist images, scriptures, and two monks. Whenever Buddhism arrived in China, it had relatively little influence on acupuncture. Although the reasons why Buddhist medicine was not acculturated to the extent of the religion itself are not obvious, Buddhist medicine met with relatively little acceptance.

The conceptual framework of Buddhist medicine suffered at the hands of the early, mostly Daoist, translators. Mistranslation occurred, and relatively little of the literature found its way into the Chinese cultural library.[70] Paul Unschuld cautions that there are so many Chinese medical works that have not been examined that an unexpected Buddhist influence could still emerge. However, as of now, there is little such evidence.

Both Sun Si-miao and Hua To are often given as examples of Buddhist influence on acupuncture. But Sun Si-miao's attempts to rationalize the Buddhist four-element doctrine with the qi paradigm found no followers, perhaps because of the mathematical error it contains. In addition, because there is no subsequent development of the anesthesiology and surgery attributed to Hua To, and his story is so similar to tales of the Indian physician Jivaka, Hua To may to some extent be an imported fable.[71]

Some historians suggest that Buddhism contributed the psychological perspective to medicine in China. Meditation, psychotherapeutic measures, and faith healing are seen as Buddhist influences. Buddha is reputed to have told Qi Bo 'You go heal his body first, I will come later to treat his mental suffering.'[72] Although this influence is uncertain, it is clear that the martial arts were influenced by Buddhism. Bodhidharma, Da Mo in Chinese, arrived in China in 527. He first visited the court of Liang Wu Di, then Wei, and then Le Yang, where he established residence. There he is quoted as saying:

The spirit should be tranquil and alert, but the body should be strong and active. Without tranquillity one cannot attain wisdom and transform into a Buddha; without health one cannot have good circulation and breathing. Hence the body should be properly exercised so that the muscles and tendons may be supple and the spirit will not then suffer from the misery of weakness.[73]

He is also the traditional creator of the 'Eighteen Le Han's Hands' exercise system, and is said to have created the Shao Lin system of martial artistry when he saw how weary the faces of the monks appeared.[74]

Acupuncture clearly continued to develop during these dynasties. The most famous text of the period was Huang-fu Mi's *Zhen Jiu Jia Yi Jing* (*The Systematic Classic of Acupuncture and Moxibustion*) of 282. That text reported 300 acupoints on the 12 regular channels, and 49 on the two midline channels — some 649 of the 670 presently accepted by modern Chinese sources.[75] The *Jia Yi Jing* is the oldest extant technical book devoted to acupuncture and moxibustion. It deals systematically with physiology, pathology, diagnosis, and therapy. It was the first text to introduce acupuncture's now-famous emphasis on disease prevention. This text's introduction of the idea that superior physicians treat disease before it arises became one of the

central ideals of the tradition. The text also established the essentials of the modern 'point book' format, describing the channels, naming the points on each, and listing their locations and how deeply each should be needled. It also records the length of time for which needles should be retained, the number of moxa cones to be applied to each point, and what each point is known to treat.[76]

Another important book of this time was Wang Shu-he's famous *Mai Jing* (*Pulse Classic*). This text expanded the ideas of pulse diagnosis from that described in the *Nan Jing*. It is the first systematic catalog of pulse patterns. In it Wang Shu-he described pulse diagnosis with reference to both acupuncture and traditional pharmaceutics, establishing one of the traditions that can be found in modern practice. When modern Chinese patients are asked to decoct and drink a so-called 'herbal' *tang* (a thick, soup-like decoction), they partake of another practice of this era. In practice, these formulas contain botanical, animal, and mineral products, not just the herbaceous botanicals to which the word 'herb' refers. Derived from the experience-centered folk tradition and eventually incorporated into the medicine of systematic correspondence, traditional pharmaceutics has been used as both an adjunct to acupuncture and as a separate internal and external medicine. Indeed, today in China it is the most popular expression of TCM. In the West, as in China and Japan, it has become a central aspect of the traditional medical marketplace, although typically in new, manufactured formats.

This period of political disunity was important for the development of acupuncture because during this time much that survives in modern acupuncture was systematized. In effect, the composition of acupuncture, both its practical and philosophical tenets, were then in place. These were to be permanent, lasting until the modern era.[77] The idea of *qi* circulation was considerably elaborated, becoming nearly modern in many aspects. The principles of correspondence, yin-yang, and the five phases were totally incorporated into the fabric of the art, affecting everything from the observations of diagnosis to the choice of acupoints in treatment. The view of the human body and its functions and their description in both natural and social metaphors became stable. For example, some of the names by which the points were then known remain in use today. The philosophical currents of Daoism, Buddhism, and Confucianism, the interplay and changing relations of which would continue to influence medical thought, were fully represented in Chinese society. Although the empire was still disunited, that too would change in the ensuing, short-lived Sui dynasty.

It was during the latter part of the Six Dynasties period that Chinese traditional medicines were exported to neighboring East Asian countries. Buddhist monks brought Chinese traditional medicines to both Korea and Japan. By some estimates the systems of pharmaceutics, acupuncture, and moxibustion were first sent to Paekche, Korea, by the emperor Wu Di in around 515.[78] Huang-fu Mi's influential *Zhen Jiu Jia Yi Jing* was among the texts known to have been brought to Paekche. But there is also speculation that acupuncture may have been practiced in Korea as early as the Han dynasty, when colonial prefectures had been established there. Although Chinese traditional medicines were absorbed and practiced in Korea, it would be many centuries before they gained official recognition, probably because Koreans had strong traditions of their own.

In 553 the Kingdom of Paekche sent Wang Yurungt'a and two masters of drug production to Japan to help reorganize medical education. However, it is commonly accepted that the most profound influence on Japan was that of the Buddhist monk Zhi Cong (Chiso), who brought 164 volumes on medicine from China, via Korea, in 562. This medical knowledge, like most of inflowing Chinese culture, was rapidly assimilated. In 562 Japan was relatively primitive compared to China. The first native government had only been in place for some 200 years. Thus, when the Japanese first officially contacted China, they tried to import as much as they could — writing, bureaucracy, Confucianism, Buddhism, Daoism, and medicine.

After its first import of medical texts, the Japanese government built free public hospitals attached to Buddhist temples, and asked every envoy to China to acquire more medical treatises. This absorption of Chinese culture and technology continued in waves until the middle of the 9th century, when contact with China was curtailed by political events.[79]

All the major Chinese medical traditions were imported during this period — herbal drugs, acupuncture, moxibustion, and massage. The earliest Japanese practitioners paid great attention to the early texts such the *Nei Jing, Nan Jing,* and *Zhen Jiu Jia Yi Jing*. Just as these early texts were important to the development of medical practice in China, so were they in Japan. In fact, the Japanese appear to have been more conservative in their adoption of this literature. For example, as the acupuncture and moxibustion literature was separate from herbal literature, the practices were kept separate, a tendency that persisted, with few exceptions, into the modern era.[80]

It is thought that Chinese traditional medical systems had an influence on Vietnamese medicine from the –2nd century onwards.[81] Thus Vietnam, like Korea and Japan, also has a long history of acupuncture and moxibustion. However, in these early stages, China's East Asian neighbors were content to import as much as possible. Japanese innovations, for example, did not begin until after contact with China had been curtailed.

Sui, 590 to 617: the period of reunification

Just after these disseminations, the first Sui ruler, Sui Wen-di, ended the political disunity of the Six Dynasties. He was an effective leader who applied principles from all three of China's religions, and thus won popular support. He reunited China militarily, recentralized the government, and rebuilt and extended the waterways and canals. He and his successor each ruled with an iron hand and conscripted huge workforces to labor on public projects, many of whom died.[82]

During this period, medicine in China continued to develop. For example, government farms for drug plants were organized. These must have been important because they were located near the capital and were assigned convenient and fertile lands. Probably the most famous medical person of this time was Sun Si-miao (581 to 682), one of the best regarded, but enigmatic, characters in acupuncture's story. To his classic education in the natural sciences and medicine, Sun Si-miao brought influences from both Daoism and Buddhism.[83] His works on prescriptions combine systematic correspondence with Daoist exorcism and some Buddhist concepts. However, his attempts to reconcile the basic principles of Buddhist medical theory and the medicine of systematic correspondence found no followers. He was a very cosmopolitan writer, and his works include a complete treatise on alchemy, descriptions of toxics to be worn as charms or burned as fumigants, and what is the oldest known collection of spells

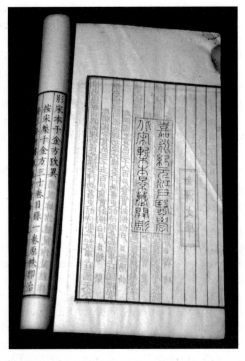

Figure 1.8 Title page of *Qian Jin Fang* (Qing reproduction of Song edition). (Courtesy of Paradigm Publications.)

for demonic medicine. In addition to these pursuits he produced works on drug therapy, acupuncture, and moxibustion: the *Qian Jin Yao Fang* of 652 and the *Qian Jin Yi Fang* of 670 (Fig. 1.8). His long-lasting fame is made evident by the fact that authors of subsequent centuries published books under his name. A famous example is the *Yinhai Jingwei* (*Reflections on the Silver Sea*), a classic text on eye diseases written no earlier than the 14th century.[84]

Probably drawing on earlier works, Sun Si-miao developed a format for acupuncture charts that is very much like what is in use today. There were three views: front, back, and side. On each of these views both the regular and extraordinary channels were set forth in five colors of ink. Sun Si-miao is regarded as having systematized the measurement system that is still used to describe the positions of acupoints. In this system the *cun*, or 'body inch,' is the distance from knuckle to knuckle of the patient's middle finger when it is bent to form three sides of a rectangle.[85]

Sun Si-miao also described many disease symptoms and treatments, the use of *a-shi* (painful points) and 'extra points' (points not located on the channels), and gave warnings against the use of particular acupoints.[86] Again, each of these concepts is found in modern acupuncturists' training. It is reasonable to suggest that the use of *a-shi* points is the original precedent for the modern concept of the trigger point. He also described 13 acupoints, sometimes called the 'ghost points,' for the treatment of demon-related diseases. Today these points are often mentioned in the context of psychological problems.

Another important writer was Yang Shang-shan, who either wrote or compiled the *Huang Di Nei Jing Tai Su*, an influential text explaining earlier ideas from the *Nei Jing* and *Nan Jing*, and other treatises that were no longer extant by this period. In general, however, like the Tang dynasty to follow, the Sui was not a period of general innovation, but a period of diffusion. Just as reunification of the empire prepared Chinese culture to receive and respond to the social and cultural forces of

China's second golden age, the Tang, the diffusion of acupuncture prepared the rest of Chinese medicine for the absorption of the principles of systematic correspondence.

Tang, 618 to 906: the period of culmination

Although most Tang rulers favored Daoist ideas, what characterizes the Tang is not the Daoist dominance, but broad social, and cultural sophistication.[87] The Tang was a period of cultural brilliance that both native and foreign historians describe as the second Chinese golden age. The empire was united; the three philosophical pillars (Confucianism, Daoism, and Buddhism) and contact with neighboring cultures created an atmosphere of intellectual richness. Like the Han following the Qin, the Tang was a collective sigh of relief for the Chinese, who were again relatively free of oppression by their imperial rulers and able to enjoy the fecund variety in which Chinese genius seems to flourish.

Buddhism achieved its greatest number of adherents during the Tang.[88] A vast interchange between arts and sciences occurred through the Indian pilgrimages of Chinese Buddhists. Like pilgrims everywhere, they returned not only with souvenirs and religious relics, but also with memories and impressions, new ideas and inspirations. Monasteries, having accumulated considerable wealth, played an economic role as sources of credit, agrarian employment, and as the seat of commercial enterprises. However, their success targeted them for a campaign of secularization by the Tang administration. Their tremendous resources were reappropriated for the state and its tax roles. In the years 841 to 845, 4000 monasteries were destroyed, 260 000 monks and nuns were returned to the laity, and 40 000 temples with a million acres of land were confiscated.[89] This vast wealth flowed into a society that was already prosperous. Populations flourished, and all the social classes enjoyed the fruits of the cultural harvest.[90]

There was a new edition of the *Huang Di Nei Jing Su Wen*. This Tang edition by Wang Bing is notable for including the first chronobiological link between acupuncture and the 60-year cycle of the Chinese calendar.[91] The system uses the concepts of *yin-yang* to name 'host' and 'guest' years, with particular seasonal expectations. It is probably the outcome of long observation of disease patterns, or even epidemics, relative to the seasons and the astronomic observations on which the Chinese calendar is based. This method became formalized as *wu-yun liu-qi* (five periods, six *qi*). Although the idea is found in earlier texts and the terms are used in the *Nei Jing*, it is probably of Tang origin. References in older *Nei Jing* editions are all in chapters of dubious age. The *Nei Jing* of 762 made a significant contribution to the form in which the *Nei Jing* is now known.

Acupuncture also had detractors; in the *Wai Tai Bi Yao* (*Important Formulae and Prescriptions Revealed by a Governor of a Distance Province*) of 752, Wang Dao would refer to acupuncture as dangerous, and recommend only moxibustion and heat treatment.[92]

Despite the innovation, creativity, and wealth of the Tang, the development of acupuncture was not very notable. Most Tang medical and intellectual investment centered on the 'elixir of life,' the alchemical source of immortality. This sought-after elixir now had its broadest and deepest effect on Chinese culture. Thousands experimented, hoping to discover the source of immortality. Seven of the 22 Tang rulers died from formulas meant to give them eternal life. This cultural obsession occupied many resources and, despite the appreciable death toll and waste of resources, resulted in a greater knowledge of medicinal substances. Pine seeds and resin, chamomile, and the *li-shi* mushroom are among the medicinals investigated, some of which retain an aura of their Tang reputation even today.

This futile search did not entirely monopolize medical activity. The base of knowledge expanded sufficiently that four specialized types of doctor were recognized — physicians (meaning herb doctors), acupuncturists, masseurs, and exorcists.[93] Doctors, however, did not achieve elevated social status.

Because there was little useful medical innovation during the Tang, the essential corpus of acupuncture knowledge remained essentially stable. For example, books continued to list 649 of the presently accepted 670 acupoints.[94] This is not to say, however, that nothing more was learned. In 670, for example, Zui Zhi-di wrote a treatise on the cure of what may have been tuberculosis, or a tuberculosis-like illness, where the acupoints known today as BL-17 and BL-19 (to which BL-15 was later added) are treated by moxibustion. These points were still indicated for this disease when Soulie de Morant prepared his significant compendium of Chinese treatments in the early 20th century. What are possibly the first references to veterinary acupuncture and moxibustion can be found in the Tang dynasty, but these do not appear to have been very commonly used or influential.

During this time, herbal therapeutics, acupuncture, moxibustion, and massage matured further and became well established in both Korea and Japan. The first Korean institute of medicine was established in 692. It taught acupuncture, moxibustion, and natural drugs as specialties. In Japan, in 702 the first Imperial medical college was established in Nara by the emperor Monmu. This college had 7-year courses, with acupuncture and moxibustion having their own specialized faculty. Here the study of the *Nei Jing*, *Nan Jing*, the *Ming Tang* (which is no longer extant) and the *Zhen Jiu Jia Yi Jing* comprised the core studies.[95] Other specialized study included herbal pharmaceutics and *anma* massage. Although, as we will see, acupuncture and moxibustion would experience periods of both growth and decline over the centuries, the formation of medical colleges in Korea and Japan established acupuncture and moxibustion as accepted systems of healing, as they remain to this day in both countries.

Five dynasties, 907 to 960, Song, 960 to 1264: the period of Neo-Confucianism

The Tang dynasty collapsed of its own inertia in 906 after a lengthy decline. A general estab-lished the Song government in 960 after 50 years of contested rule, a period known as the 'Five Dynasties' for its discontinuity of government. Although China remained united, it was now surrounded by aggressive foreign states, some of which already held Chinese territory. The Song rulers appeased their neighbors at considerable expense, but avoided war. A trade deficit, lowered tax revenues, and the circulation of paper money contributed to inflation, and their fiscal power eroded.[96]

Social and economic differentiation and specialization grew as the population continued its urban and southern shift. Guilds were formed, agricultural and commercial production expanded as new technologies came on line. Interdependence increased as cities, regions, trades, and professions became more and more specialized. As Paul Unschuld explains, the period's interest in details and refinements was matched by an increasing awareness and attention to the interrelatedness of the whole and its components.[97] Thus, in addition to the progress of secular studies, Confucianism and Daoism adopted this new scientism, while Buddhism declined relative to their success. In particular, the emerging *qi*-centered neo-Confucian model successfully countered the Buddhist idea of the material world as pure illusion. What achieved intellectual supremacy was the notion proposed by the doctrine of *qi* that *qi* had always existed and that all things came in and out of existence as gatherings or dissolutions of *qi*.[98] Medicine paralleled these events; in Paul Unschuld's words:

First, we can observe the fragmentation into specialized fields, as well as a tendency toward pronounced reductionism in notions about the cause, nature and treatment of illness; second, there were intensive efforts to verify the validity of the medicine of systematic correspondence by extending it to practical drug therapy.[99]

Thus Daoist and Buddhist exorcisms as well as drug therapy joined acupuncture in being founded on systematic correspondence. Where, for example, at the beginning of the Song period there were nearly 100 acupuncture texts, 50 physiological texts, and even 70 books devoted to the pulse alone, less than 10 works had followed Zhang Zhong-jing's ordering of drug treatments according to the principles of systematic correspondence.[100] Thus, it is only in this period, a millennium past the *Nan Jing*, that the qi paradigm achieved dominance over all the branches of Chinese traditional medicine. Yin-yang, the five phases, the celestial stems and terrestrial branches, and the six climatic influences permeated every branch of Chinese medicine.

In line with this development of systematic correspondences, the *Nan Jing* received greater attention, even eclipsing the *Nei Jing*. In fact, by 1155 the author of a preface to a new edition of the *Ling Shu* wrote that the text had been lost for a long time and that hardly anyone studied it.[101] By 1058 the *Nan Jing* had reached Korea. When the Mongols of the following Yuan dynasty decided to translate important Chinese texts into their own language, it was the *Nan Jing*, not the older *Nei Jing*, that they chose. Another indication of this text's importance during this era is the appearance of a Persian edition.[102]

Another of Japan's contributions to acupuncture was foreshadowed in this era, a refined art of moxibustion. Export to Japan saved Wen Ren Qi-nian's text of 1226, the *Bei Ji Jiu Fa* (*Moxibustion Methods for Use in Emergencies*). This work describes the treatment of 23 diseases exclusively by moxibustion. The text was nicely illustrated; it was lost in China, but was preserved in Japan until 1890 so that it is available today (Fig. 1.9).[103]

Massage, which probably dates to antiquity, was, according to Soulie de Morant, perfected during the 11th to 12th centuries. He notes that the Ming classic *Zhen Jiu Da Cheng* reproduces the most important passages of works by a children's doctor, Chen Wenzhong (Wen Xu): *Xiao Er An Mo Jing* (*Massage of Channels for Children*) and *Xiao Er Bing Yuan Fang Lun* (*Discourses and Prescriptions on the Origin of Illnesses of Children*).

The *wu-yun liu-qi* chronobiological concept introduced in the Tang edition of the *Su Wen* achieved enough status to become an examination topic. In 1241 Dou Han-jing published *Zhen Jing Zhi Nan* (*Compass Bearings*) for acupuncture

and moxibustion. This text described *zi-wu*, or noon and midnight cycles, and monthly, seasonal and annual cycles of *qi* according to which acupuncture could be performed.[104]

Even with the neo-Confucian influence, government investment played no particularly notable role in medicine. During the Song dynasty there would be a brief attempt to establish charitable drug dispensaries. However, this resulted in nothing of significance.[105] The emperor ordered a life-size bronze statue of a human, which was constructed in 1026. The metal walls of this statue were holed at acupoint locations and the statue covered with yellow wax. When students selected and needled the appropriate location, they would be rewarded by drops of water that indicated they had passed their exam.[106] Accompanying this statue was a now well-known text by Wang Wei-yi, the *Tong Ren Shu Xue Zhen Jiu Tu Jing* which, following the *Zhen Jiu Jia Yi Jing*, further systematized and clarified the location and indications of acupuncture points.

During the Song dynasty there were several other notable publications and developments in acupuncture and moxibustion. There were

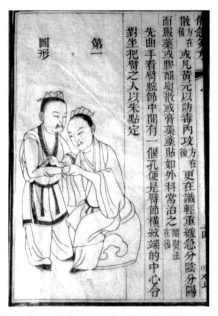

Figure 1.9 Moxibustion prescriptions for emergency use. (Courtesy of Paradigm Publications.)

several moxibustion-only treatises such as Dou-zhe's *Huang Di Ming Tang Jiu Jing*, which helped permanently establish the tradition of moxibustion. There was also the first published text describing the systematic structure of *nai jia fa*, a 10-day biorhythmic cycle used in acupuncture treatment. He Ruo-yu's *Zi Wu Liu Zhu Zhen Jing* established biorhythmic treatment as a permanent fixture in the practice of acupuncture. It was further elaborated in the Ming dynasty, and remains in use today.[107]

Also in the Song dynasty Yuan Ti's book *Tai Yi Shen Zhen* appeared (1125). This began the 'Shen Zhen' school of moxibustion, where poles of moxibustion with various herbs admixed were ignited and then applied to acupuncture points. This is probably the precursor of the Japanese *onkyu* moxa, a method that persists in modern practice. The Song was also the dynasty in which anatomical charts of the body and internal organs were first published. These anatomical speculations were based on observations made in the vivisection of the rebel Ou Xi-fan (1045) and several other studies done in the early 1100s.[108] These charts were later adopted by both Chinese and Japanese authors in the 1300s. They were used until the 18th and 19th centuries, when more precise and accurate Western anatomical information was imported.

Although these refinements of the practices of acupuncture and moxibustion are notable, it is primarily the developments in drug therapy for which the Song dynasty is best remembered. In essence it was the broad social and intellectual climate of the period between the Song and Ming that produced specialization and refinement of the qi paradigm. These refinements were expressed in the ideas of individual physicians whose work was so seminal that their reputations survive to the present day. Among these is Liu Wan-su, a physician who lived between 1110 and 1200. Li Wan-su proposed a further elaboration of the five-phase model and incorporated this into herbal therapy. Because of his concentration on fire and heat, his work is the start of what would become known as the 'school of cooling.'

His treatments also featured the consistent use of acupuncture and drug therapy in combination, as well as the application of Buddhist charms.[109]

Zhang Cong-zhen (1156 to 1228), also known as Cong Zheng, also combined herbal drugs, acupuncture, and a variety of other techniques, but used these techniques to eliminate evil influences through the skin, or through tears, vomit, urine or feces.[110]

Another of the famous Song physicians is Zhu Dan-qi, known as Chen Yan. He is most remembered for the text *San Yin Ji Yi Bing Zheng Fan Lun* (*Prescriptions Elucidated on the Premise That All Pathological Symptoms Have Only Three Primary Causes*) of 1174.[111] Chen Yan's ideas contributed to the Jin-Yuan revival of the Zhang Zhong-jing's Han era works, *Shang Han Lun* and *Jin Gui Yao Lue*. Until then, as mentioned earlier, these texts had been effectively ignored.

Li Gao (1180 to 1251), often known by his pen name Li Dong-yuan, contributed his own innovations based on his reading of statements in the *Huang Di Nei Jing Su Wen*. He attributed many illnesses to digestive malfunction. He thus categorized external damage to the spleen and stomach (i.e. that arising from poorly chosen food and drink and exhaustion), and internal damage (i.e. that resulting from emotional excess) as principal sources of disease. He recommended supplementing the spleen and stomach, an approach to treatment adopted by his contemporaries, and many thereafter, to the extent that it is still a school of thought in Chinese traditional medicine.[112]

Although the writers most remembered for having adapted Chinese drug therapy to the medicine of systematic correspondence lived and worked during the Song dynasty, the intellectual effort they began forms a movement that historians label as Song-Jin-Yuan. Indeed, until questioned by later medical writers, the ideas of this period would form a steady orthodoxy within the always mixed and various medicines of China. Throughout the Song-Jin-Yuan period the materia medica grew, older literature was re-examined, and clinicians continuously observed and explored. Although acupuncture can fairly be said to have developed during these centuries only in so far as its details are concerned, the expansion of herbal therapy was significant, and its resulting categories and etiologies have come to influence acupuncture today.[113]

During this period, Japanese society continued to develop and was beginning to show its own specializations and innovations. After contact with China was curtailed in the mid-9th century, Chinese thought had less influence on the development of Japanese acupuncture. Although contact with China was eventually re-established and more literature was undoubtedly imported, distinctly Japanese traditions began during this period. However, by the late 12th century, acupuncture and moxibustion had become less popular. This decline in popularity persisted until the mid-16th century, when traditional literature, techniques, and ideas with a distinctly Japanese flavor once again began to flourish.[114] The most notable book to appear during this period was the *Ishin Po*, by Tamba Yasuyori. This book was commissioned by the Emperor in 982. It described the diversity of traditional medical practices of the time. Of its 30 scrolls, one is devoted to acupuncture and moxibustion. This book is notable, not only because it is still extant in its original form, but also because it is an encyclopedia of lost Chinese and Japanese medical literature. It preserves books that no longer exist in any other form.

In Korea, the most notable developments also concerned traditional medicinals. There was a significant trade of natural drugs from Korea to China, and a consequent exchange of medical information. This also included acupuncture literature. By the 11th century, a text like the one that accompanied the bronze statue was in constant use in the training of Korean acupuncturists. There are also records of an influx of medical knowledge from China to Vietnam. In the early 12th century, Gao Dai-yun of the Nan Zhao kingdom (now part of northern Vietnam), returned from the Song court with 62 medical treatises.[115]

Yuan, 1264 to 1368: the period of Mongol control

The Yuan dynasty marked a period when China came under Mongol rule, initially under Ghenghis Khan and then his grandson Kublai Khan. The period is particularly important because it marked the beginning of Western impact on China. Kublai Khan ruled China as part of a vast empire. From Vietnam and Tibet in the south, to Mongolia, Korea, and Manchuria in the north and Europe in the West, the Khan ruled most of the Eurasian landmass. Everywhere the light cavalry of the nomadic Mongols was feared and victorious. For the first time in history a traveler could move from the coast of China to the frontiers of Europe within a single domain and without impediment. In fact, many Western impressions of China come from this period because one traveler — Marco Polo — did walk from Europe to the court of Kublai Khan where he served as an advisor. By 1263, there are also reports of a European physician at the court of Kublai Khan, and by 1272 the same doctor, Isaiah, who was also a linguist and a scholar, opened a hospital, called 'Broad Charity', in Beijing.[116] He was the first trickle of what would later become a torrent of Western medical knowledge.

The Mongol rulers were neither Westernized nor Sinicized; they retained their own language, and kept important government posts for their own people. They despised cities and urban life, and were universally feared for their unrelenting destruction of urban centers that refused to surrender — the ruins can still be seen today. However, persuasive Chinese officials dissuaded them from undoing China's urbanization. Although China was a subject state it was neither horribly oppressed nor financially ruined. Agriculture and commerce flourished, intellectual life was unhindered, neo-Confucianism continued to spread, and traditional education was preserved.

The Yuan dynasty saw the founding of the Tai Yi Yuan, or Imperial Academy of Medicine. During the Jin this had been subordinate to the Court Ceremonial Institute. In the Yuan it became an independent government agency with responsibility for medical standards and the training of physicians for government services and, although perhaps only in name, treatment of the Emperor. This reflects both an increase in importance and a growth of scope, with medicine becoming increasingly specialized.

In 1329 Wang Guo-rui produced the *Bian Que Shen Ying Zhen Jiu You Long Jing*, a manual in verse of 'Bian Que's marvellously successful principles.' It was a treatment manual where information was transmitted by mnemonic verse.[117] The Yuan was also a period of bronze acupuncture statues, devices that symbolize the relative stability of acupuncture's base of data. Hua Shuo's *Shi Si Jing Fa Hui* (*An Elucidation of the Fourteen Channels*) was published in 1341. That text places 303 points on the 12 regular channels, and 51 on the two medial channels – a total of 657 of the now-accepted 670 acupoints.[118] Hua Shou realized that the governing vessel and conception vessel were the only extra channels to have their own points, and created many of the modern waterway analogies used to describe the circulation of *qi*. Interestingly, he also coined the term *jing xue*, or 'channel point,' indicating a new degree of theoretical import for the channels. His edition of the *Nan Jing* is considered by some to be the best of those that survive.

There was also a further development in the specialized practice of moxibustion with the publication of Dou Cai's *Bian Que Xin Shu* and Zhuang Zhuo's *Gao Huang Shu Xue Jiu Fa*. These were small but influential moxibustion classics. The first compilation book, the *Zhen Jiu Si Shu*, by Dou Gui-fang, appeared during this era. This method of publication for acupuncture texts became commonplace as authors edited other people's works. The treatment of domesticated animals with acupuncture and moxibustion also appears to have taken root during the Yuan.

Few developments of note were made during this period in neighboring East Asian countries. One notable exception is the *Nam Duoc Than Hieu*, by Tue Tinh of Vietnam. This work compiles information about the practice of Vietnamese traditional medicine. There was also a continued exchange between China and her neighbors, as exemplified by stories of the Chinese physician Zou Geng treating the Vietnamese crown prince in 1340. However, it would not be until the Ming dynasty that acupuncture and moxibustion became revitalized throughout the region.

Ming, 1368 to 1643: the period of restoration

Beginning in 1325, the Chinese people began to rebel against their Mongol rulers. Busy fighting among themselves, the once-united tribesmen were unable to contend effectively with these rebellions, and by 1368 Chinese troops once again controlled the capital of Beijing. The man named emperor was Zhu Yuan-zhang, a low-born military leader who had become the most important rebel commander. Zhu Yuan-zhang ruled absolutely. At the expense of the Confucian bureaucracy, he concentrated power in himself and in the imperial office he controlled. Indeed, the bureaucracy lost power not only upward to an autocratic ruler, but also downward and outward to an emerging civil service.[119]

Both of the major characteristics of the Ming government directly affected medicine, as Paul Unschuld states:

Two aspects of early Ming politics are of particular significance ... the rise of the Neo-Confucianism of the brothers Cheng and Zhu Xi to orthodox political and social policy, and the 'democratization' of the civil service.[120]

In effect, not only did a Confucian education become available to many more people, but the bureaucracy was also open to a far broader subset of the population.[121] It was as if, in modern terms, a demanding essay-type examination of unlimited scope had been replaced by a multiple-choice test with questions taken from a published list. Those who were merely literate now qualified for positions that had once only been open to those with an advanced education. People with only a basic education reached unprecedented levels in society.

This popularization affected acupuncture. Greater opportunity came from reduced limits. This resulted in greater prosperity for many more people. There were also more books, more readers, and a better chance for any writer to achieve publication. In modern terms, the Ming saw an 'information explosion.'[122] This explosion was able to spread even further, because neo-Confucianism was so permeated with Daoist and Buddhist thought as to be transformed. It represented no impediment to innovation. With the dominant philosophy so open, intellectual diversity flourished. In Paul Unschuld's words:

While an obsolete Neo-Confucianism covered the empire like a hard crust, beneath the surface a vigorous intellectual life developed, increasingly distancing itself from orthodoxy and underlining the growing contrast between the state and its claims, on the one hand, and the expectations and desires of the people and scholarly community on the other hand.[123]

It was a time of broad and deep intellectual ferment, unrestrained by either the self-interested autocrat at the head of the state or the dominant philosophy. Orthodoxy lost its power and diversity took its place. Indeed, the Ming ferment was of such breadth that, apart from the proven classics, all Ming works must be regarded with caution. The selection is so great that a Ming author may be found to support almost any proposition. Later in the 20th century, as before in the imperial past, there were attempts to decree one-and-only medical practices, but heterogeneity is the central character of Chinese medicine and the Ming is its extreme.

Like the society, medicine was a turmoil of diversity, although its ranks were perhaps less democratized. From 1368 there had been a significant distinction among the classes of physicians. There were the *cao ze ling yi*, roving practitioners who had a familial, experiential knowledge of medicine. They went from house to house, village to village, like peddlers. There were also *yi guan*, or medical bureaucrats. This rank was composed largely of *Ru Yi*, or scholar physicians, although it was not impossible for a successful *ling yi* to attain this official status.

Medical thought stayed with the trends of the Song-Jin-Yuan, in particular with regard to the incorporation of natural drugs into the medicine of systematic correspondence. However, it continued with the fervor of the Ming. There were even attempts to incorporate demonology into the qi paradigm. But the most noteworthy Ming contributions to medicine came from the continued flowering of individual approaches and interpretations.[124]

Among the many adaptations of the Ming era all the Song-Jin-Yuan schools found adherents. Through his student Dai Si-gong, Zhu Zhen-heng's notion that an inadequacy of *yin* was at the root of most illness became the central dogma of the *yang-yin* school. Another writer, Xue Ji, carried forward the emphasis on the spleen and stomach originally proposed by Zhu Zhen-heng and Li Gao. In contrast, Zhang Jie-bin proposed that *yang* could not possibly be in surplus because *yang qi* sustained life. In his terms, yang was hard to get, easy to lose, and, once lost, hard to regain. There was also a compromise school whose members did not accept only one theory but rather selected appropriate therapies from the entire medical literature. In a very Chinese response to diversity, practitioners used what worked.[125]

In 1641 to 1644 there was a widespread epidemic for which the followers of Li Gao's spleen and stomach school were completely ineffective. Amidst the general belief that this method should have excelled at treating this condition, the public failure was magnified by Wu Hu-xing's appreciable success. His ideas were recorded in the *Wen Yi Lun* (*Theory of Warm-Induced Disorders*). His therapies were based on the idea that evil influences must be expelled to reduce fever. These treatments made considerable use of aggressive measures that induced elimination. Thus another approach joined the heterogenous mix of the period.[126]

During the Ming dynasty, acupuncture continued to be relatively stable. However, by the end of the Ming dynasty, criticism of the formerly dominant *yun-qi* stem–branch biorhythmic system had eroded the popularity of acupuncture. Although Jin Yi-sun's *Zhen Jiu Ze*

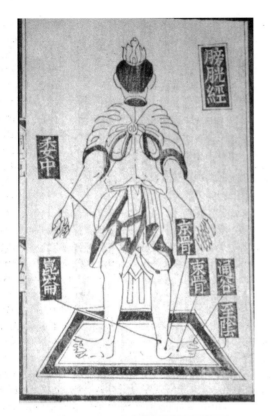

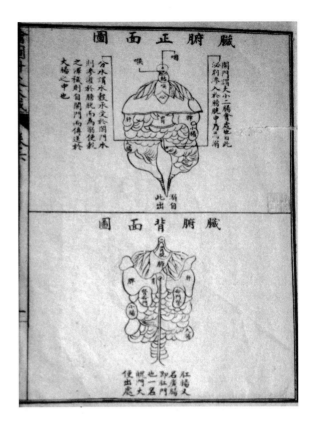

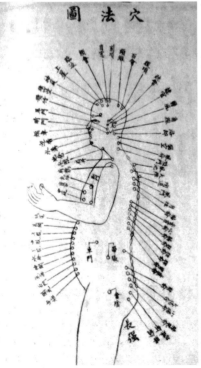

Figure 1.10 Illustrations from the *Great Compendiums.*
(Courtesy of Paradigm Publications.)

Ri Bian (1447) was so generally accepted during the Ming that its ideas appeared in the popular texts of the period, criticism of the supporting ideas of Juan Xun-yi, Wang Ji, and Zhang Jie-bin nonetheless led to a loss of intellectual dominance and a decline in the social role of acupuncture.[127]

In medical literature, however, the Ming was a high point. There were several important texts, some of which are still used and respected. Compilation treatises such as the *Zhen Jiu Da Quan* by Xu Feng (1437), the *Zhen Jiu Ju Ying*, by Gao Wu (1529), and the *Zhen Jiu Da Cheng*, by Yang Ji-zhou (1601), were very influential. Xu Feng's *Zhen Jiu Da Quan* was important because it was the first text to systematically describe the eight extraordinary vessels and the daily, 10-day and 60-day biorhythm treatment methods. Each of these survives in modern practice, and can be seen as the basis of some treatment ideas used today. Gao Wu's *Zhen Jiu Ju Ying* systematized useful and time-tested treatments, and introduced the use of supplementing and draining acupoints. These too are routinely used today, as is his systematization of the *Nan Jing* five-phase treatment. However, it is Yang Ji-zhou's *Zhen Jiu Da Cheng* that is the most famous acupuncture treatise of the Ming period, and perhaps of any era.

The *Zhen Jiu Da Cheng* (1601) was produced in at least 30 editions prior to 1900, and in about 50 more since then. This, the *Great Compendium of Acupuncture and Moxibustion*, notes 308 points on the 12 regular channels and 51 on the two medial channels. This total of 667 acupoints almost exactly matches the 670 now accepted.[128] Acupoint names catalogued in the *Great Compendium* remain in use today, as are the treatments it describes. Produced in the midst of the tremendous diversity of the late 1500s, Yang Ji-zhou's *Great Compendium* and Li Shi-zhen's *Ben Cao Gang Mu* are the outstanding medical events of the Ming (Fig. 1.10).

Both these important works introduce the innovation of giving exact sources, just as in modern scholarship. Both compile not merely the ideas of a single teacher or individual school of thought, but a relative orthodoxy derived from clinical consensus. Although they contain no statistical justifications, they are similar to what we know today as 'meta-studies,' because they compile information that is thought to be validated by many practitioners in a variety of clinical settings. Both preserve information from many texts and represent the epitome of scholarship in their respective fields. Each preserves what was found clinically useful in the past. The codifications each develops, such as the *Great Compendium's* system for describing acupoint locations, survive to the present. Each is still considered the surviving high point of the written tradition, and the strongest representative of classical clinical acupuncture. Yang Ji-zhou's *Zhen Jiu Da Cheng*, and Soulie de Morant's seminal French work *L'Acuponcture Chinoise* that is based on it, are still described as the finest clinical manuals.[129]

But there were other influential texts of the period. Li Shi-zhen's treatise on the extraordinary vessel system, the *Qi Jing Ba Mai Kao* (1578), has influenced the theory and practice of the extra vessels ever since. Like his *Ben Cao Gang Mu*, this text exemplifies Li's scholarship. There were also a number of influential *Nei Jing* commentaries, such as Zhang Jie-bin's *Lei Jing* (1624) and the *Nei Jing Zhi Yao* by Li Zhong-zi (1642). There were also *Nan Jing* commentaries, such as the *Nan Jing Ji Zhu* by Wang Jiu-si (1505) and the *Tu Zhu Ba Shi Yi Nan Jing* by Zheng Shi-xien (1510).

We also find important treatises concerning Chinese traditional medicines other than acupuncture. Some simultaneously describe acupuncture, moxibustion, and herbalism. Examples of these are Li Ting's *Yi Xue Ru Men* (1575) and Zhang Jie-bin's *Jing Yue Quan Shu* (1624). One author of the period went so far as to state that the 'ancients' had believed one who knew drugs but not acupuncture, or acupuncture but not moxa, could never be a true physician. Although we clearly see a blending of acupuncture, moxibustion, and the practice of pharmacotherapy in these texts, this approach never achieved dominance. There were strong traditions of acupuncture and moxibustion in combination, and of acupuncture or moxibustion alone, and all were practiced with or without the use of natural drugs from herbs, minerals, and animal products.

The use of veterinary acupuncture and moxibustion seems to have become even more commonplace for the treatment of domesticated animals (Box 1.1). We find, for example, texts devoted to the treatment of specific animals, the *Ma Niu Yi Fang* (1399) being a good example. This text is devoted to the treatment of horses and oxen. One of its distinctive features is that the animals are shown to have points with precise effects, but not systems of channels.

During the Ming dynasty there were also developments in neighboring East Asian countries. In the early 1600s an influential encyclopedia of herbal pharmaceutics, the *Tong-Eui-Po-Gam*, was published in Korea. However, the most notable Korean contribution was probably Sa-Am Do-In's 1500s text the *Chimkyu Yokyol*. In this text, the monk Sa-Am described a systematization of five-phase treatment based on the ancient *Nan Jing*. His four-acupoint treatment formulas for replete and vacuous conditions are still famous today.[130] These treatments

---

Box 1.1   Veterinary acupuncture

Although there were references to the treatment of animals in the *Shen Nong Ben Cao*, and in texts in the later Han dynasty, it was not until the 6th century that the first veterinary acupuncture book, Bai Le's *Bai Le Zhen Jing*, was written. By this time, this and the *Bai Le Liao Ma Jing* and *Qi Min Yao Shu* described the treatment of more than 40 diseases in the farm animals: horse, cow, sheep and pig.

In the Sui dynasty, more than 30 veterinary acupuncture books specializing in diagnosis, treatment, or herbal pharmaceutics were written. Among these were the *Lei Fang Ma Jing* and *Ma Shu* specializing in horses, the *Shui Niu Jing* specializing in water buffalo, and more general texts such as the *Qi Bai Dui Zheng* and the *Niu Ma Tuo Jing*, together with texts focusing on the detailed description of acupoint locations, such as the *Ma Jing Kong Xue Tu*. These texts described the anatomical locations of acupuncture points for each animal and the combinations and techniques of point stimulation for various diseases.

In the Tang dynasty one of the better known texts was the *Si Mu An Ji Ji*, by Li Shi. Further treatises were written during the Song and Yuan dynasties, but the most famous treatise was the typical Ming-style compilation, the *Yuan Heng Liao Ma Ji* (1608), by the veterinarian brothers Yu Ben Yuan and Yu Heng. This text detailed the treatment of horses, cows, camels, cattle, and water buffalo, and is very influential even today. It is generally believed that veterinary acupuncture arrived in Japan during this era.

During the Qing dynasty, little innovation in veterinary acupuncture can be found, just as all traditional medicine declined in the Qing. After 1911, veterinary acupuncture suffered further setbacks, as did acupuncture in general. However, with the publication of the *Zhong Shou Yi Zhen Jiu Xue* in 1959, traditional veterinary acupuncture underwent a resurgence. Since the early 1970s, various new techniques such as electro acupuncture have been integrated into its practice. The most recent texts

describe the use of acupuncture, moxibustion, local injection, ear acupuncture, iron branding, bloodletting, and electro acupuncture for diseases in a variety of animals. Acupoint locations for the horse, cow, pig, goat, sheep, camel, dog, rabbit, cat, chick, and duck are mapped. Animals typically present different arrangements of acupoints than do humans, and also differ by species.

As a visitor to Hidetaro Mori's Osaka Acupuncture and Moxibustion College, Stephen Birch was delighted when Mori showed him his library, including his rare book collection, among which were two court medical scrolls (each about 20 feet long) devoted to the acupuncture treatment of hunting hawks. These were beautifully crafted documents with ornate illustrations and text. In Yoshio Manaka's private book collection, Birch found several treatises devoted to the treatment of animals, including a lengthy and detailed text in Chinese on the treatment of horses. These texts were profusely illustrated and very elegant. In Tokyo, Birch also met Meiyu Okada, a well-known *keiraku chiryo* practitioner, who, a number of years before, had written a specialized text on the treatment of horses by acupuncture. Clearly, the use of acupuncture in veterinary practice is alive and well, and has a long tradition of practice in East Asia.

In the West there is a growing interest in veterinary acupuncture. Racing tracks in various locations around the USA have acupuncturists working on horses. Veterinarians are specializing in acupuncture for both small and large animals. Specialized training courses for veterinarians are available and the International Veterinary Acupuncture Society has been in existence since the mid-1970s.

Source: Bossut D 1990 Development of veterinary acupuncture in China. Paper presented at the 16th International Veterinary Acupuncture Society Congress on Veterinary Acupuncture, Holland

survive not only in Korea, but also in Japan, Europe, the UK, and the USA. They are tested in the licensing examinations in Korea and the USA. A century before, traditional medical practices that had first come from China were officially sanctioned in Korea. This helped Korean traditional medicine, including indigenous systems of acupuncture, moxibustion, and pharmaceutics, to flourish.

During this period, acupuncture and moxibustion underwent a resurgence in Japan, and uniquely Japanese contributions continued to appear. In the late 1500s the court physician Isai Misonou began the Mubunryu school. This style of practice was unusual in that diagnosis was accomplished almost exclusively through palpation of the abdomen and lower chest. This style of diagnosis persists today throughout Japan.[131] Known as 'abdominal palpation' or 'hara diagnosis,' it is used in all aspects of Japanese traditional practice. Isai Misonou also introduced a unique treatment method. He used large, nearly blunt, gold and silver needles that were tapped with a weighted wooden mallet on

reactive points of the abdomen and chest. This, his whole treatment, is still considered effective for many conditions.

In the early 1600s, Tokuhon Nagata wrote a now-famous poem describing the uses of moxibustion, furthering the tradition of moxibustion as a sole practice. At the same time, Japanese commentaries on the *Nei Jing* and *Nan Jing* flourished, beginning a tradition that survived to the end of the 19th century. In Japan, as in China, it was considered a sign of status for a traditional physician to explain the *Nei Jing* or *Nan Jing*. There were so many such commentaries from this period that acupuncture must have been a 'growth industry' in Japan. There was also a continued influx of medical knowledge from China. For example, it is thought that the emigration of Zheng Yi-yuan to Nagasaki in the late 15th century helped improve Japanese medical learning.[132]

However, one of the most influential events of the period was the arrival of Dutch traders in Japan. In 1639, the Tokugawa Shogunate named the Dutch as its principal European

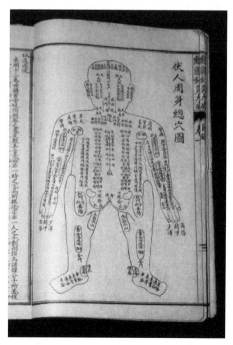

Figure 1.11 Acupoints and proportional measures. (Courtesy of Paradigm Publications).

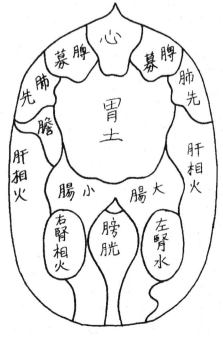

Figure 1.12 Mubunryu abdominal patterns. (Courtesy of *Chasing the Dragon's Tail*, Manaka, Itrya, Birch.)

trading partner. From this time Dutch medicine exerted a powerful influence on acupuncture and moxibustion, which, as we will see, nearly destroyed traditional medical practices in the eras that followed.

Qing, 1644 to 1911: the end of the empire

The Ming dynasty ended in dissolution. Although the newly united Manchu nation had made inroads at the periphery of China, the empire's internal bureaucratic strife, natural disasters, and weakness lead to popular uprisings. These could not be contained, and the Mongol-aided Manchurian invasion of 1618 could not be restrained. Chinese aristocrats, preferring subjugation by foreigners to losing their heads to Chinese rebels, surrendered, and the Qing dynasty commenced in 1636.[133]

The Manchu had appropriated the Confucian social model prior to their conquest of China. This cultural continuity, along with the continued presence of the now subject Chinese aristocracy, made their rule relatively benign. Between 1662 and 1796, three particularly effective Manchurian rulers established not only a cultural merger, but also a genuine peak of civil and economic well-being. Then, after this 100-year interlude the philosophical diversity of the Ming produced a conservative rebound that permeated all of Chinese culture.[134]

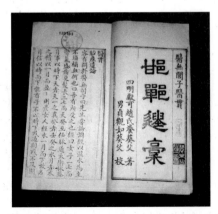

Figure 1.13 *Yi Guan* or 'Thorough Knowledge of Medicine' of 1687. (Courtesy of Paradigm Publications.)

The conservatives saw a cheapened Song neo-Confucianism as responsible for the empire's subjugation. However, in the retrospect of secular history, what probably doomed the Qing was the economic and political realities of the 19th century – a vastly increased population that could not be effectively fed, the opium trade and opium war, the devastations of two rebellions, and, finally, the Sino-Japanese war. Although there were attempted reforms, and the government undertook to acquire Western weapons and materials,[135] these attempts were ineffective, and the last emperor abdicated on February 12, 1912. The new Chinese Republic was thus born in confusion and helplessness, while Chinese intellectual life was mired in an intellectual anticlimax to the Ming.[136]

Although the diversity of medical approaches that blossomed during the Ming continued during the Qing, their bloom lacked luster and the tree was wilting from the root. With the ever-increasing presence of Western medical knowledge and techniques, traditional practices declined. The influence of the Jennarian smallpox vaccination beginning in 1805,[137] the first missionary surgeon in 1835, the first translation of Western medical texts in the 1850s, and the establishment of China's first Western medical school in 1886 were omens portending the demise of traditional medicine. The introduction of the germ theories of List, Koch, and Pasteur in the late 1890s was the intellectual *coup de grace*. With more public clinical failures like those of the spleen and stomach school in the previous era, the population lost faith. By the middle of the 19th century even Chinese practitioners abandoned their own medicine.[138]

By the end of the era, only one traditional medical school remained, the Imperial college; there, instruction consisted of reciting the classics.[139] Secular support for traditional medicine was nil, and in 1914 the Minister for Education announced that he intended to abolish Chinese traditional medicine altogether. Attempts to establish new schools in the period 1910 to 1920 failed because the same bureau refused them recognition.[140] One particularly critical Western observer noted that Chinese traditional medicine had become 'one grand free-for-all profession, with no registration or code of ethics whatsoever.'[141]

Intellectually, the period is characterized by a division between the liberals, who sought to incorporate Western knowledge, and the conservatives, who rejected medical innovations since the Song, searching for purity in the past. This trend is mirrored in Japan. These trends did not lead to functioning schools of thought but to cliques built around the few surviving skilled physicians. In the end, it would be Western scientism, not traditional healing, that acquired the faith both of the Chinese people and their medical practitioners. No single view held together the vision of medical thinkers. The diversity of schools of thought had reduced the qi paradigm to a tangled web of details and complexities.[142]

It is not surprising that those who still valued Chinese traditional medicine looked backward. Fang You-zhi was one of the first proponents of the Han-Xue movement. Han-Xue proponents proposed a return to the Han dynasty medical sources. He devoted his life to seeking the truth of the *Shen Nong Ben Cao* and the *Shang Han Lun*, because he felt that these texts had been misunderstood and their meaning lost by recent generations. However, it would be Xu Da-chun, a highly educated scholar from a family of physicians, who would best and most articulately represent the Han-Xue movement.

In his *Yi Xue Yuan Liu Lun*, Xu Da-chun (pen name Xu Ling-tai) described the problems of this period as a result of deviations from what the 'Sages of the past' had established in the Han, his choice of a classic age.[143] Xu was uncompromising and had only cynical prose for the so-called 'Four Masters,' the famous Song physicians. Whether or not the loss of tradition was as profound as Xu Da-chun believed it to be, the loss of technical skill had to have been considerable. What Xu mentions as forgotten in acupuncture are matters of essential knowledge without which today's students cannot pass their exams. He also criticizes acupuncturists of the era for incorrect channel and point location, overreliance on formula acupuncture, ignorance

of the generic five-phase points, loss of supplementation and draining theory and technique, loss of needle technique, and ignorance of seasonal correspondences and the methods of internal medicine.[144]

Although Soulie de Morant reported witnessing the successful use of acupuncture against cholera in 1901, and recounts his studies with two traditional practitioners of great skill, indeed, of academic rank, other Western writers found only street-vendor acupuncturists, men described as nothing short of 'walking infestations.'[145] Apparently, at least by the end of the empire, traditional pharmacotherapeutics stood largely alone against the onslaught of the medicine of the West. By the 1930s, the Chinese practitioner Tin Yau So would write that there was only one acupuncturist in all of Canton.

Traditional herbal medicine was also unable to hold its own against the accomplishments of early 20th century biomedicine. Suffering from discontinuity, Chinese traditional medicine was crushed by the growing faith in Western science that would eventually dominate China. Zhao Xue-min, who collected hundreds of prescriptions from itinerant doctors and other travelers, gives us a clear view of the disparity between the theories of the establishment and the rank-and-file doctors who treated the masses. His collection, the *Chuan Ya*, is remarkable as, in Paul Unschuld's words:

What first strikes the reader of the more than 1000 drug prescriptions and guidelines of the *Chuan-ya* is the virtually complete absence of yin-yang theories and of the five-phase doctrine.[146]

Not only was there disparity, the population's faith in traditional herbal medicine was all but gone, medicine being considered 'an avocation, a side occupation, or else purely a business.'[147] Herbal doctors were known as 'Mr Drug-Seller' and were called to their patients serially, with pleas to one or another of the medical gods as a last resort. Magico-religious medicine and demonology persisted. To avoid the plague of 1896, Daoist leaders arranged for soldiers to fire their weapons in all directions to scare away the plague demon.[148] By 1934, when statistics are first collected, China's death rate was so great that the number of Chinese who died — merely in excess of deaths in similarly sized European populations — was twice the death toll of the entire First World War. It would be enemies of traditional medicine who would write its epitaph thus:

...medicine in this country has become rigid in the fetters of tradition. Our task, however, is not so much to dwell upon this traditional non-progressive state of thought as to utilise it as a background for an attempt to picture the victorious entry of modern medicine into this ancient land of Cathay.[149]

Biomedicine is still referred to as 'modern medicine' in China today.

It should thus be no surprise that, during the two and a half centuries of the Qing dynasty, there were few influential books on acupuncture written in China. *Nei Jing* and *Nan Jing* commentaries such as Yao Zhi-an's *Su Wen Jing Zhu Jie Jie*, Xu Da-chun's *Nan Jing Jing Shu*, and Ye Lin's *Nan Jing Zheng Yi* are the exceptions. The Tai Yi school of moxibustion resurged, exemplified by Fan Yu-qi's *Tai Yi Shen Zhen* (1727). This book had appeared in at least 20 editions by the end of the Qing. *Yi Jing* acupuncture practice also returned after its presentation in the *Zhen Jiu Yi Xue*, by Li Shou-xian (1798). This text too had numerous editions that continued to the modern era. *Yi Jing* acupuncture traditions are continued today by the American Academy of Medical Acupuncture, which teaches Western-trained physicians practicing acupuncture an extended form developed by Maurice Mussat of France. There was still a school of independent moxibustion practice exemplified in the *Shen Jiu Jing Lun*, by Wu Yan-cheng (1851). The best-known compilation of the period is probably Wu Qian's *Yi Zong Jin Jian* (1742). This work compiled much information about the practice of acupuncture, moxibustion, andpharmaceutics.

Regardless of these exceptions, the Qing was a period of tremendous decline for acupuncture and moxibustion in China. China was without a strong medical model. It was not until the mid-19th century, some 100 years after the acculturation of biomedicine in Japan, that Western medicine achieved credibility in China.

Although Wang Qing-ren argued in the early 19th century that a functional model of the body was meaningless without understanding the actual structures, foreign ideas were still assimilated very slowly. Thus for a long time China suffered from a lack of a strongly rooted medicine, either indigenous or foreign.

The same clash between the traditional and modern that occurred in China also influenced Vietnam during this period. In the 1700s, an eminent physician, Lan Ong, compiled the influential *Y Ton Tam Linh*. However, under French colonial rule traditional medicine was cast aside for French medicine. Traditional medicine was able to survive in the rural areas and, ironically, Vietnamese practitioners would later help establish acupuncture in France. However, it would only return to more general use after the advent of communist rule in the 20th century.

Possibly the most significant Korean development came at the end of the 19th century when Lee Jaema formulated four-constitution medicine. His ideas have held continuous and significant influence over the practice of acupuncture, moxibustion, and herbal pharmaceutics. Lee Jaema's theories and methods are still taught in modern Korean schools.[150] In both Korea and Japan, however, acupuncture and moxibustion remained relatively robust until the end of the 19th century. Many texts, theories, and innovations can be found in Korea and Japan during this period. This was also the period when Western scientific medicine began to impact on traditional medical practices in Japan. Despite Japan's limited foreign contact, most of the books and articles on acupuncture and moxibustion published in Europe during the mid-17th century had their roots in Japan.[151]

In Japan, this two and a half century period included the Edo-Tokugawa and Meiji periods. The two periods together marked a swing away from isolationism and toward radical modernization and industrialization. With the industrialization achieved in Meiji Japan, and particularly with the militarization of the late 19th and early 20th centuries, came the decreed extinction of traditional medicines and the legislated adoption of biomedicine.[152] Western anatomical–physiological medicine was openly and quickly assimilated in Japan.[153] Many practitioners of acupuncture and moxibustion discarded traditional explanatory models in favor of anatomically based models. Thus in the 18th century a rift developed between those who accepted and those who rejected traditional theories — a rift that persists today.

However, until that time, Japanese traditional practitioners advanced. Waichi Sugiyama, who is still known as the father of acupuncture in Japan, left his mark in the late 1600s. Sugiyama invented the *shinkan* (insertion tube), which revolutionized the practice of acupuncture.[154] With the needle inside the hollow *shinkan*, a slight tap is sufficient for insertion. This, combined with industrial technology, made thinner and thinner needles practical, with a tremendous impact on modern acupuncture. The Japanese, like Westerners, prefer thinner needles because thin, tube-inserted needles are virtually painless. In fact, today almost every acupuncturist in Japan, the USA, and increasingly in Europe uses insertion tubes because modern Japanese-style needles are so thin — often half the thickness, or less, of other needles — that patients can hardly feel the insertion.

The insertion tube also helped emphasize the role of palpation in diagnosis and point location by freeing one hand. Sugiyama is thought to have invented the insertion tube because he was blind and the tube made it easier for him to practice. After publishing his famous book *Sugiyama Ryu Sanbusho*, he established the first acupuncture school for the blind, thus founding a tradition that has survived for 300 years. Today some 40% of Japanese practitioners (approximately 20 000 acupuncturists) are blind.[155] However, the role of the blind in Japanese acupuncture extends far beyond these numbers. Without sight, the sense of touch often becomes extremely acute. Thus blind practitioners have been responsible for discoveries in palpatory diagnosis and have developed many highly refined methods of practice. Not only would blind acupuncturists preserve the art through the difficulties of the later Meiji Restoration, but the developments that

Sugiyama began have affected nearly every acupuncturist working today.

In the early and mid-1700s we find further refinements of the tradition of moxibustion in Konzan Goto's *Mokyu Susetsu*, and Shutoku Kagawa's *Ipon Do Kyusen* and *Kagawa Kyuten*. Again, in the early 1800s the *Meika Kyusen*, by Waki and Hirai, helped develop moxibustion for modern times. Another important development of the mid-1700s was the introduction of the unique Japanese pediatric acupuncture called *shonishin* ('children's needle') therapy.[156] This system began in the Osaka region, where it is still very popular. The use of rounded, blunt, or smooth-edged instruments applied by rubbing, scraping, or tapping is especially effective for young children, who dislike inserted needles. These systems survived into modern times almost exclusively as an oral tradition.

But, for the Japanese in the 18th century, the most influential development was probably Sugita Gempaku's *Kaitai Shinso*. This was a translation of a Dutch anatomical text by Kulms, *The Anatomische Tabellen*. This text had a huge impact because for the first time medical practitioners could observe anatomical structures.[157] This landmark publication is still remembered in Japanese high-school courses. It immediately brought European anatomical knowledge into conflict with tradition. In the words of Gempaku: 'I understand that true medicine consists of the detailed investigation of the human body's internal structures' and, even though the ancient traditional physicians had performed anatomical dissection, they could not 'sweep away the foggy obscurity… their eyes and ears were confused by turbid traditions.'[158] From this time on, scientific medicine would dominate acupuncture, moxibustion, and traditional pharmaceutics.

After the initial shock this new medicine created, there was a flurry of activity as authors tried to rationalize traditional models with the new knowledge. One example is Mitsutane's *Kaitai Hatsumou* (1813). In another important and influential text, *Shinkyu Setsuyaku*, by Soutetsu Ishizaka (1811), acupuncture and moxibustion were justified in terms of Western anatomy. As we will see, conflict between traditional and modern models, and the attempt to find a middle ground between the two, remains a major theme in modern practice.

Mixed in with these trends was an entirely clinical approach — repeating what has worked before. Known effective acupoints and combinations were used for specific problems. This formulary acupuncture has always existed wherever acupuncture was practiced. In Chinese history the literate scholar-physicians have always been a minority, and it would be surprising if the majority of treatments had not always been composed this way. But nowhere else did this approach become as firmly established as in Meiji Japan. When acupuncture and moxibustion were all but banned by the Meiji government, this pragmatic approach was all that remained, an arrangement with precedents in 18th century events concerning traditional herbal pharmaceutics. Although this pragmatic approach is often disdained by acupuncture's modern proponents, it has contributed to the survival and acceptance of acupuncture by providing a basic formulary.

In the mid-1700s there were two major schools of herbal medicine: the Koho school, championed by Todo Yoshimasu; and the Gosei school of Dosan Manase. The Koho school was based on ideas from the Han classic, *Shang Han Lun*. It rejected more recent developments. The Gosei school was based on the *yin–yang* and five-phase doctrines. Yoshimasu's approach became very popular, and probably encouraged the Meiji 'compromise school' of pragmatic acupuncture. There was also a new scientific approach precipitated by Gempaku's work. This became a third major approach to practice, the so-called 'Rampo school.' All three schools have influenced the modern period.

By the middle of the 19th century, Japan was desperately trying to modernize. With the beginning of the Meiji period in 1868 radical change became the rule throughout Japanese society. Fearful that Western nations would monopolize resources Japan needed, the new government tried to industrialize and militarize

in order to compete with the West. In medicine the changes were drastic. German medicine was adopted wholesale, in part because Japan had watched German military and political success with admiration. Traditional herbal pharmaceutics, called *Kampo* ('Han [Chinese] methods') was all but outlawed. Only biomedical physicians were allowed to practice. This ruling persists today but is less restrictive, and a sizable over-the-counter trade thrives. Before the Meiji Restoration, acupuncturists could, if they wanted, practice *Kampo*, although numerically few did, but by the mid-19th century they were legally restrained. Acupuncture and moxibustion were also banned during the Meiji Reformation. However, in addition to Western-trained physicians, the blind were allowed to practice.[159] Whether this was meant as a forward-thinking social policy or not, it had an enlightened effect, as acupuncture became a preferred profession for the blind.

All traditional explanatory models were banned in the curricula of schools. The idea of anatomically discrete and separate points with known empirical effects became legal dogma. Essentially, acupuncture and moxibustion were stripped of their theoretical foundations. In 1894 Tesai Okubo published his *Kyuji Shinso*, in which he claimed that acupuncture and moxibustion were nerve stimulation therapies.[160] This is now called *shigeki ryoho* or 'stimulation therapy.' Another example is Michi Goto's claim in 1912 that acupoints are related to the Zones of Head (now known in relation to neural dermatomes). Other examples are the numerous pharmacological studies on the effects of moxibustion. Between 1900 and 1941 many studies were performed to understand the action of moxibustion, putting it on more solid scientific ground.[161]

This period is considered by many to have been terrible for Japan's traditional medical systems, a shock treatment. However, eventually it generated a powerful conservative backlash, which reformed traditional approaches. Although traumatic at the time, it soon triggered a powerful growth phase for traditional acupuncture in modern Japan.[162]

NOTES

1 Lu Gwei-Djen, Needham J 1980 Celestial lancets: a history and rationale of acupuncture and moxa. Cambridge University Press, Cambridge, pp 3–4

2 Campbell J 1962 The masks of god: oriental mythology. Penguin, New York, pp 375–376

3 See note 2, p 380

4 See note 2, p 380

5 See note 2, p 396

6 See note 2, p 397

7 Unschuld PU 1985 Medicine in China: a history of ideas. University of California Press, Berkeley, p 19

8 See note 7, p 25

9 See note 1, p 70

10 See note 7, p 29

11 See note 7, p 35

12 See note 1, p 70

13 See note 7, p 35

14 See note 7, p 31

15 Wong KC, Wu L T 1985 History of Chinese medicine, 2nd edn. Southern Medical Materials, Taipei, p 39

16 See note 7, p 63

17 See note 7, p 64

18 See note 7, p 73

19 See note 7, p 52

20 See note 7, p 57

21 See note 7, p 67

22 See note 7, p 101

23 See note 15, p 70

24 See note 7, p 111

25 See note 7, p 32

26 See note 2, p 429

27 See note 7, p 80

28 See note 7, p 33

29 See note 7, p 34

30 Cohen AP (ed) 1979 Selected works of Peter A. Bodenberg. University of California Press, Berkeley, p 11

31 See note 15, p 260

32 See note 7, p 454

33 See note 7, p 13

34 See note 2, p 431

35 See note 2, p 431

36 See note 7, pp 94–95

37 See note 1, p 78

38 Translation by Paul Unschuld. Personal communication

39 See note 7, p 14

40 See note 7, pp 94–95

41 See note 7, p 55

42 See note 1, p 175

43 See note 1, p 110

44 See note 7, p 38

45 See note 15, p 68

46 See note 7, p 75

47 See note 7, p 54

48(a) See discussions in: Manaka Y, Itaya K, Birch S 1995 Chasing the dragon's tail. Paradigm, Brookline, MA. (b) See also: Matsumoto K, Birch S 1988 Hara diagnosis: reflections on the sea. Paradigm Publications, Brookline, MA

49 See note 1, p 100

50 Wiseman N, Boss K 1990 Glossary of Chinese medical terms and acupuncture points; Paradigm Publications, Brookline, MA, pp x–xi

51 See note 50

52 See note 15, p 38. Liao, Acupuncture for low back pain, in Huang Di Nei Jing Su Wen

53 Hillier SM, Jewell JA 1983 Health care and traditional Chinese medicine in China 1800–1982. Routledge & Kegan Paul, London, p 150

54 See note 15, p 38

55 Unschuld PU 1986 Medicine in China: *Nan Ching* the classic of difficult issues. University of California Press, Berkely, pp 29–34

56 See note 55, p 18

57 See note 55, p 4

58 See note 7, p 179

59 See note 55, p 7

60 See note 55, p 15

61 See note 55, p 65

62 Wiseman N, Ellis A 1985 Fundamentals of Chinese medicine. Paradigm, Brookline, MA, p 145

63 Birch S 1995 On the development of Japanese style acupuncture in the US. Ido no Nippon Magazine, 7, 11: 84–90

64 See note 7, pp 168–169

65 See note 7, pp 168–169

66 For example, line 96 of the text describes the modifications of *Xiao Chai Hu Tang, 'Minor Bupleurum Formula.'* Mitchel C, Wiseman N, Feng Y 1999 *Shang Han Lun*, Paradigm Publications, Brookline, MA

67 See note 66, lines 16, 119, 221, 267

68 See note 7, p 133

69 See note 7, p 133

70 See note 7, p 150

71 See note 7, p 151

72 See note 15, p 72

73 See note 15, p 72

74 See note 15, p 73

75 See note 1, p 100

76 See note 1, p 119

77 See note 7, p 154

78 See note 1, p 263

79 See note 1, p 264

80 Birch S 1989–1991 Acupuncture in Japan; an introductory survey. Review: Part 1, 6:12–13, 1989; Part 2, 7:16–20, 1990; Part 3, 8:21–26, 1990; Part 4, 9:28–31, 39–42, 1991

81 See note 1, p 267

82 Needham J 1954 Science and civilization in China, vol 1. Cambridge University Press, Cambridge, pp 123–124

83 See note 7, p 43

84 Unschuld PU. personal communication

85 See note 1, pp 124–125

86 See note 1, p 127

87 See note 7, p 155

88 See note 7, p 156

89 See note 2, p 444

90 See note 7, p 160

91 See note 7, p 160

92 See note 1, p 177

93 See note 15, p 75

94 See note 1, p 100

95 See note 1, p 265

96 See note 7, p 162

97 See note 7, p 162

98 See note 7, p 165
99 See note 7, pp 167–168
100 See note 7, p 168
101 See note 1, p 89
102 See note 55, p 40
103 See note 1, p 155
104 See note 1, p 139
105 See note 7, p 150
106 See note 1, p 131
107 Liu Bing-quan 1988 Optimum time for acupuncture. Shandong Science and Technology Press, Jinan
108 See note 15, p 196
109 See note 7, pp 173–174
110 See note 7, pp 174–175
111 See note 7, p 175
112 See note 7, pp 177–178
113 See note 7, p 167
114 See note 80
115 See note 1, p 263
116 See note 15, p 261
117 See note 1, p 155
118 See note 1, p 100
119 See note 7, p 190
120 See note 7, p 190
121 See note 7, p 191
122 See note 7, p 191
123 See note 7, p 191
124 See note 7, p 195
125 See note 7, p 203
126 See note 7, p 205
127 See note 1, p 149
128 See note 1, p 100
129 See note 1, p 159
130 Zmiewski P, Feit R 1990 Acumoxa therapy. Paradigm, Brookline, MA
131 See, for example, note 48(b)
132 See note 1, p 266
133 See note 7, p 192
134 See note 7, p 193
135 See note 15, p 143–144
136 See note 1, p 160
137 See note 53, p 3
138 See note 7, p 195
139 See note 53, p 4
140 See note 15, p 145
141 See note 15, p 141
142 See note 7, p 197
143 Unschuld PU 1990 Forgotten traditions of ancient Chinese medicine. Paradigm, Brookline, MA, p 3
144 See note 143, pp 244–246
145 See note 53, p 6
146 See note 7, p 211
147 See note 15, p 178
148 See note 53, p 7
149 See note 15, p 257
150 Song Jang-Heon 1985 The role of Korean oriental medicine, Korean Oriental Medical Association, Seoul, p 5
151 See note 1,
152 See note 80
153 Kuriyama S 1992 Between mind and eye; Japanese anatomy in the eighteenth century. In: Leslie C, Young A (eds) Paths to Asian medical knowledge. University of California Press, Berkeley, pp 21–43
154 Birch S, Ida J 1998 Japanese acupuncture: a clinical guide. Paradigm, Brookline, MA
155 See note 154. Sonoda K 1988 Health and illness in changing Japanese society. University of Tokyo Press, Tokyo, p 78
156 Mori H, Yoneyama H 1983 *Shonishin Ho*; acupuncture for children. Ido no Nippon Sha, Yokokusa
157 See note 153, p 23
158 See note 153, p 24
159 See note 80. Matsumoto H 1994 Acupuncture and moxibustion in Japan. North American Journal of Oriental Medicine 1(2): 11–17
160 See note 80; note 48(a), pp 13–14
161 See note 48(a), pp 353–354
162 See notes 80 and 159. See also note 48(a) pp 353–354

2

The acculturation and re-acculturation of acupuncture

Considering the history of traditional Chinese medicines, finding a diversity of techniques and ideas in modern practice should be unsurprising. The scope of the tradition is so great in age and extent that scholars have concluded that clinical techniques cannot be accurately applied, or even translated, without considering their historical context. The reputation of a medicinal in a Tang source, or a Ming theoretical notion, cannot be unquestionably applied without considering their generative context. For example, merely knowing the acupoints used to treat a particular pattern is insufficient because we must also know the qualitative criteria by which the pattern was recognized and the stimulus sought in treatment.

Although this does mean that some Western notions need re-thinking, knowledge of this diversity helps us understand acupuncture. Viable human skills evolve, change, and adapt to circumstance. Knowing that acupuncture has often successfully met the challenge of adaptation is a far stronger demand on our attention than are fanciful histories and faith-like notions of purity. Consider, for example, the often-expressed idea that the holism of Asian medicines derives from a lack of anatomical exploration. Not only does this obscure Chinese history, but it also prejudicially assumes that the Chinese were a uniquely rigid and uncurious people. Although acupuncture's history is complex and often indistinct, it does reveal a vibrant system of practice that has served vast populations for nearly 2000 years. That which we can learn from it, including holistic techniques, is rooted in the practical experience of that history, not in Chinese peculiarities.

We also must re-think Western impressions that are based on assumptions which history does not confirm. For example, if we were to imagine that all the known medical colleges and all the centers of literate learning had graduated scholar-practitioners at unimaginable capacity, it would still be impossible to think that the Chinese people were primarily treated by *ru yi*, scholar-doctors. There were never enough classically trained doctors to serve entire populations. Medicine was not a high-status profession in China, indeed even now-famous physicians like Sun Si-miao were once disdained for following a medical career. The vast majority of treatments were performed by people who trained as apprentices, like trades-men. Many, if not most, were illiterate. Because apprentices are trained to replicate exactly their teacher's skills, this led to teacher–student lines of specialized practice. Thus there were perhaps thousands of lineal specializations of greater or lesser import.

Again, diversity; again, ways of thinking and learning different from our own. Even today, Chinese physicians who have learned the expectations of Western students will warn: 'Never ask, "What is a slippery pulse?" Instead ask: "What do you call a slippery pulse and what do you do when you find one?" Only then will you learn what your teacher actually does.' In essence then there is no more a single, universal 'traditional Chinese acupuncture' than there is a single, universal 'traditional European art.' Tradition is not a synonym for unchanging truth, lack of innovation, or a dogmatic fixity of ideas. It is a vast source of experience, opinion, and information that must be understood in context. One of Yoshio Manaka's many stories clearly illustrates these issues:

Let us imagine that it is nearly four hundred years ago in China and I am a good friend of Yang Ji-Zhou, the author of the *Zhen Jiu Da Cheng*. Because of this, he might have included these [(e.g. Manaka's)] treatments in his text of 1601 [*The Great Compendium*], despite the limited experience of my two cases.

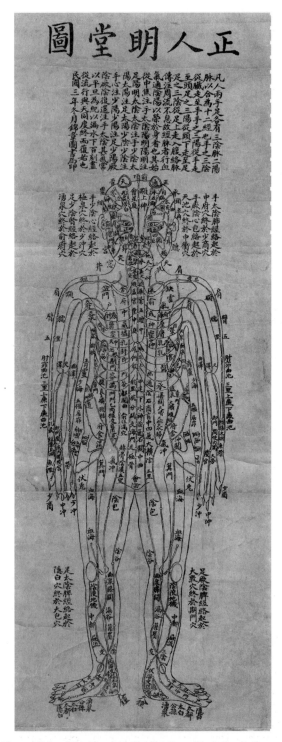

Figure 2.1   Qing Dynasty Acupuncture Chart, front view. (200 × 530 cm; ink on paper, courtesy of Paradigm Publications.)

Today, almost four hundred years later, practitioners and students reading his text will place great trust in my results because they were included in this great and revered text, and because my friend's reputation in later centuries is excellent. Is this a sufficient criteria for making general proclamations about the treatment of asthma and trigeminal neuralgia?

What if these treatments were to go through the mill of heuristic adaptations and later authors transmitted my results by saying only that CV-22 is good for asthma, or TB-5 is good for trigeminal neuralgia, without including the method I used (moxa) or the theory of the extraordinary vessels? What if translators then simplified the terms with which I diagnosed these conditions? Would these points reliably produce the desired results or would there be only a statistical percentage of patients who were helped?[1]

Methodology is lacking in traditional literature because books were used in a different way. They supplemented hands-on, naked-sense teaching. Once understood, once set in context, once the assumptions of the compilers and translators are known, Chinese literature can be of tremendous value. Unavoidably, the story of acupuncture's westward flow has too often been a tale of partial information taken as the whole. Because acupuncture was simultaneously re-acculturating in every Asian nation, rising from the ashes of traditional cultures forever changed by war and other vast political and cultural events, it has been difficult for Western researchers to examine the generative context of many ideas.

This was true from the first. News of acupuncture and Chinese traditional medical practices arrived in Europe early in the Qing dynasty (Box 2.1). There were already references to, and descriptions of, pulse diagnosis, acupuncture, and moxibustion in Germany, Holland, and England by 1700. But by 1718 it was described as a remedy that had gone out of fashion. In 1755 the Dutch physician Gerhard van Swieten anticipated modern developments in acupuncture by nearly 2 centuries when he speculated that acupuncture and moxibustion were neurological phenomena. This idea was to appear again in 1798 — when Rougement would label acumoxa treatment as

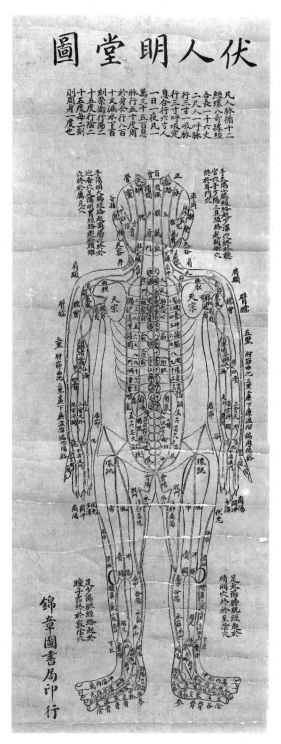

Figure 2.2   Qing Dynasty Acupuncture Chart, back view. (200 × 530 cm, ink on paper, courtesy of Paradigm Publications.)

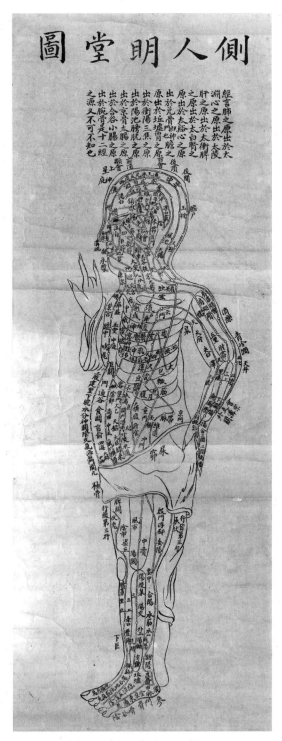

Figure 2.3 Qing Dynasty Acupuncture Chart, side view. (200 × 530 cm, ink on paper, courtesy of Paradigm Publications.)

'counter irritation therapy' – an idea that would resurface in Japan a century later.

Acupuncture was primarily used in the treatment of pain through methods that were void of traditional theories (Box 2.2). The first and most common Western adaptation was needling pressure-sensitive points near a patient-reported pain. As we saw in Chapter 1, this method was first described in the 6th century by Sun Si-miao, who referred to these as *a-shi* ('it's there' or 'ouch') points. Nineteenth century uses were neither fully traditional nor very broadly based. More importantly though, they clearly reflected the biases of the Western physicians who adopted acupuncture.

THE ASIAN REVIVAL

If Western physicians took too much for granted, the Chinese lost too much to circumstance. By 1912, acupuncture and moxibustion were in precipitous decline, barely able to counter the growth of biomedicine in Japan and China. In other East Asian countries, for example Vietnam, the same decline was also evident. In Europe and North America, acupuncture and moxibustion had gained a finger-hold, but were far from accepted. A simplified form of acupuncture had been adopted by a few physicians, but Soulie de Morant spent another decade in China before he returned with a vision of acupuncture that would take hold in Europe. Of course, acupuncture and moxibustion were practiced by Asians living in Europe, especially ethnic Chinese and Vietnamese in their own communities. Islands of traditional practice remained in Asia; the blind practitioners of Japan never ceased to preserve and innovate. But, as the world stood at the brink of the First World War, the traditional arts of acupuncture and moxibustion were close to cultural extinction.

In China the supports of traditional medicine had shattered. The failure of the traditional bureaucracy, the indifference of European powers, the abject poverty and misery of the population, and the rapidly increasing influence of Western medicine, all contributed to its decimation. It met the 20th century as isolated

Box 2.1	Cross-fertilization
1658	Jacob de Bondt published the first reference to Chinese pulse diagnosis
1682	The German Andreas Cleyer wrote a treatise on Chinese pulse diagnosis
1683	The Dutch physician Willem ten Rhinje published an essay on acupuncture, including the first illustrations of the acupuncture channel system
1693	The English physician William Temple wrote about the use of moxibustion
1712	The German physician Englebert Kaempfer wrote essays on acupuncture and moxibustion
1718	Acupuncture was mentioned in a surgical text as a remedy that had gone out of fashion
1755	The Dutch physician Gerhard van Swieten speculated on the possible neurological basis of acupuncture and moxibustion
1798	C. J. Rougement wrote of acupuncture and moxibustion as a form of 'counter-irritant' therapy
1774	Sugita Gempaku translated a Dutch anatomical text into Japanese, signaling the beginning of a strong Western influence on Japanese traditional medicine
1805	The Jennerian smallpox vaccine was introduced to China
1835	The first medical missionary–surgeon arrived in China, with techniques that fascinated the Chinese at that time
1851–1858	The first six Western medical texts appeared in China
1880	Gray's Anatomy first appeared in China
1886	The first missionary medical school was established in China
1894	In Japan, Tesai Okubo declared acupuncture and moxibustion to be 'stimulation therapies'
Late 1890s	The European germ theories of Koch, List, and Pasteur start to arrive in China. By the 19th century, acupuncture and moxibustion were more widely used in Europe and their use spread to the USA. For example, in 1892, acupuncture was described in Osler's landmark medical textbook

and competing forms. In Japan, acupuncture was held hostage. With each successful modernization and industrialization, and with the growing therapeutic repertoire of biomedicine, it was restricted further. In Europe, acupuncture was also in decline. It had a few strong supporters, and would resurge significantly only after George Soulie de Morant had spent 20 years tirelessly working against indifference and hostility. In North America acupuncture began this era as a footnote. A simplified form of acupuncture was recommended for low-back pain in Osler's *Principles and Practice of Medicine,* but this endorsement apparently influenced few physicians. Although fascinating stories have undoubtedly been lost by historical inattention to the lives of Chinese immigrants to western USA, among European Americans, acupuncture was barely practiced at all.

Despite these unimpressive beginnings, the modern story of acupuncture is nonetheless its rise from impotence at the beginning of the 20th century, hiatus and persecution through the Second World War, to resurgence in East Asia and expansion throughout the West. Yet, from this loss of place, this lack of social or political influence, it gained its freedom.

Unfettered by now-defunct traditional forms and prejudices, and thought to be of little economic value, acupuncture was carried forward only by those whose attachment was either to the art itself or to one of its practical applications. Orphaned by the old establishment, it was adopted and put to work. Because it did well, today, at the turn of the 20th century, it enjoys what may be its greatest popularity to date. An estimated 1–1.5 million people practice acupuncture somewhere on the planet, and as many as a quarter of the Earth's population has ready access to an acupuncturist.

THE PRE-SECOND WORLD WAR DECLINE

We are presenting this part of acupuncture's story in two major sections: its radical decline everywhere before the Second World War and its recovery since. Again, this is a convenient way to tell the story, but the country-by-country exposition understates the many complex interactions. Because there are so few formal histories concerning acupuncture in the West, our recounting is often, of necessity, based on interviews. We have thus surely understated the

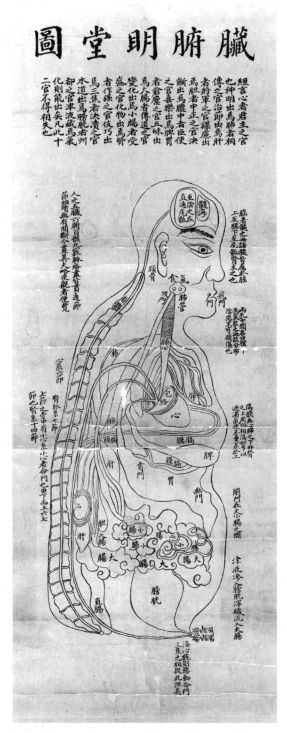

Figure 2.4 Qing Dynasty Acupuncture Chart, *Zang Fu*. (200 × 530 cm; ink on paper, courtesy of Paradigm Publications.)

contributions of many, to whom we apologize. Although modern Asian medical history has been professionally explored, and those works are cited herein, there are very few scrutinizable sources for the Western acculturation of acupuncture. Thus the following presentation is preliminary. Nonetheless, we think it reasonable to assert that, after the Second World War, and particularly after 1970, the explosive acceptance of acupuncture in the West has made it a truly international field, and that this is the central trend of the period. Thus, because what most modern acupuncturists do took shape in the second half of the 20th century, acupuncture today encompasses an enormous diversity of practices, with roots in several countries. Although many of these practices can fairly identify earlier texts and traditions as their source, acupuncture has effectively become a modern art that can be understood in the modern social, political, and economic context.

Again, it is China that has been the leading player. The story of medicine in China in the 20th century is the story of a new social and political order in which both Eastern and Western medicine were applied. China's view of its own medicine must be seen in the context of its new faith in ways of thinking that were close enough to the Chinese mindset to encourage adoption but different enough to allow hope for a better future. China, like the rest of Asia in the early 20th century, was flooded with European and American influence. However, what Europeans first brought to China was not medicine or culture; it was a narcotic drug. China had been 'opened' largely through an imposed trade in opium. European and American merchants promoted the demand for opium to acquire previously unavailable Chinese products for resale in the West. Between 1821 and 1854, opium deliveries to China would increase by 1600%.[2] It was a trade in agony and human suffering, twisted to typify the Chinese and not the Westerners who organized it for their own profit. Still indistinct in Western histories, the opium trade was a social horror that very aptly reflects the subhuman status in which many Westerners held the Chinese. This

Box 2.2		Nineteenth-century uses of acupuncture in the West
1802	England	W. Coley wrote about the uses of acupuncture
1816	France	L. Berlioz wrote a book on acupuncture
1820	Italy	S. Bozetti wrote a book on acupuncture
1821	England	J. M. Churchill wrote on the use of acupuncture for rheumatalgia
1822	USA	First favorable comments on acupuncture in a US medical journal
1825	France	J. B. Sarlandiere first wrote on the uses of electro acupuncture
1825	Italy	A. Carraro wrote on the uses of acupuncture
1825	USA	F. Bache started using acupuncture for pain relief
1826	England	D. Wandsworth wrote on the uses of acupuncture for pain relief
1826	Germany	G. E. Woost reviewed the status of acupuncture
1827	England	J. Elliotson wrote on the uses of acupuncture for rheumatalgia
1828	Germany	J. Bernstein wrote on acupuncture for rheumatic pain
1828	Germany	L. H. A. Lohmayer wrote on acupuncture for rheumatic pain
1828	France	J. Cloquet and T. M. Dantu wrote a book on acupuncture
1833	USA	W. M. Lee wrote on the use of acupuncture for rheumatism
1834	Italy	F. S. da Camin reproduced Sarlandiere's electroacupuncture ideas
1871	England	T. P. Teale wrote on acupuncture for pain relief
1880	England	S. Snell wrote on acupuncture for pain relief
1892	Canada	W. Osler described the use of acupuncture for lumbago in his influential *Principles and Practice of Medicine*

chauvinism, naturally, biased Western opinions of the creations of Chinese culture, including acupuncture.

In the political arena, China fared no better. Between 1853 and 1865, during what is known as the 'Taiping Rebellion,' a rebel leader occupied Nanjing for 12 years. He was displaced only when British troops resolved the conflict. The Qing government's impotence in the face of this rebellion — during which as many as 20 million Chinese may have died — is an effective symbol for the end of the governmental system that had served China for nearly 2000 years. Although French and British forces did occupy Beijing, and treaty ports or concessions were occupied by colonial powers, China was never actually colonized. Governmental efficacy was nonetheless lost. In 1877–1878 there was a famine that left 9 million people in horrifying condition. Parents sold or killed their children, people maimed themselves because begging, other than suicide, seemed the only escape from starvation.[3] There was no public sanitation; open sewers and refuse-strewn streets were the standard urban vista. In this atmosphere of decline and loss of self-determination, the Republic of China was formed in 1911. The last dynastic ruler's abdication was the prelude to a struggle for power among those who differed

in their views of how China should be rebuilt in the image of the West.[4]

When the Qing dynasty ended, general Xuan Shi Kai, friend of the well-known Western medical doctor Sun Yat Sen, became the first president of the Chinese Republic. However, democracy had no root in Chinese culture and did not survive. It was not until 1926 that Jiang Jieshi (Chiang Kai-shek), by force of arms and not politics, united the country. Meanwhile, another Western import, Communism, had already taken hold. The Chinese Communist Party (CCP) was formed in 1921. Although briefly allied with the Nationalist Guomindang (GMD) until 1927, violence rooted in political discord would set it on a solitary course. The CCP established itself in guerrilla bases after the invasion by Japan. The period beginning in 1937 with that invasion and the Second World War, and ending in 1949 with successful revolution, left China in ruins.

For China, the first half of the 20th century was a period of nearly unimaginable human suffering. A horrifying drama of starvation and acts of human desperation played against the terror of the Japanese invasion. The Japanese brought nothing of their own earlier and more rapid scientization except weapons of total war aimed at a population only barely prepared to deal with the previous century. Some of the crimes of the Japanese occupation are only today being revealed. The industrialized cities were places of awful working and living conditions. The countryside was an ocean of impoverished peasants. Infectious diseases were endemic and epidemic.[5]

Traditional medicine was not in a position to exercise its abilities. Could acupuncture, which had long offered vermifugal treatments, have cured these millions? Perhaps, but no empire survived to organize the effort, and many Chinese probably knew nothing of the possibility. Those who did might have searched in vain for capable acupuncturists, as many Chinese traditional practitioners were lost in the plagues that raged through China.[6] The Chinese were looking to modernize as much as possible and were turning to Western medicine. Thus the beginning of the 20th century was theoretically, as well as practically, devastating for acupuncture and traditional Chinese pharmaceutics.

Although the history of the conflict between China's old and new philosophies would be written by the CCP and the eventual communist government of China, that conflict was not essentially created by communism. Both communism and biomedicine were being acculturated in a shift from the now-repudiated traditional values to newly adopted concepts that had found favor in the West. The Marxist theory of dialectical materialism was seen by many as a scientific expression. No less an authority than Mao himself would proclaim that communist culture was based in science.[7] Thus it interested many, not just those politically active as Communists.[8] In effect, Western ideas that seemed rooted in science were replacing the Three Pillars as the foundations of Chinese medicine:

Modern science assumed the role of the doctrine of systematic correspondence, whose magic-derived concepts of *yin-yang* and the five phases were now spurned as fully inadequate for the solution of new technological problems.

Marxism, which appeared in China claiming to be a scientific social theory, replaced Confucianism, whose socio-theoretical concepts and view of history had been closely associated with the old 'natural science' of systematic correspondence.[9]

Thus from the Republic's first days the intellectual elite were prepared to abandon traditional culture. Everywhere, the qi paradigm was rebuked. When traditional practitioners sought registration from the Minister of Education, they were informed that he had already decided to prohibit their practice. As early as September 1915 an order was issued demanding that medical, pharmacy, and veterinary students meet the qualifications established by Western nations.[10] In 1922, the Minister of the Interior licensed both Western and traditional practitioners. Then, in 1929, the Ministry of Health finally ceased registration of traditional doctors, and announced an explicit proposal to abolish traditional medicine. China repudiated its own medicine, taking faith in its Western rival.

However, faith in the new medicine and its encompassing science were not sufficient to create a working medical system. Although both the national government and the European concessions made constructive attempts, these were so small, so poorly funded, and so late as to have no effect. When the Japanese invaded in 1937, there were only 77 health centers and 144 rural care stations in a nation that consisted of 2000 cities and 100 000 villages.[11]

Chinese medicine was not without its heroes. The *zhong yi* movement proposed innovations that would later be incorporated into what is now called Traditional Chinese Medicine (TCM). During the 1920s a number of traditional practitioners — among them Qin Bowei, who would later contribute to the modern technical description of TCM[12] — sought to salvage traditional medicine. They attempted to reconcile many traditions under a single banner, *zhong yi*, creating a solid front that could resist the encroachment of *xi yi*, Western medicine.[13] Although not then successful, this movement laid the foundation of the modern development of traditional medicine after the Second World War.

In Japan, scientific validation of acupuncture and moxibustion was also everywhere encouraged. Technically, 120 *koketsu*, discrete acupuncture points, were defined by underlying, usually neurological, structures. The only acupuncture points now considered valid were those that had empirically observed clinical effects. Traditional concepts, *qi, yin-yang*, and channels were entirely discarded. Acupuncture was seen as a practice based on the stimulation of discrete anatomically-defined points with scientifically-demonstrated effects. Provided this was the model taught and practiced, acupuncture and moxibustion were allowed to survive. The movement that was started by Sugita Gempaku and was promoted by the Rampo school achieved dominance. In the several decades after 1868, the basis of acupuncture practice shifted from the coexistence of modern and traditional explanatory models to a purely scientific rationale.

Traditional medical practices in all of Asia followed the trends in China and Japan. In Korea during the first half of this century there was little innovation or development. Acupuncture, moxibustion, and traditional pharmaceutics lost ground to biomedicine, and suffered appreciably in the violent political upheavals of the time. The Japanese invasion of Korea devastated Korean culture, including traditional medicine. Acupuncture and moxibustion in Vietnam were also slow to develop, compared with the post-war years. Not much information is available. Under French colonial rule biomedicine was actively promoted and traditional medicines suffered except in areas that could not afford Western-style clinics.

Little can be found about acupuncture in Europe and North America during this period. Probably the most significant events were the return of Soulie de Morant to France in 1917 and his subsequent publications. But these did not find a receptive audience until after the Second World War. It is probable that acupuncture was practiced in the Asian communities of Europe and North America, but little information survives.

THE POST-SECOND WORLD WAR RECOVERY

After the Second World War, there was a dramatic resurgence of acupuncture around the world, particularly in China. In the period before the Japanese invasion of China, there had been many debates about the future of traditional medicine; but it was the war experience of Mao Ze-dong that gave traditional medicine a firm commitment. The communist official Ma Hai-de stated this clearly:

The witch doctors are banned, they are dangerous. We got rid of them by introducing them in the 'yangko' plays so that the people laughed at them and we got them better jobs – gave them farms – anything, as long as they would stop harming the people. The herb doctors, the acupuncturists and the midwives we kept but we gave them training in the essentials of Western medicine. Chinese herb-doctors have done an enormous lot of good.[14]

Thus, as the communists under Mao promoted traditional medicine, they set about changing it to make it more acceptable, more scientific.

In the first days of the People's Republic, among the first orders of business was health care for a huge society, the already threadbare fabric of which had been reduced to an unraveled mass of disconnected threads. The social structures that had supported traditional medicine were in ruins. The Three Pillars could not support their own weight, much less a model of medical reality under constant attack. The islands of traditional skill that Soulie de Morant had known, the last physician scholars, the current generation of lineal apprentices – so many had drowned beneath violent waves of war, social collapse, epidemic, and famine.

China's political leaders were faced with the seemingly insurmountable problems of serving a half billion population with less than 40 000 Western physicians and upwards of 500 000 disorganized and discursively trained traditional practitioners. This is the health-care crisis that the United Nations Relief Organization called 'the greatest and most intractable public health problem of any nation in the world.'[15] Here was the clear, pragmatic reason for the CCP to promote traditional medicine; there was no other choice.

Although the experience of war and providing health care to a vast nation would make Mao Ze-dong the most reliable political advocate for traditional medicine, even admired members of the CCP would continue to oppose it. Mao would need to purge party leaders and state officials in defense of TCM.[16] However, in the CCP generally there was a strong feeling for preserving the essence of Chinese culture against the onslaught of Western creations. These feelings helped save traditional medicine from outright abandonment or prohibition. But in the CCP's political environment traditional medicine could not survive without being scientized. This was the political compromise that evolved between conservatives who saw it as an aspect of Chinese culture to preserve and modernists who saw it as, at best, a collection of empirical tricks, some of which might be useful.

Starting in the 1950s traditional medical schools with standardized curricula were established to teach basic biomedical sciences, traditional pharmacotherapy, and acupuncture. To accomplish this the theoretical basis of acupuncture and herbal medicine had to be standardized and adapted to classroom training. For the first time in history a united medicine was abstracted from the materials of tradition. The *zhong yi* movement, which had begun to describe a coherent mode of practice in the 1920s, triumphantly re-emerged. Their work is the foundation of treatments used today. In the process, however, political compromise would guarantee the exclusion of many traditional ideas that did not fit party doctrine. As historians Hillier and Jewell state it:

The Communist Party sought to achieve the objectives the Guomindang government had failed to reach in 1935; to unify and regulate traditional practitioners and incorporate them with doctors of Western medicine into a single federation under state control. Such unification was necessary to utilize in the most efficient way every available medical resource to combat the huge burden of infectious and parasitic disease in China, to build up the ramshackle health care system, and to exert ideological control over both the 'bourgeois' tendencies of modern doctors and the 'feudal superstitions' of the traditional ones.[17]

Traditional medical practice was saved, but the qi paradigm was its ransom. As Paul Unschuld notes, it was now the branches of a tree, the philosophical roots of which had been severed.[18] Nonetheless, for the first time in the 20th century, Chinese medicine had a firm cultural position, a clear economic role, and a powerful political patron.

Meanwhile, many Western medical schools were established. Creating a Western medical system was such a priority that today only 30% of China's medical colleges are traditionally oriented,[19] and Western physicians outnumber traditional practitioners two to one.[20] These pressures changed acupuncture and traditional herbal medicine profoundly, because it was the increasing demand for medical services, not the preservation of traditional methods, that occupied the nation's resources. Better training, the supervision of apprentice programs, prosecution of medical drug smuggling, and the policing of ineffective herbal remedies were the priority undertakings. By providing doctors of TCM with an opportunity to research and publish, the government gave them status. However, the state exercised control, and biomedical doctors earned five to ten times greater salaries, a policy which continues to direct China's best students away from TCM.[21]

There have been a number of important developments since. In the Great Leap Forward (1958–1959), besides a number of general political changes, some of which were economically catastrophic, Mao pursued the integration of traditional and Western medicine even further. In 1958, Mao made the famous statement: 'Chinese medicine is a great treasure-house! We must make all efforts to uncover it and raise its standards.'[22] In the 1950s a month of traditional medical study was required of all Western medical students. This created a large population with an exceedingly cursory training in acupuncture. The impact of this policy would be felt 2 decades later when Western scientists would turn to these medical-school graduates, and the English-language derivatives of the Chinese literature created to train them, to develop their clinical trials of acupuncture. Thus, these studies were often inadequate.

During the Great Leap Forward, in an environment of prominence for rural public health issues, the integration of traditional and modern medicine was to become an even more significant priority. In politics, the CCP was walking a tightrope between the preservation of a low-cost, available, and native expedient, and support for practices that were far too obviously rooted in China's feudal history. TCM too clearly rested on a non-materialist philosophy — correspondence rather than material logic. The techniques were useful, but the qi paradigm was a political liability. This quandary called for a political resolution; it would be called the 'Three Combinations:'

- medical education and productive labor, mass campaigns and traditional medicine
- leading functionaries, teachers, and students under Party leadership
- teaching, scientific research, and treatment with prevention.

In the end, economic need and political expedience, not theory or science, determined the outcome. That outcome was not that traditional medicine was honored as an intellectual treasure to be preserved. Instead, it was Mao's 'treasure-house' from which the useful was to be culled, sorted, scrubbed, and polished by science in service of the state.

Yet, by the end of the Great Leap Forward this unification of traditional and Western medicine was pleasing none. Traditional practitioners feared eventual elimination as they had neither money nor prestige. Furthermore, they were not themselves united. To make matters worse, popularization and expansion had further diluted what had never been a homogenous system. Despite this, CCP pressure for

integration continued, and the system expanded like a tidal wave.

From the viewpoint of many Western scientists, one of the most important developments began in this period. This was the utilization of acupuncture as an anesthetic and analgesic during surgery. During this time aggressive acupuncture techniques were developed and became a routine part of TCM. When Westerners started flooding China after Nixon's visit, it was these techniques they were shown. They brought these back to the West, where they were popularized and became a primary focus for research. Even today, Western books derived from Chinese writings of this period evidence deeper insertions, stronger needle stimulus, and a greater use of minor surgical techniques (Tables 2.1 and 2.2).[23]

Once again, everything in China would change as the political unrest resulted in the 'Great Proletarian Cultural Revolution.' Although TCM did not inspire the Cultural Revolution, its roots in the qi paradigm, which was still considered feudal superstition, would be a political focus. Traditionalists outside the state system would be labeled as 'witch doctors.' Some who are today 'living treasures' in China, were then banned. For example, Cheng Tan An, whose treatments are now widely recognized, was persecuted.[24] However, TCM would continue to be popularized, because acupuncture, moxibustion, and natural drugs were still inexpensive and useful.[25]

Indirectly, however, the Cultural Revolution had significant consequences for all medicine. Among the millions of its victims were physicians, scientists, and many of the intellectuals

Table 2.1 Depth of insertion (in *cun*, or 'body inches') and number of points at each needle depth given in historical acupuncture textbooks

Book	Mean (median) depth	No. of points				
		0.1–0.3	0.35–0.6	0.65–1.0	1.1–1.5	1.6–3.0
Zhen Jiu Jia Yi Jing (282)	0.49 (0.4)	171	113	51	5	9
Tong Ren Shu Xue Zhen Jiu To Jing (1027)	0.42 (0.3)	182	94	47	1	1
Zhen Jiu Ji Sheng Jing (1220)	0.41 (0.3)	196	89	50	0	1
Zhen Jiu Ju Ying (1529)	0.41 (0.3)	186	99	45	1	2
Zhen Jiu Da Cheng (1601)	0.41 (0.3)	191	96	48	1	1

Table 2.2 Depth of insertion (in *cun*, or 'body inches') and number of points at each needle depth given in modern acupuncture textbooks

Book	Mean (median) depth	No. of points				
		0.1–0.3	0.35–0.6	0.65–1.0	1.1–1.5	1.6–3.0
Essentials of Chinese Acupuncture (1980)	0.57 (0.5)	58	151	136	12	1
Chinese Acupuncture and Moxibustion (1987)	0.60 (0.6)	25	165	158	8	2
Acupuncture A Comprehensive Text (1981)	1.03 (0.85)	18	41	138	121	41
Fundamentals of Chinese Acupuncture (1988)	0.54 (0.45)	74	156	117	8	1

on whom both the modern and traditional health-care systems depended. Training stopped and students continued to graduate, although their colleges had not held classes for years. Political ideology ruled where modern science had once held sway. Politically incorrect traditionalists were forced to hide and could not teach. Some fled to the periphery of China, some to America or Europe, where they began to impart their views and clinical systems to Western students.[26]

Order was restored after the initial unrest of the revolution. The party began to rebuild, and by 1969 Mao had regained control of all Chinese health care policy. Under his direction, both rural and urban populations saw improvements in the availability of care, but by far the most recognized phenomenon of the era, perhaps even to an extent greater than it may objectively deserve, was the Barefoot Doctor movement. Just as it appealed to the people-to-people ethic of the Red Guards, it also appealed to populist sensibilities in Western democracies and generated a powerfully positive reputation in the West.

In theory, Barefoot Doctors were worker-doctors. Their salary, education, and repertoire of medicines and equipment were financed

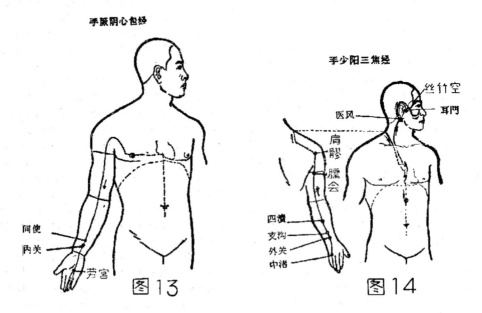

Figure 2.5 Pages from a Barefoot Doctor-era Manual (the manual was equipped with a single filliform needle inserted through the last page). (Courtesy of Paradigm Publications.)

through the local work units that each Barefoot Doctor served. These units, called 'brigades,' were thus freed of the bourgeois burden of fee-based medicine and the state was freed of the need to pay for its rural medical operations. In theory, the utilization of acupuncture and traditional herbal medicines would reduce expenses to a level that rural populations could afford. Practice did not prove the theory. Acupuncture requires physical and sensory skills that are not quickly or easily achieved. Quality control in the selection and preparation of herbal drugs has always taken time to acquire. These facts, coupled with the popular bias expressed in labeling biomedicine 'modern medicine,' meant that the Barefoot Doctors had a tendency to mostly use biomedical drugs, disrupting the delicate finances of the brigade.

From a Western perspective, events of this period are bizarre — unskilled hospital staff treated patients, peasants worked in scientific laboratories, nurses operated while physicians cleaned toilets and floors, and Barefoot Doctors prescribed scientific medicines. However, these more dramatic excesses should not overwhelm the successes. By 1975 the Barefoot Doctors could be credited with the treatment of 70–80% of all illnesses, and an increased reliance on traditional medicinals did allow both a reduction of costs and an expansion of services.

Simultaneously, TCM was changing. In the period between 1970 and 1976, CCP leaders decided that, because TCM theory was merely medieval superstition, research in TCM needed to be no more than repeated practice. Yet, despite any commitment to fund what the West might recognize as valid research, the stated goal of this period was to raise TCM 'to the plane of modern science.'[27] Although the development of TCM and its subsidiary branch TCM acupuncture were on the whole very successful, the enormous political forces behind those changes so undermined research that acupuncture became more vulnerable than ever to Western skeptics.

Following the Cultural Revolution, traditional medicine stabilized. In the 1970s, under programs sponsored by the World Health Organization (WHO), physicians from many countries came to China to study in one- to three-month acupuncture programs. Since the early 1980s many two- to three-month programs have been established for non-physician acupuncturists from around the world. Today, many Western acupuncture schools have ties to traditional medical schools in China, and their students go there to study in pre- or post-graduation programs. Since the 'three roads' policy of the 1980s, whereby traditional medicine, biomedicine, and their combination, 'integrated medicine,' were permitted to develop on their own, more than 2000 Chinese physicians have graduated with a thorough training in both traditional and modern medicine. The WHO programs considerably contributed to acupuncture's westward migration.

The situation for the scientific study of traditional medicine has also improved, although it is still under political controls. Although much of the newer work is better by Western standards, the bulk of Chinese studies still fail to convince Western scientists. Because the studies are so often poorly designed and controlled, entirely absent of biostatistical technique, researchers in the West take little Chinese work seriously, some believing it to be politically doctrinaire.[28]

In Japan the same nearly instantaneous Westernization had different effects, because the social structure was more quickly restored. The Meiji restrictions had already caused a backlash in favor of more traditional approaches, and by the 1920s traditional approaches had found effective cultural supports. In 1926, Tadanao Nakayama, a journalist friend of the famous moxibustionist Takeshi Sawada, published an influential book promoting traditional medicine. Other prominent practitioners such as Sorei Yanagiya and, later, Shinichiro Takeyama became effective critics of the restrictive approach. The essence of their protest was that the grain had been discarded with the chaff. Although they admitted that there were problems with blindly following the classics, they argued that there was nonetheless valuable information in those texts. Yanagiya, for example, promoted the idea of a critical re-evaluation of the classics in order to determine what was clinically valid.[29]

Although this re-evaluation was not based on scientific testing methods that would meet all the requirements of a modern research institution, it did come very close for the era and the extent of the attempt to recognize traditional concepts. It was in many ways similar to the empirical testing of acumoxa therapies and herbal medicines performed in China since the 1950s. It concluded successfully. By 1930 Yanagiya had become the center of a group of like-minded people such as as Sodo Okabe and Keiri Inoue. From this center he sounded his now-famous call for a 'return to the classics,' a theme that echoes the centuries-earlier rallying cry of the Koho school in Japan and the Han Xue school in China.

Often it seems that, when scientific thinking gains the upper hand in Japan or China, there is a conservative backlash that re-invigorates traditional medicine. But, importantly, as the modern era progressed, each of these re-invigorations has been increasingly tempered by a critical view of tradition, each has been centered on a more carefully structured approach. Regardless of whether that structure is a direct Western influence, the reassertion of a longevous strand of indigenous logic, or a combination of those trends, it is clearly at work. The works of both Xu Da-chun and Sorei Yanagiya exemplify this profoundly, despite their separation in time and location.

Yanagiya published many books and is regarded by most as the leader of the Japanese classicist movement. By the 1930s other conservative movements would arise. Takeshi Sawada, for example, was central to the development of another group. Many associations and trends that have survived into modern practice emerged. Of particular import is the movement called *keiraku chiryo*, after its concentration on 'meridian (channel) therapy.'

The *keiraku chiryo* movement grew throughout the 1930s, culminating in the creation of a formal association in 1940. The movement, as with everything traditional in Japan, was interrupted in 1943. The association resurfaced in 1946 during the American occupation.[30] This carefully structured return to the traditional methods of practice was distinguished by two features. First, the leaders of the *keiraku chiryo* movement were famous clinicians who subjected their classical interpretations to scrutiny in clinical practice. Secondly, the classic of choice was the *Nan Jing*. For developing palpation methods and for refining delicate needle techniques, the *Nan Jing* was the richest source. Keiri Inoue, for example, was well known for 'needling' points without actually inserting a needle.

The *keiraku chiryo* movement also became a focal point for blind practitioners such as Kodo Fukushima. In the early 1930s Fukushima had been an anti-war activist, opposing the Japanese government's aggressive foreign adventures. For this he was punitively conscripted and sent to the Manchurian front line. There, in 1932, he received a head wound. But, known as an anti-war activist, he was denied proper treatment and allowed to go blind. Discharged, blinded, and judged ineligible for veteran assistance because of his anti-war protests, he studied acupuncture, graduating from acupuncture school in 1938. Dissatisfied with what he learned in school, he approached Yanagiya and his group in 1940. At first he was rejected, but he was then encouraged to begin his own study group for other blind practitioners. This eventually led to the establishment in 1959 of the association known as *Toyohari*, 'East Asian needle therapy group.'[31]

At the end of the war, Japan was in shambles. The American occupation forces under US General Douglas MacArthur were overseeing the reconstruction of Japan. Everywhere the country pieced itself together. Acupuncturists who had survived the conflict began to regroup and, despite desperate shortages, in October 1945 Soichiro Tobe, the long-standing senior editor of the *Ido no Nippon* magazine, was able to publish an issue of this important acupuncture journal.[32] Survivors of the Hiroshima and Nagasaki atomic bombings would provide a further impetus to traditional medicine, as

Japanese traditional medicines were employed to counter the effects of radiation.[33] Among these were practitioners such as Yoshiharu Shibata, a physician whose lifetime research in acupuncture, herbal, and diet therapies for radiation-related problems would eventually be applied to improving cancer therapies. In 1947, in a political move not unlike those launched by Western physicians in China, Japanese physicians who opposed traditional medicine convinced MacArthur's headquarters to eliminate traditional practices completely. This became a rallying point for the acupuncture community. A group of prominent acupuncturists, including Soichiro Tobe, encamped MacArthur, becoming a regular feature at his headquarters in protest of this decision. Other prominent acupuncturists and physicians also pleaded the case for acupuncture.[34] Probably the most influential event was a mass rally of blind acupuncturists in Tokyo. Organizing quickly to preserve the profession, they became the catalyst of acupuncture's salvation.[35]

There was already a growing sympathy for traditional medicines at the American headquarters, but this protest was the 'last straw.' It would have been politically devastating for MacArthur to eliminate a traditional social institution for Japan's blind. Thus, as a direct consequence of these protests, MacArthur withdrew the original announcement and issued a notice of his intention to allow the continued practice of traditional medicine. However, this continuance would require the establishment of those institutions thought necessary for medicine in a modern Western society. There would be centralized and standardized curricula and licensure laws.[36] As in China, a political leader decided the future of acupuncture. Ironically, it would be the American general who was every bit as dramatic as Mao.

In 1948 the licensure laws for acupuncture, moxibustion, and massage were passed, and committees were formed to structure the core curricula of schools.[37] There would be significant training in biomedical sciences, at that time approximately 35% of the classroom hours. As there had been separate traditions of practice in

acupuncture, moxibustion, and massage, each of these practices was provided with a separate license, but individuals who earned more than one license were allowed to combine their practice. This policy continues today in Japanese acupuncture education. Students can learn in one of four tracks: only acupuncture; only moxibustion; acupuncture and moxibustion; or acupuncture, moxibustion, anma, and shiatsu massage.[38] The law restricting the practice of Kampo to Western-trained physicians and pharmacists has been retained.

This approach had the advantage of allowing specialization in a socioeconomic environment that encouraged adaptation, research, and development. By, perhaps inadvertently, recognizing the diversity of approaches and preferences that have always characterized the practice of traditional medicines throughout Asia, the new laws gave acupuncture a chance to adapt to a new era. Acupuncture could meet new needs in the diffuse and organic way that had characterized its many historical adaptations. In essence this approach preserved pluralism by forcing economic competition. Instead of politically eliminating practices by excising them from curricula and examinations, every idea had to survive the marketplace. This, particularly as the dominance of biomedicine grew stronger, demanded specialization, research, and competition. Thus, in Japan, acupuncture and herbal medicine grew independently within an increasingly sophisticated Western medical economy, acquiring considerable technical specialization.

Progression has been consistent. In the late 1940s there were about 60 acupuncture and moxibustion schools for the blind and a few schools for the sighted. The new regulations encouraged an influx of sighted practitioners; thus there are today about 40 schools for sighted students and 20 for blind students.[39] With the licenses established encouraging diversity and specialization, the blossoming of ideas, methods, and techniques that began in the 1950s has continued to the present. Once free of active government suppression and able to compete in an economy dominated by biomedicine, acupuncturists and moxibustion-ists proved studious and inventive. Those who were not failed.

Because the population became more and more accepting of Western medicine and scientific methods, and because physicians could also practice acupuncture without any special training, acupuncture and moxibustion adapted to the needs of the entire population, rich and poor, laborer and intellectual, as practitioners specialized in the resulting competition for patients. These and other historical pressures fostered one of the most significant periods of growth and development for acupuncture and moxibustion in all of Japanese history.

The traditionally oriented trend that had coalesced into the *keiraku chiryo* movement of the early 1940s became a number of different schools based on slight variances in the interpretation of classical passages as well as specializations of technique. These allied schools today represent about 20% of the acupuncturists in Japan. The scientifically oriented trends derived from the earlier Rampo school continued to receive government support. Today, scientific approaches represent another 20% of Japanese acupuncturists. The remaining 60% do not stand beneath any one banner, but utilize a variety of approaches and explanatory models.[40]

In general, the post-war period was one of considerable fecundity for acupuncture in Japan. In the 1950s Kobei Akabane invented the channel-balancing method of practice as well as the *hinaishin*, or 'intradermal needle.' Both these creations, but especially the latter, are popular in Japan today. Yoshio Nakatani, with the assistance of his friend Yoshio Manaka, invented the *Ryodoraku* electrodermal measurement method to objectify diagnosis. Manaka invented the 'ion pumping cords' and performed surgical analgesia for appendectomies in his hospital in Odawara as early as the mid-1950s. Manaka's reputation among Chinese political leaders resulted in a personally mediated international exchange, even when diplomatic relations were closed.[41] Japanese publishers provided Japanese editions of Chinese texts.

In this period many practitioners started to apply electro acupuncture methods. All the schools of thought flourished, and a significant dialogue between Japanese practitioners and interested Westerners began. For example, the arrival in Japan of the German physician Herbert Schmidt was much heralded because it was seen as increasing the prestige of acupuncture in both Japan and Europe.[42] There was an exchange of ideas between European physicians and Japanese practitioners that provided the foundation of several European and American systems of practice. Some of these are still active today. At this time China was closed to the West, open only to its Soviet allies. Thus Japan was the center of acupuncture's dissemination because information from China flowed only through those who had fled the revolution, many of whom practiced pre-TCM forms of acupuncture.

In the 1960s, while these various schools continued to flourish, the newly developed statistical clinical research methods known as 'biostatistics' arrived in Japan. This led to the first controlled clinical trials of acupuncture by Haruto Kinoshita and Sodo Okabe.[43] The arrival of these powerful research methods also armed scientifically oriented practitioners with a new method for challenging traditional approaches. Although some good research was done, some tried to put traditional methods to 'do or die' tests that heated the debate, bred distrust, and nonetheless failed. Some of this tension remains today.

In the 1970s acupuncture and moxibustion underwent the same boom in Japan as it did elsewhere around the world following the reopening of relations between the USA and China in 1971. Significant growth in the numbers of practitioners and approaches came during the 1970s, but the work of Japanese practitioners was eclipsed by the world's attention to newly innovated TCM. The Japanese expansion continued almost unnoticed in the 1980s and 1990s, as did individual Japanese acupuncturists' influence around the world. Today acupuncture in Japan can be reimbursed under the National Health Insurance plan for the following six conditions: whiplash, low-back pain, neuralgia, rheumatism, cervico-brachial syndrome, and periarthritis of the shoulder, only after failed biomedical treatment. However, not all acupuncturists routinely make claims against this coverage.[44]

After the Second World War, traditional medicines regained ground in Korea (at least in the South, as little is known about the North). In 1948, traditional herbal medicine was recognized and absorbed by the Ministry of Health and Social Affairs. Regulations passed in 1952 legitimized the practice,[45] but actual licensure was never achieved. This remains as a problem for Korea's current generation of traditional practitioners. In Korea the trend towards the unified practice of traditional pharmaceutics, acupuncture, and moxibustion was institutionalized by the 'Doctor of Oriental Medicine' degree.[46] This degree was officially recognized and Oriental medical schools were established. Generally the trend in Korea had been similar to that in China — pharmaceutical medicine was the dominant traditional system. Thus, when acumoxa therapy was integrated with Oriental medical curricula, acupuncture became an adjunct to pharmaceutics. Acupuncture and moxibustion are becoming increasingly popular, especially in the treatment of stroke patients. However, Korean methods are as yet less well known in the West than are Japanese and Chinese approaches.

The teaching of Oriental medicine in Korea includes basic biomedical science as well as traditional theories and techniques. Among the latter are the Korean-founded four acupoint combinations of Sa-Am of the 16th century and the four constitutional patterns of Lee Che-ma of the late 19th century. Although there appears to be a diversity of ideas expressed in the clinical practice of acupuncture, a system of practice not dissimilar to Chinese TCM is standard.[47] As in China, validation of practice and theory through scientific research is an important goal. One of the important figures in this research was Kim Bong Han. He announced the discovery of an anatomical basis for the channels and acupoints in a correlated corpus-

cular system.[48] However, because others were unable to reproduce his findings, they are no longer considered valid.

Another interesting development occurred in Korea during the 1970s. This was Tae Woo Yoo's discovery of Koryo Sooji Chim. Known in the West as 'Korean Hand Acupuncture,' this system is similar to the auricular acupuncture systems of the French doctor Paul Nogier, in that it maps all parts of the body to a corresponding region — in Tae Woo Yoo's case, regions of the hands. In his system the hands are exclusively treated.

After North Vietnam entered the Chinese sphere of influence, its leader Ho Chi Minh adopted Chinese health policy, probably in response to the same political and public health pressures operative in post-liberation China. In 1955, he proposed that 'medical cadres should build on our own medicine, harmonizing Eastern and Western medicine,' a clear reflection of contemporary Chinese policy. By 1960 the National Congress of the Vietnamese Communist Party advocated the combination of traditional and modern medicines in all fields. Supportive policy revisions were added in 1961, 1966, and 1967.[49]

In 1973, John Levinson glimpsed traditional medicine in North Vietnam and found that, like China and Korea, traditional pharmaceutics was the dominant practice. Trends in education were similar to those in China. There were short courses of study available, all medical students were taught some traditional medicine, and more extensive training was available for those who wished it.[50] Today, Vietnamese variations of acupuncture and moxibustion reach the West primarily through Vietnamese-born French nationals. Nguyen Van Nghi of France, for example, has written several books on acupuncture that reflect Vietnamese influences. He has also interpreted Vietnamese editions of famous Chinese texts.

After the exodus to Taiwan following the Guomindang's defeat in 1949, medicine in the Republic of China was dominated by biomedicine. As the country modernized, establishing itself as a powerful economy, the popularity of biomedicine increased. However, the Republic of China also managed to retain much of the richness and plurality of traditional medical practice. Today, traditional pharmaceutics is used more than any other traditional medicine, but acupuncture and moxibustion remain relatively popular. Wu Huiping, a personal friend of Jiang Jieshi (Chiang Kai-shek), advocated for acupuncture, and thus it was never suppressed. As in the People's Republic, physicians in Taiwan can practice acupuncture and moxibustion with less training than traditional practitioners. However, unlike the People's Republic, practices such as shamanism and geomancy are not forbidden, and adherents in the general population practice openly.[51]

Economically, Taiwan is more like Japan than China. Acupuncture and moxibustion must survive as discretionary services in a medical economy dominated by biomedicine. There are an estimated 7500 Chinese medical doctors practicing in Taiwan. Of these, an estimated 10% routinely practice acupuncture and moxibustion. These traditional physicians are licensed by one of two means. They can graduate from an established program such as that of China Medical College, or they may study less formally and pass both a basic and a specific examination.[52] Graduates of the China Medical College learn both Chinese medicine and biomedicine. Around 38% of the 7-year program is devoted to the study of traditional medicine, a small portion of which is acupuncture training. After completing the program, graduates are admitted to licensing examinations in both Western and Chinese medicine, but many graduates do not choose to sit for the Chinese medical examination. Even those who focus almost exclusively on Chinese medicine must also learn biomedicine, much as do students of acupuncture in Japan.

The system in Taiwan provides public and private insurance coverage of acupuncture and moxibustion. Labor Insurance (what is usually termed 'Worker's Compensation' in the USA) has reimbursed acupuncture providers since 1983, and government employee insurance since 1988. In all, acupuncture and moxibustion are relatively popular in Taiwan, but are dwarfed by both biomedicine and traditional pharmacotherapy. The 'leading edge' of acupuncture and moxibustion in Taiwan, as in mainland China, is research. Many physicians who practice acupuncture and moxibustion are involved in research. Institutions like the China Medical College are famous for their research. Indeed, some of the best research published in the West has been done at this college.

WESTWARD TRANSMISSION

With what must now be a familiar caveat regarding the arbitrariness of chronological narrative, we propose that acupuncture journeyed westward in rough parallel to its reacculturation in East Asia. For this reason current Western understandings are often partial, and are often keyed to a particular person, place, or time of transmission. As acupuncture recovered social status, economic utility, and political sponsorship in China, Japan, and the other Asian nations where it had traditionally been practiced, it became more apparent to travelers and more worthy of mention. Its first modern transmissions thus came from Japan, where the American occupation, a growing political and social amnity with Western nations, and rapid economic development increased the points of contact. At first, Chinese influence was sporadic, as it was carried by Chinese of varying skills who were escaping China for political or economic reasons. However, as soon as Chinese interchange with the West was reestablished and a political resolution for acupuncture evolved within the CCP, it would again be Chinese ideas and innovations that dominated Western attentions.

Acupuncture in the USA

Prior to 1971, with Nixon's opening of China and James Reston's *New York Times* article detailing his experience with acupuncture for post-surgical pain control, there was little acupuncture available in the USA. People in Asian communities, especially the Chinatowns of the east and west coasts, were certainly practicing acupuncture, mostly for their fellow Asians. Little was known, and only a very small group of Americans was studying acupuncture in California by 1969.[53] The same was true on the east coast, where only a few people, largely members of the Boston macrobiotic movement, had begun to study with local Chinese and Japanese teachers. Following Japanese management techniques, a young educator, Dr Nakamura, who is today President of Meiji Acupuncture College in Japan, was sent to Boston to teach and become acquainted with American ways. Hiroshi Hayashi, a master of the O Zen Dai, a lineal Japanese medicinal cooking tradition, operated a training program (Box 2.3) in which dozens of Americans and Europeans became apprenticed. Graduates of these programs often figured in the westward transmission of the Japanese traditional health professions. Toshi Hasegawa, a young Japanese surgeon, encouraged Japanese–American communications through Japanese-language articles on the American holistic health movement in the mainstream Japanese press.[54]

In retrospect, however, these activities produced a distinct cycle of interest and acceptance in the USA. In the first half of the 1970s acupuncture was a darling of the American media, but in the second half of the decade there was a sharp decline in popularity. This was followed by another slow but steady increase in the early 1980s. Why this cycle? There are probably several reasons. Among these is the fact that the 1970s was the decade in which 1960s student activists came of age. Many were completing graduate and undergraduate degrees. Others were looking for nontraditional ways to support their young families. As the strong feelings of the protest era were still very much alive in Europe and America, many of its veterans were effectively unemployable, either by choice or due to employer bias. Thus there was a ready audience for new ideas and new careers, and there were literally thousands of activists trained in the demanding schools of grass-roots political protest. The bridge between student

---

Box 2.3 The nervous *deshi*

At three in the morning, a young American is sitting with the Master, his teacher's teacher, the 'Emperor of a Thousand Chefs.' One thousand being symbolic for all, the title describes a *Dai Sensei*, Great Teacher. His own teacher, himself a *sensei*, is the Grand Master's principal *deshi*, a word that implies not merely the condition of being a student, but also that of owing an unpardonable debt, a responsibility that involves life-long submission to a something greater than oneself. He is in the presence of two men, one who now leads, and one who will next lead, a lineal tradition that has lasted generations.

The meal his teacher has prepared was more than merely delicious, it was beautiful, art for a moment, a work of skills earned by long practice and tireless discipline. Even well-picked its remains show a delicate mastery. But, despite an empty bottle of Napolean Brandy, an offering to the Great Master bought at the expense of 3 weeks' pay, the young *deshi* is still on edge, afraid to embarrass his teacher with some *faux pas* of language or custom.

He is profoundly aware that he is an imposter. It takes years of disciplined life and demonstrations of rigorous skill for a Japanese to earn a place at this table. He is here because he is a novelty, an interesting diversion. Strongly constituted and only a few years from athletic training, he can learn by example and make sensory distinctions that his fellow American and European students seem not to perceive. He can survive this initiation of excessive drink, sleep on the floor, live through a ritual cold shower, and be at work on time, more or less capable. Hardly the stuff of a full-fledged adept, but good enough for a *gaijin*, a 'foreigner.'

As Sensei teases sensei about the deficiencies of his copy book, notes copied character by character, teacher to student, for unimaginable years, the foreign *deshi's* curiosity gets the best of his caution. He asks to learn something from this treasure, something found nowhere in his own own culture. They laugh and play act a story in English:
Deshi: Sensei, I must prepare a meal for our Lord and the Chinese Ambassador. They come to speak of war and peace. What should I prepare?
Sensei: 'What do you want, war or peace?'

Maybe it is truth, maybe it is not, maybe it is a story older than any of them. But who cares, it is a good night to talk of how mind is *qi*, of how *qi* arises from food, and how food is transformed by fire and the *qi* of the chef, of the difference between men's food and women's food, of how food is the foundation of health and the highest expression of medicine.

leader and organizer, war resister and entrepreneur, was short, broad, and well traveled.

Professional politics probably also played a role. Paul Root Wolpe of Yale University has argued that the decreased interest in acupuncture during the latter half of the 1970s was due to a systematic effort by the biomedical community to reestablish professional authority or cultural dominance over acupuncture.[55] In 1973, the US Food and Drug Administration (FDA) classified the acupuncture needle, and thus acupuncture, as experimental. In 1974, the American Medical Association asserted that, as acupuncture was experimental, it should only be practiced in the context of established research protocols by physicians and not at all by so-called 'lay practitioners,' including the expert Asians of the time. Wolpe argues that the singular successes of acupuncture in the early 1970s were perceived by many physicians as a threat to their authority, just as Western medicine was seen as a threat when it first arrived in China and Japan. He proposes that, by placing acupuncture in the 'holding cell' of experimental status, that threat was eliminated.

For those who participated in acupuncture licensure efforts, it is clear that both physician opposition and internal conflict among acupuncture's philosophical and ethnic divisions retarded those efforts. However, the extent of any physician-funded opposition is unclear. And, regardless of what future in-depth research will reveal regarding the political role of physicians, the contribution of individual physicians should not go unmentioned. It was they who provided the medical supervision without which early acupuncturists could not have practiced legally. Thus there are many individual physicians who have made important contributions to acupuncture's development. For example, it is certain that the first US acupuncture school would not have survived without the pioneering support of James Doyle, a Massachusetts osteopath.

Contests concerning who could or could not practice acupuncture under the restrictions of the experimental label did not always go the way of physicians. In 1980 a Texas judge ruled on a restriction allowing only physicians to practice acupuncture by saying that acupuncture 'is no more experimental as a mode of

---

Box 2.4   The grateful patient

Licensure in Massachusetts came relatively late considering that some of the first classes, native acupuncturists, and the nation's first school were near the capitol city of Boston. Delays came from internal struggles, conflicts between Asian and American supporters over a proposed English language requirement, and a variety of political problems. But, thanks to the steady efforts of volunteers from the New England School of Acupuncture, the Massachusetts Acupuncture Society, the Chinese community, practitioners, and patients, acupuncture finally got its 'day in court,' a public hearing before the appropriate legislative committee.

This meeting came to its defining moment when a handsome, grey-haired, physician, the senior neurologist at one of Boston's prestigious medical centers, stepped forward to testify. Speaking directly to the legislators, the fingers of his hands tapping lightly together as if to contact the gods of medicine in prayer, he urged them to save the residents of Massachusetts from this impending curse. He was ill informed, the bulk of his factual information being an overstatement of a 1977 study by George Ulett. Yet, the power of his bearing, the tone with which he

delivered words like 'protoscience,' his rhetorical skill, had force. He smiled at the committee members as he left, thanking each personally, no doubt just as he did when they were guests at his hospital's fund-raising dinners.

As he left, a slender man passed him coming forward. Unannounced and uninvited, slowly limping on his cane, he worked his way through the crowded aisles until he stood directly before the committee's table. He raised the cane, not threateningly, but deliberately and rapped the table as if it were he who held the chairman's gavel – rap! rap! rap! There was silence. rap! rap! rap! 'Don't listen to that man' rap! rap! 'These arrogant doctors' rap! 'They said I would never drive.' rap! 'They said I would never walk.' rap! 'They said the only thing for my pain was their expensive drugs.' rap! 'I drove here today.' rap! 'I walked here to tell you, don't listen to that man, acupuncture saved my life, and you're not going to take it away from me.'

He lowered his cane, and walked back to his chair. The meeting slowly returned to more mundane testimony. But, for many there, this was the moment that acupuncture came to Massachusetts.

medical treatment than is the Chinese language as a mode of communication. What is experimental is not acupuncture, but Westerners' understanding of it and their ability to utilize it properly.'[56] Turf wars between physicians and, specifically, trained acupuncturists have come and gone, but today they are transforming to collaborative efforts based on common goals. Pennsylvania is a model state in this regard. There, with the careful work of the physician Pat LaRiccia, considerable cooperation has been achieved. In New York, the Mercy College Acupuncture Program operates with the co-operation of the medical staff in the hospital where its clinical training occurs.[57]

Although it is true that the 'experimental' label imposed a stigma of quackery that was exploited in anti-acupuncture lobbying, it is difficult to find any evidence that supports the commonly held idea that an inimicable FDA deliberately created that barrier. At the April 1994 FDA Workshop on Acupuncture, FDA officials revealed that acupuncture was classified as experimental only after noone stepped forward with positive evidence. After the FDA realized that it was required to do something about acupuncture because there was no evidence of safety and efficacy, the periods set aside for public and professional comment expired without anyone offering evidence. Although this was clearly an opportunity that the acupuncture community failed to recognize, there were very few practitioners and very little research available in 1973. An organized defense of acupuncture would have been difficult, even had the existing organizations undertaken the effort. However, classifying the acupuncture needle as a class III (experimental) device hardly retarded the grass-roots movements that had already begun.

Perhaps unknown to those physicians who tried to assert their authority over acupuncture in the early 1970s, acupuncture had already taken hold. By the mid-1970s it had started to establish itself through home-grown teaching programs, books, and increasingly formal schools. By 1974, the few acupuncture books available were selling in quantities that would not be matched until new schools would begin in the 1980s. Classes based on Soulie de Morant's work were being taught in the USA and Canada, and acupuncture training had already begun to move from teachers' living rooms to the storefronts and storerooms from which the first professional schools would begin.

Bill Prensky, an acupuncturist and now Dean of Mercy College's acupuncture program, helped pioneer acupuncture's move from informal to professional training. In 1969 Bill and his colleagues Steven Rosenblatt and David Bresler founded the Institute of Taoist Studies in Los Angeles, where they studied acupuncture with Ju Gim Shek. In 1973 they brought the well-known acupuncturist James Tin Yau So from Hong Kong, where he was not only a famous clinician but also a sought-after teacher. They arranged for Dr So to be teacher and senior acupuncturist at the Acupuncture Research Project of the UCLA School of Medicine, which they had begun that year. After working on the project for a year, they all moved to Boston in 1974. This core group founded the two seminal US acupuncture schools: The New England School of Acupuncture in Boston, and The California Acupuncture College in San Francisco. Following the founding of these two schools, both of which obtained state approval, other state-approved education programs began around the USA. Acupuncture training became firmly established. These developments laid the foundation for the rapid growth of acupuncture in the 1980s.[58]

Another factor that contributed to the resurgence of acupuncture was the return of young Westerners who had gone to Asia to study acupuncture. Among the first to become well known were Ted Kaptchuk, John O'Connor, and Dan Bensky. After studying together in Macao in the mid-1970s, with Bensky studying further in Taiwan, they produced influential books. Largely for the first time, Westerners were hearing from students who had studied in Chinese settings. Kaptchuk's 1983 book, *The Web That Has No Weaver*, is still a popular presentation of traditional medicine practiced in modern China. Dan Bensky and John O'Connor's

Acupuncture: A Comprehensive Text (1981) was the first publicly available translation of a modern Chinese acupuncture textbook. These books provided not only the substance of many early acupuncture courses, but also the data on which license examinations would be based.

Although it was Chinese TCM that would eventually dominate acupuncture in the English-speaking world, those who were finishing a decade of education and apprenticeship in Japan would also contribute. Miles Roberts, Dan Kenner, Peter Thompson, and others graduated from the Meiji Oriental Medicine Institute in Kyoto, completing not only the 3-year program but also the demanding Japanese national licensure examination entirely in Japanese. Returning after 7- to 10-year apprenticeships with experienced teachers, they continue to promote and support the technical development of acupuncture with their practices, writing, and research.

The most recent estimates are that some 50 acupuncture or Oriental medical schools operate in the USA, with smaller but proportional numbers in Europe and the Commonwealth nations. There are also several programs for training physicians. The early acupuncture schools formed a national council, now called the Council of Colleges of Acupuncture and Oriental Medicine, (CCAOM), which in 1982 formed the National Accreditation Commission for Schools and Colleges of Acupuncture and Oriental Medicine, (NACSCAOM), now known as the Accreditation Commission for Acupuncture and Oriental Medicine, (ACAOM). The ACAOM produced an accreditation process. The Department of Education accepted that program to the professional master's degree level in 1988. At present, 24 schools have been accredited and 10 are candidates.[59] This accreditation gives eligible students access to US student-loan programs, a benefit that has resulted in a continual increase in the number of students. The length of training in these programs is 3–4 years.

Training for physicians is available through programs such as those at the New York University School of Medicine and Dentistry, and the American Academy of Medical Acupuncturists, (AAMA), originally through UCLA. These programs have trained some 3000 physicians, osteopaths, and dentists in Medical Acupuncture, which by the mid-1980s had become distinct from what is taught in ACAOM schools. Joseph Helms, founding president of the AAMA, was instrumental in establishing a training program for physicians that parallels that for acupuncturists in extent. He adapted a model of practice developed by France's Maurice Mussat. This differs in several seminal technical details and clinical strategies from the TCM model. The AAMA training program satisfies the minimum educational standards established by the World Federation of Acupuncture and Moxibustion Societies, an international acupuncture organization.

Most schools and colleges followed the curriculum used in China in the 1960s, 1970s, and early 1980s, combining acupuncture with traditional pharmaceutics. Although this approach has been replaced in China by specialized training in either acupuncture or traditional pharmaceutics, many US schools prefer the integrated curriculum, hence the designation of schools as teaching 'Acupuncture' or 'Oriental Medicine.' Among US acupuncture educators there is some friction between those promoting the integrated approach and those promoting specialized training. This, as well as other factors, led to the 1994 separation of a National Acupuncture and Oriental Medicine Alliance (NAOMA) from the original US practitioner organization, the American Association of Acupuncture and Oriental Medicine, (AAAOM) — now the American Association of Oriental Medicine (AAOM). As seen in our review of history, factionalization is nothing new. Acupuncture, moxibustion, traditional pharmaceutics, and their several permutations of combination have long been matters where individual choice and political and social constraints have mixed. Professional structures in Asian nations were equally fragmented until their current structures were politically determined.

Although the establishment of formal training programs helped spawn a revival of acupuncture from the early 1980s onward, the issues of who can do what, and who makes which practice-governing decisions, are far from settled. There are significant discrepancies in laws determining the scope of practice, the inclusion of traditional pharmaceutics, and the extent of training and practice independence. There are also significant differences in the degree of physician supervision required and the training demanded of physicians who wish to practice acupuncture. However, this issue is mostly confined to the USA. Most countries use national regulations. With federal as well as 50 state regulatory bodies, it is possible to have up to 51 different rules on any practice issue.

This makes US acupuncture laws uniquely confusing and sometimes simply strange. California, which was so liberal as to require state insurance reimbursements in advance of most published efficacy research, nonetheless bans a number of non-Chinese techniques for which the research is good. States such as Connecticut and New York refuse to recognize individuals who were trained prior to the ACAOM era. For example, for an established practitioner like Birch to be licensed in these states he would need to regraduate from the school he helped develop, where his former students would train him to pass examinations that are partly based on the textbooks he has written. Although humorous and moot in Birch's case, such circumstance are not laughing matters. For example, one of the health-care organizations that has most aggressively pursued complementary approaches in the eastern USA, Oxford Health Plans, Inc., must legally exclude from service providers those who have the most experience.

Although US acupuncture has seen both growth and decline during the last 20 years, it is currently surging, as ever more schools open up and more jurisdictions legitimize its practice. The jurisdictions that regulate or license acupuncture and the year in which the law took effect are shown in Box 2.5.[60] Although each state has its own educational and license requirements, a majority have adopted an examination promulgated nationally as the generic standard of minimum competence. This examination was devised by the National Commission for the Certification of Acupuncturists (NCCA) — now the National Commission for the Certification of Acupuncture and Oriental Medicine (NCCAOM), which was formed and funded by US acupuncture schools in 1985.

One estimate sets the number of acupuncture licenses issued in the USA by July 1993 at

---

Box 2.5   Acupuncture licensure approved state-by-state in the USA

1973 Nevada, Oregon
1974 Hawaii, Montana
1975 Louisiana
1976 California
1978 New Mexico, Rhode Island
1981 Florida
1982 Maryland
1983 New Jersey, South Carolina, Utah
1985 Vermont, Washington
1986 Massachusetts, Pennsylvania
1987 Maine
1989 Colorado, Washington DC, Wisconsin
1990 Alaska
1991 New York
1993 Iowa, North Carolina, Texas, Virginia
1994 Minnesota
1995 Connecticut

In 1996 and 1997, five more states have achieved licensure: Arizona, Illinois, New Hampshire, Tennessee, and West Virginia

6476.[61] An FDA report of the same year by David Lytle estimated that there are probably around 9000 acupuncturists in the USA, of which physicians are thought to comprise between 2000–3000 and while a comprehensive survey has yet to be conducted, recent conservative estimates suggest that there are now some 10 000 practitioners in the USA, one for every 25 000 people.[62] The same FDA report estimates that 9–12 million treatments are administered every year, a 0.5 billion dollar micro-economy.[63] Although Eisenberg and colleagues' recent studies of 'unconventional' medical practices shows that only a small percentage of Americans currently use acupuncture, the 1993 study indicated that visits to acupuncturists per patient are more frequent than for any other complementary therapy, and that there are signs of significant growth.[64]

To understand these trends, it is useful to look at the diversity of methods and approaches found in the USA, and some specialized uses that are having a profound impact on US health care. Although most acupuncture schools focus on the TCM acupuncture that evolved between 1950 and 1970 in China, a diversity of approaches is actually practiced. The USA has long been known as a 'melting pot' of cultures and ideas, and as regards acupuncture this is still certainly true. European acupuncture, having begun with the heritage of Soulie de Morant, now evidences a similar diversity within a growing TCM plurality.[65]

Besides the dominant TCM approach, other Chinese systems are also practiced. These include methods taught by James Tin Yau So, Tung family-style acupuncture, and other familial or lineal forms imported from Taiwan, Hong Kong, or pre-liberation China. There are also a variety of Japanese approaches, such as yin–yang balancing, keiraku chiryo, and toyohari, currently taught in the USA. Birch, his wife Junko Ida, and their associates began the first American branches of the Toyohari Association in 1992. Other forms of keiraku chiryo include the yin–yang channel-balancing therapy of Yoshio Manaka and modern forms, such as those taught by Miki Shima. Nakatani's Ryodoraku

system is practiced worldwide, often among physicians. The traditional acupuncture begun in the UK by Jack Worsley is also taught in US schools. A number of modern approaches from France and Germany, in particular Paul Nogier's auriculotherapy, and Rheinhold Voll's EAV (electro acupuncture according to Voll) are transmitted through programs for working acupuncturists. Yves Requena's Terrain system is taught through seminars at the largest acupuncture school in the USA, the Pacific College. Korean and Vietnamese systems, for example, Korean constitutional acupuncture or Tae Woo Yoo's hand acupuncture, are also taught and practiced.

The fastest growing acupuncture program in the USA was pioneered by Michael Smith at the Lincoln Hospital in Bronx, New York. It applies acupuncture as part of a comprehensive drug rehabilitation program. First used by H. L. Wen of Hong Kong in 1972, this treatment has proven to be a valuable part of a comprehensive therapy for drug addiction. Just as the systematized use of acupuncture in China served a necessity for which Western medicine was unprepared, acupuncture is now playing a growing role in this critical problem.

Drug abuse is one of the largest public health problems in the West, especially the USA. There are an estimated 18 million people who abuse or are addicted to alcohol, 12 million who abuse prescription drugs, and approximately 1 million heroin addicts in the USA alone. An estimated 2 million people use cocaine every week.[66] Drugs that cost pennies to produce have huge street values, so the largest proportion of crimes are committed in order to be able to afford illicit drugs. A recent study of 573 hard drug abusers in Miami found that in 1 year their crimes were as follows:[67]

- 6000 robberies and assaults
- 6700 burglaries
- 900 automobile thefts
- 25 000 acts of shoplifting
- 46 000 other larcenies or frauds.

This is a total of 84 600 crimes, an average of 148 crimes per addict per year. Clearly, substance abuse is an immense burden on public health and safety.

Standard treatments for substance abuse have clearly proven inadequate. Among those receiving standard treatment for drug addiction there is at least a 60% recidivism – 60% return to use driven by their addiction. For example, one of the standard therapies for heroin addiction is the daily administration of methadone. Recent studies have found that upwards of 60% of these so-called 'maintained addicts' were abusing cocaine and other drugs, despite methadone treatment. There is essentially no standard treatment for cocaine or crack-cocaine abuse, the worst of inner-city problems.

It is here that the pioneering work of practitioners such as psychiatrist Mike Smith in the Bronx, Pat Culliton in Minneapolis, Ana Olivera in New York, Janet Konefal in Miami, David Eisen in Oregon, Lianne Audette in Los Angeles, Joe Kay in Boston, and their colleagues in more than 600 centers have had a significant impact. In fact, what is sometimes called 'acupuncture detoxification' has been so successful that various state authorities have adopted acupuncture as a rehabilitation tool.

The US Attorney General Janet Reno and First Lady Hillary Clinton's brother Hugh Rodham were involved in establishing the drug diversionary program in Metro-Dade County, Florida, together with judges Herbert Klein and Stanley Goldstein. In Metro-Dade County, as in many places, courts and prisons are overwhelmed with repeat drug offenders. In 1988 the failure of the system inspired the Chief Justice of the Florida Supreme Court to send Associate Chief Judge Herbert Klein to tour the USA looking for answers to the crack-cocaine problem. He found Mike Smith and the program at the Lincoln Hospital in the Bronx. Agreeing that it would be more useful to rehabilitate rather than punish drug offenders, Klein and his associates set up an experimental drug diversion and treatment program with Judge Goldstein on the bench.[68]

Starting in 1989, drug offenders were offered the choice of prison or rehabilitation. Rehabilitation involves four phases: I, detoxification (featuring acupuncture); II, counseling (with follow-up acupuncture); III, education or vocational assessment and training; and IV, graduation. Successful completion of the program, 'graduation,' requires 'clean urines' (no chemical signs of drug use) and no re-arrest for any reason for 1 year. The program coordinator Tim Murray estimates that, between June 1989 and March 1993, 4500 entered the program and that 60% graduated or are still in the program. Of those who have graduated, only 11% have been re-arrested on any criminal charge. With normal recidivism rates six times higher, this is an unqualified success.[69]

This is not the only accomplishment. An Institute of Justice study found that the Metro-Dade County program (between June 1989 and March 1993) had to drop fewer cases, had lower incarceration and re-arrest rates, and had a significant increase in time before re-arrest. Those not re-arrested increased from the standard 45% to 52–67%. Time before re-arrest rose from 75–88 days to 235 days.[70] This implies that half of those who entered the program refrained from all criminal activity. In simple terms this is a reduction of 330 000 crimes per year just among the 4500 persons in the Miami diversion program. Whether or not this estimate is accurate, it is clear that no other program has come near to these results and that the social benefits are immense. Tim Murray estimates that the program costs about $800 per client per year, the cost of 9 days in jail.[71]

An innovative pilot study at the Santa Barbara County Jail explored the role of acupuncture in preventing 'post-acute withdrawal syndrome,' which is thought to contribute to re-arrests following release from jail. Alex Brumbaugh and his colleagues treated inmates during the 30-day period prior to their parole. They treated 51 inmate volunteers, 85% of whom had a history of abusing alcohol or another drug. Inmates who received 24 or more treatments during their last 30 days of incarceration were two-thirds less likely to be re-arrested in the 2 months following release than were those who received six treatments or less.[72] Although this is a pilot study from which sweeping conclusions should not be drawn, the potential it indicates is clearly important.

Currently, both state and federal prison officials, courts, and judges are interested in acupuncture rehabilitation programs. In mid-1994 there were 30 documentable programs, operating in, for example, California, Minnesota, Alabama, Oregon, Texas, Missouri, Nevada, New York, Arkansas, and Washington, DC, with plans for many more in process. Although a crime bill submitted by the Clinton administration contained substantial funding for these programs, these funds would never reach those in need. That bill became the center of a national partisan conflict in which it was defeated.

Despite political failures, several major developments have occurred in the USA. These involved major government acceptance of acupuncture at a level unprecedented in the West. Since 1973 the US FDA has classified the acupuncture needle as an experimental device.[73] This meant that acupuncture needles could only be used in experimental studies. This has been a major impediment to mainstream acceptance of acupuncture. Pressure to change this classification began in the early 1990s, and resulted in a major Workshop on Acupuncture in April 1994. The workshop was jointly sponsored by the FDA and the Office of Alternative Medicine at the National Institutes of Health. Leading US and international researchers assembled to present the best evidence of acupuncture's efficacy. FDA researchers then scrutinized the data in preparation for a citizens' petition to classify the acupuncture needle as safe and effective.

Five major areas of effectiveness were identified for which reasonable data from clinical trials existed: pain, respiratory disease, substance abuse, rehabilitation from central nervous system damage, and emesis. After waiting for more than a year, the FDA reclassified the acupuncture needle as safe and effective. However, this approval was not based on the weight of evidence, as none of the indications of effectiveness was approved. Rather it was 'grandfathered' by long-term use[74] (see Ch. 5). Birch, who was the principal author of the

'pain' submission and helped compile the other four submissions, suggests that the workshop was successful despite its less than ideal conclusion, in part because it was needed for the next step of approval.

In November 1997, a Consensus Development Conference on Acupuncture was convened at the National Institutes of Health. This conference also involved evidence on the nature, practice, and effectiveness of acupuncture for a variety of conditions. A panel of independent experts reviewed and weighed the evidence. They issued a finding very favorable to acupuncture, simultaneously calling for more and better research.[75] The full implications of this conclusion and the FDA approval are too recent to be fully understood. However, it is clear that a door has opened to the wider acceptance and practice of acupuncture, a topic we will revisit later in this text.

Acupuncture in the UK

Acupuncture began to emerge in the UK in the 1960s. There were two major movements. The first focused on physicians, the second on those specifically educated as acupuncturists.[76] Physician practitioner Felix Mann had begun to write about acupuncture. This helped found a medical acupuncture movement that is still present in the UK today. Mann described traditional theories, concepts, and practices, helping to popularize acupuncture for English-speaking readers. But he eventually rejected traditional explanatory models in favor of scientific explanations that he proposed. His books have been influential; they were arguably the most comprehensive English-language works until the early 1980s.

The acupuncture movement in the UK primarily centered around three individuals who initially studied and formed a school together, but then, after disagreements, each started their own schools. These were Messrs Worsley, Van Buren, and Rose-Neil. Worsley began the movement called 'traditional acupuncture,' which is still popular today in both the UK and the USA. It is estimated that most of the acupuncturists in the UK were trained at Worsley's school at Leamington Spa.[77] Van Buren and Rose-Neil's schools have perhaps been less influential, except within the UK. Since the early 1980s when practitioners and students started going to China to study, a number of TCM-based schools have also begun.[78] These schools sponsor a seminar circuit for popular authors that is making ideas about acupuncture relatively more homogeneous in the English-speaking nations.

The various UK schools, although initially in conflict with each other, have begun the same process that the US schools began — that of accreditation, as well as a movement towards certification and licensure.[79] Currently there is no license for acupuncture in the UK; its practice is allowed by common law. Thus the legal pressures operative in Asia and the USA have played a lesser homogenizing role. There are practitioners who are not graduates of any school, graduates of correspondence courses, and practitioners with various amounts of apprentice training. Today, UK schools are generally following the non-academic accreditation strategy used in the USA. However, some schools are academically accredited and offer academic bachelor's or master's degree.[80]

In an effort to organize as better educated practitioners, and to unite in the face of possible European Economic Union rules that could potentially restrict the practice of acupuncture, graduates of these acupuncture schools have formed an umbrella register. Today there are an estimated 1500 members.[81] Yet, there is no clear estimate of the total number of UK practitioners. Assuming that UK and US attitudes are broadly similar, we can guess that the practitioner ratio in the UK is similar to that in the USA (i.e. about one practitioner per 25 000 population).

Acupuncture is partially covered by the British National Health Service (NHS). Practitioners who work within an NHS clinic, for example physicians working in a hospital, receive NHS reimbursement for acupuncture. However, since the early 1990s restructuring of the NHS, acupuncturists receive NHS funds only if they work through a general practitioner's clinic.[82] A recent survey of members on the National Register found that as many as 18% of respondents were working in NHS-based practices; 55% receive referrals from physicians working within the NHS.[83]

There are also organized efforts towards more and improved research in the UK. George Lewith and Julian Kenyon's Center for the Study of Complementary Medicine in Southampton, the academic center at the University of Exeter, the Centre for Complementary Health Studies, started by Simon Mills and Roger Hill, and recently joined by Edzard Ernst, and the London-based Research Council for Complementary Medicine are actively pursuing this goal. Some of the best research on acupuncture has come from these centers, notably the work done by George Lewith and Charles Vincent. The Prince of Wales, Prince Charles, initiated an exploration of how complementary medicines, including acupuncture, can be moved towards further integration with biomedicine. The group he commenced recently published a report that discusses research strategies to assist that integration.[84]

Generally, acupuncture is relatively popular in the UK, with significant cultural and political support. The Queen has a personal acupuncturist, Prince Charles and the late Princess Diana have used acupuncture. Rumors abound that even the Conservative Party ex-leader Margaret Thatcher uses acupuncture. Today, acupuncture is a slowly growing but firmly rooted system in the UK, with levels of utilization similar to those in the USA and no powerful political or economic disincentives.

Acupuncture in the Commonwealth countries

In Commonwealth countries such as Canada, Australia, and New Zealand the situation is somewhat similar. There are both physician and acupuncture groups in each country that are to some extent competitive. Recent sociological research from Australia traces a history of acupuncture, particularly acupuncture schools, that is very similar to that in the USA.[85] In Australia three acupuncture schools operate within university programs and provide their graduates with a formal degree. There are plans for more university programs. Over 4500 practitioners have been identified in Australia,[86] which, with a population of less than 20 million, gives an approximate ratio of one practitioner for every 3800 persons, a higher use of complementary medicines than Eisenberg reports for the USA. MacLennan et al[87] estimate that half the Australian population (as compared to over one-third of the US population[88]) have used an alternative medicine. Thus, there are several evidences of a greater utilization of acupuncture in Australia than in other English-speaking nations.[89] The physician acupuncture groups such as the Australian and the New Zealand Medical Acupuncture Societies have growing memberships with well organized training programs. In Quebec, where there is a large French-speaking population, French influence is, of course, strong. Yet, at present it is Chinese TCM that appears to be the most influential trend. French writers such as Nogier, Soulie de Morant, Chamfrault, and Requena, and Quebequois such as Oscar and Mario Wexu remain influential.

Acupuncture in European nations

The situation for acupuncture in the rest of Europe is somewhat different than in the English-speaking countries. Each country in Europe generally has both a different set of rules and a different level of extra-legal tolerance. Many countries only allow physicians to practice acupuncture, for example, France, Belgium, Denmark, the Scandinavian countries, and Italy. However, acupuncturists are tolerated through unambitious enforcement of these exclusionary laws.

The oldest and most established school in the Netherlands, the Anglo-Dutch Institute for Oriental Medicine, was established in 1972. This school has primarily trained physicians and physical therapists in acupuncture. This emphasis arose not only because the founders

thought it more practical to train people who already possessed a medical training, but also because until recently the practice of acupuncture was legally restricted to physicians and physical therapists. However, when the Dutch government realized that there were thousands practicing who were neither physicians nor physical therapists, and that more than 20 schools existed to train them, laws governing the practice of acupuncture were liberalized.[90] With a population of 16 million and an estimated 5000 practitioners or more, there is about one practitioner to every 3200 people in the Netherlands. Birch currently practices in Holland, teaching throughout Europe.

Not all European nations have tried to restrict acupuncture practice to physicians. For example, in Germany there are estimated to be 20 000 to 30 000 physicians who practice acupuncture (somewhere between 10% and 20% of practicing physicians),[91] and possibly as many as 2000 who trained as *heil-praktikers* or natural therapists (*Heil-praktik*, 'health practice,' is a movement that began in the 1930s and allows a broad choice of healing disciplines). The practice of acupuncture in Germany was influenced by acupuncture in Japan, just as Japanese medicine was influenced by German medicine before the Second World War. In the 1950s, Sorei Yanagiya taught there, paving the way for the introduction of a variety of Japanese approaches, particularly *Keiraku chiryo*. In fact, one of his students, Herbert Schmidt, who also studied in Japan with Yoshio Manaka, was one of Worsley's teachers. This lineage resulted in a significant Japanese influence in the traditional acupuncture movement that Worsley began, a fact that has only recently been made public through Peter Eckman's research.[92] Europe's colonial history also contributed to acupuncture's European acculturation. As a French colony, Vietnam influenced European acupuncture both through Vietnamese practitioners who lived in France and the French who lived in Vietnam.

The opening of relations with China in the early 1970s attracted the same attention in Europe that it attracted in the USA and UK.

However, because acupuncture was already established in Europe, a more rapid assimilation was accomplished within the established medical systems. With a larger percentage of physicians practicing acupuncture, some as a medical specialty, acupuncture appears to be more widely used in Europe than in the USA and UK. In France, where physicians have been able to study acupuncture as a medical subspecialty for about 4 decades, there are now an estimated 10 000 physicians practicing acupuncture. Over 20% of the population of France has used or continues to use acupuncture.[93] This is much greater than the approximately 1% utilization in the USA and the UK.[94] Taken as a whole, the situation in Europe is comparable to that in the USA, where each state has its own set of rules and regulations, sometimes in contradiction. Part of the reason for the wider European acceptance is that more literature has existed for a longer time, and East Asian information has thus been more directly available. Many of the most noted sinologists and acupuncture experts have been European. We have noted George Soulie de Morant's instrumental work in several instances. However, writers such as Marcel Granet, the author of *La Pense Chinoise* (*Chinese Thought*) also contributed to the acculturation of acupuncture in Europe by making Asian philosophies more available.

However, it is important to note that European acupuncturists did not simply copy; rather they innovated, fully participating in the ongoing adaptation of acupuncture. Investigating the healing effects resulting from cauterizing a region of a patient's ear led Paul Nogier to discover a system of ear acupuncture.[95] This system was adapted by the Chinese who then created their own elaboration. During the 1950s, while Yoshio Nakatani was making electrical measurements of the channel and acupoint systems in Japan, developing the system now known as *Ryodoraku*, Rheinhold Voll was conducting similar experiments in Germany. Voll's system differs from Nakatani's (which will be discussed later in the text) and is known now as EAV (electro acupuncture according to Voll).[96] Just as Manaka and others

such as Tsugio Nagatomo were researching the effects of two-metal contact in Japan, similar work was performed in Germany by Gerhard Bachmann.[97] At the same time that the heavier needling techniques that are typical of TCM acupuncture were being developed in China, much lighter needling techniques were being developed and utilized in Europe, simultaneous with similar developments in Japan.

Although often unnoted outside of Europe, considerable basic and clinical research has also been conducted. When it became acceptable for physicians to practice acupuncture in France (the first regulations were formulated in 1952), physicians and researchers also began to investigate acupuncture. Researcher-practitioners, such as Niboyet and de la Fuye in France and Bischko and Kellner in Austria, have made significant contributions. European centers of sinological research have long been active, for example Joseph Needham's institute at Cambridge. Paul Unschuld has established a project for the collation, philological study, and translation of the *Nei Jing* at the Institute for the Study of the History of Medicine at the University of Munich Medical School. There, working with Asian and European scholars and the generation of PhD candidates for whom he is an inspiration and advisor, Professor Unschuld has helped advance the standards of Chinese medical collection, translation, and study throughout the world.

Acupuncture in the former USSR nations

Acupuncture arrived in the USSR in the mid-1950s. After the 1949 revolution, the isolated Chinese could only turn to their communist neighbors for assistance. Political ties with the Soviet Union began in 1953, and not long thereafter medical methods and techniques were exchanged.[98] The Soviets had already established a three-tier system of medical training. This system influenced the Chinese, who adopted versions of it for both modern and traditional medicine. In China there were 4- to 5-year programs for physicians or traditional doctors, 2-year programs for assistant doctors and assistant traditional doctors, and 3- to 6-month programs for paramedics. Later there were somewhat longer programs for Barefoot Doctors (in the USSR these rural health workers were called *feldshers*).

What the Soviets imported was a 'scientifically scrubbed' acupuncture that became known as 'reflexotherapy.'[99] It was and is practiced by physicians. Although acupuncture is practiced by those specifically trained as acupuncturists it is not officially recognized; rather it is tolerated. 'Reflexotherapy' became the neutral term chosen to label the wide variety of acupuncture approaches imported from China, Japan, and Europe. Generally, however, it incorporates those systems of practice that have been judged 'scientifically validated,' and is thus essentially void of traditional explanations. It is generally taught to physicians in postgraduate medical colleges, but is only partially centrally controlled or researched. It is used for a reasonably broad range of conditions. For example, it was reportedly used in military front-line medical centers during the Soviet army's tenure in Afghanistan.

Acupuncture is also practiced in Russia as part of what is called 'Traditional Medicine,' and is one of the many traditional methods of therapy that are practiced there.[100] Currently there are over 30 centers in Russia that teach specialized courses in Traditional Medicine to medical students and postgraduate physicians. There are more than 30 large research institutions investigating these therapies. Eugene Bragin of the Institute of Traditional Methods of Therapy in Moscow is a leading Russian proponent of acupuncture. He reports that acupuncture and other traditional methods are being increasingly selected by both physicians and patients. Most hospitals and medical centers have departments of Traditional Medicine for both in patients and outpatients.[101] Viktor Praznikov of the same institute notes that this increased utilization is largely the result of problems in the distribution of biomedical care in Russia.[102]

From the USSR, acupuncture was also quickly disseminated to East European countries. There too it has typically been practiced by physi-

cians. It is used in Romania, East Germany, Hungary, Czechoslovakia, Poland, and virtually all the former Soviet bloc. It was officially acknowledged as a medical treatment in Romania in 1958 under the leadership of Dr Bratu. It is now taught in 3-year postgraduate training programs as a medical specialty, and is thought to be practiced by as many as 1000 physicians, with approximately 5% of physicians practicing acupuncture alone.[103] In December 1996 the Polish News Agency estimated that over 1000 physicians have 'learned to cure illnesses using traditional Chinese acupuncture and moxibustion.'

With the lifting of the iron curtain, acupuncture has also been adopted into public health programs. Substance abuse is a significant problem in Eastern Europe and Russia, just as it is in the West. After practitioners in Eastern Europe, especially in Hungary, heard of the National Acupuncture Detox Association (NADA) movement in the USA, senior acupuncturist Paul Zmiewski, who had already helped found a US school,[104] moved to Hungary to establish substance abuse programs. Before his untimely death in 1993, the program Paul began in Budapest was adopted by the Hungarian government as a national model.

The trends of medical practice in the former Soviet bloc mirror the broader trends of recent history. Acupuncture was assimilated only when it was labeled as 'scientifically validated.' This was true regardless of the level or system in which acupuncture was eventually settled. This was determined by economic factors. In the Soviet bloc there were already sufficient numbers of mid-level health workers and paramedics. Thus acupuncture was assimilated as a physician's specialty. In China and North Vietnam, where poverty, insufficient resources, and massive pre-existing health problems demanded government attention, acupuncture was adopted to different extents at each level of practice. In Japan, where biomedical dominance of the medical system was more complete, both politically and practically, acupuncture was not so much assimilated as given a chance to compete at something of a disadvantage.

A summary of westward transmissions

The principal events that occurred in the acupuncture field after the end of the Second World War are summarized in Box 2.6.

MODERN WESTERN INTELLECTUAL TRENDS

If any modern Western history of acupuncture is preliminary, the intellectual history of its Western transmission is at best an outline.

Box 2.6	The principal events in the field of acupuncture since the end of the Second World War
1947	Following Douglas MacArthur's attempt to eliminate acupuncture and moxibustion in Japan, effective personal and public protest resulted in proposals for testing and licensing procedures
1948	Licensing procedures were enacted in Japan
1948	Traditional medicine including acupuncture and moxibustion, was promoted in Korea
Early 1950s	Chinese traditional medicines received support from Mao and others sympathetic to Chinese cultural demands. Political committees were formed to scientize and standardize traditional medicine, so that it could contribute to the country's vast primary-care needs. The major traditional medical schools were established. Soulie de Morant's publications become available in French
1950s	Acupuncture and moxibustion developed in France, Germany, Austria, and other European countries
1952	The first official ruling on acupuncture and moxibustion in France limited the practice of acupuncture to physicians
Mid-1950s	Acupuncture and moxibustion were exported to the USSR and from there to other Eastern bloc countries. For example, Romania officially adopted the practice in 1958
1957	The treatment repertoire of Soulie de Morant's influential text *L'Acuponcture Chinoise* was published posthumously.
1958	Mao declared 'Chinese medicine is a great treasure-house! We must make all efforts to uncover it and raise its standards'
1958–1959	The 'Great Leap Forward' in China; traditional and modern medicine began to be integrated
1960	Acupuncture and moxibustion were integrated into the health-care system in Vietnam
1960s	Acupuncture and moxibustion started to be promulgated in the UK through the works of Mann, Worsley, and others
Late 1960s	Proponents of traditional and scientific schools of thought concerning acupuncture and moxibustion competed in Japan
1965–1966	The first controlled clinical trials of acupuncture were conducted by Kinoshita and Okabe in Japan
1969	The Barefoot Doctor program in China began
1971	James Reston wrote about his postsurgical acupuncture experiences; acupuncture made headlines in the West
1972	American President Richard Nixon visited China. Starting in this year acupuncture and moxibustion were either introduced to, or strongly developed in, many countries: the USA, the UK, Australia, France, Germany, Austria, Italy, Finland, Norway, Denmark, Sweden, Spain, Eire, Portugal, Greece, Belgium, the Netherlands, Canada, New Zealand, South Africa, Ghana, Nigeria, Pakistan, to name but a few
1972 onward	Acupuncture and moxibustion grew on all continents, either as a newly introduced therapy or from indigenous ethnic Chinese and Asian communities
Post-1972	Many clinical trials of acupuncture began to be conducted around the world, especially in the USA and Europe
1972	Dr Wen of Hong Kong described the first use of ear acupuncture as a drug detoxification therapy
1977	The WHO adopted the 'health for all by the year 2000' policy
1978	The WHO began advocating the use of traditional medical practitioners to aid in the dissemination of health care to all, 'including the promotion of acupuncture/moxibustion, provided that the therapies are adequately tested and shown to be safe and effective, and so long as the skills and knowledge of the traditional practitioners are upgraded'
1980	The Chinese Government put forward the principle that 'traditional medicine, Western medicine and the combination of the two are three parallel forces,' and that therefore attention should be given to ensuring their coexistence and development
Early 1980s	The first authentic texts on acupuncture, based on the work of influential practitioners who went to China to study the medicine, were published in English. TCM was introduced into the USA and UK. These texts spawned significant developments for acupuncture in the USA and elsewhere
Mid- to late 1980s	Increasing numbers of texts on acupuncture were published, including the first of recent Japanese acupuncture texts. As TCM continued to expand in the USA, other systems such as Japanese and Korean acupuncture methods established a firm foothold

Foremost, it is far from complete. It is also largely unexamined. However, acupuncture cannot be understood until we recognize the intellectual trends of its acculturation. The westward transmission of acupuncture has most often been the work of enthusiasts and entrepreneurs whose only interest was clinical application. With notable exceptions, academic sinology has played a lesser role. Acupuncture would never have become as broadly and successfully introduced without this narrowly focused transmission. However, what is today commonly believed has only rarely been subject to academic methods or open critique.

In Western acupuncture communities the fact that acupuncture is adapting to the West, just as it has adapted in East Asian cultures, has yet to be incorporated into acupuncture education. As we have seen, acupuncture theory was reformulated in China to assure political survival. In Meiji and post-Meiji Japan it was scientized; in the USA and other Western nations it is also subject to the modifying force of political, economic, and cultural demands. Yet this is rarely noted in the training of either specifically trained or physician acupuncturists.

There are also important transmission issues that have only begun to be scrutinized. Western students are trying to understand traditional practices that are transmitted with Asian terminologies that are so old and specialized that even native Chinese speakers require translations into modern characters and idioms. So too, the philosophical orientations that Westerners identify as inherent to being Chinese are in reality as specialized in China as in the West:

Each new generation in China finds the ancient philosophies increasingly alien. The doctrines of yin and yang and the five phases have lost their rank as the obvious way of understanding reality; they are no longer part of school or family education, and have to be painstakingly learned. The medicine these doctrines serve is today cognitively isolated. In contrast, the modern sciences and technology, physics and mathematics, are part of the education of every Chinese child. They have made their imprint over the whole of private and professional life, making modern medicine automatically, as it were, appear to be true.[105]

Thus, without discipline in selection and translation, and without secure means of judging the clinical efficacy of adapted ideas, some mistransmission is highly likely.

During the early years when acupuncture pioneers defied law and convention to give acupuncture force in numbers and the credibility of success, little attention could be paid to technical issues, understanding alien concepts, or the need for developing appropriate systems for insuring clinical validity. Because many hoped that acupuncture would provide what they found lacking in modern medicine, acupuncture's development concentrated on the elements that most encouraged those hopes. The philosophical unity of traditional concepts was often seen as a solution to the fragmentation and alienation of modern society; thus acupuncture's traditional and sometimes mundane role in day-to-day symptom resolution is still largely ignored by writers, who concentrate on its holistic features. In the same way, loose translations of Asian literature make it easier to propose loose parallels to modern science, sometimes at the expense of traditional ideas.

In the simplest sense there are two main issues: authenticity and clinical validity. Determining whether an idea is authentic, when and where it fits into the massive literate and oral traditions, is no simple feat. It requires a specialized knowledge of language and literature, a broad understanding of cultural and philosophical developments, as well as a familiarity with history, politics, and economics. As we will discuss in much greater detail later in this text, ideas of how to determine what is clinically valid are only beginning to mutually serve the needs of both scientists and acupuncturists. Importantly, both of these issues are so large that their resolution is neither individual nor field-specific. Rather, it depends upon the development of multidisciplinary methods and cooperation.

Because the largest transmission of modern Western ideas about acupuncture occurred without either scrutiny by Western academic systems or the master–apprentice safeguards of the East, anomalies in how acupuncture is understood were certain. For example, those writing on acupuncture rarely note that there is a difference between cultural continuity and technical equivalence when discussing the medicine of ancient dynasties. Although such issues may seem mere academic niceties, scholarly method is in fact of considerable importance to working acupuncturists. A good example of how mistransmission has affected both the conception and practice of acupuncture is a recently promulgated model of the *qi jing ba mai*, or eight 'extraordinary vessels' (which are discussed briefly in Chs 3, 6, and 7). Although technical in detail, you need not know much about the extraordinary vessels to understand this transmission problem. Furthermore, this example is interesting because it results not in a single clinical error, but in the loss of the clinical variety and adaptability that has contributed to acupuncture's success. In effect, it eliminates or waters down an entire set of clinical tools.

Some English-language authors propose that the extraordinary vessels store and circulate the *jing* (essence)[106] and *yuan qi* (original *qi*),[107] or both.[108] We will discuss these concepts later in greater detail; they are qualities essential to human life. Many of these authors propose a close connection between all the extraordinary vessels and the *shen*, or kidneys,[109] and through the kidneys to the *jing qi* and/or the *yuan qi*. These too are entities with critical importance for human health. Each describes a quality that is easily lost and hard to regain. Simply put, this particular set of channels is said to play a significant role in the distribution of energies that is critical to human health. Because Western writers think of all these entities as energy, and energy is a straight-line phenomenon, they assume that needling the extraordinary vessels must deplete these essential energies. Put simply, the extraordinary vessels are conceptualized as a circuit that can drain the battery of human life without regard to the metaphoric quality of the traditional concepts.

As we will discuss in Chapter 3, this materialization of *qi*-related phenomena is itself a problematic trend. However, what is important here is that this concept is novel. The traditional literature concerning the extraordinary vessels is very diverse and often contradictory.[110] This likely indicates that these theories and their clinical applications developed after those of the regular channels, the *jing mai*.[111] However, even within this considerable variety, there are no primary sources that support this description, nor is there an obvious literature of contraindication and restorative treatments for the iatrogenic damage this idea implies.[112]

A review of passages concerning the extraordinary vessels in the principal texts that discuss them, the *Huang Di Nei Jing Su Wen*, *Huang Di Nei Jing Ling Shu*, *Nan Jing*, *Shi Si Jing Fa Hui*, *Zhen Jiu Da Quan*, *Zhen Jiu Ju Ying*, *Zhen Jiu Da Cheng*, and *Qi Jing Ba Mai Kao*,[113] reveals no explicit mention of any association between the extraordinary vessels and *jing qi* or *yuan qi*. Only one of the extraordinary vessels was traditionally described in relation to the kidneys, although two, in some descriptions three, intersect the kidney channel. Interestingly, two authors who claim to be transmitting the modern TCM system also claim these associations,[114] despite the lack of such claims in Chinese-language TCM texts.[115]

When naive students and other authors uncritically accept these associations,[116] and use them to extrapolate clinical principles, the implications become profound. In this case, clinicians are told that needling the extraordinary vessels expends and damages *jing*.[117] Logically then, treatment of the extraordinary vessels with any regularity would be harmful to human health. What well-meaning clinician would consider their use or study the means and methods of treatments that employ them?

Ironically, a clinical alternative that has a positive reputation in a broad selection of authentic traditional East Asian literature has begun to acquire a negative reputation in the West. Thus, the work of many practitioners, in many eras, will not be consulted because of assumptions that stand upon no firm traditional ground. Because of this misunderstanding, students ignore, practitioners fail to learn, and patients are denied potentially effective treatments.

Where did these misconceptions come from? The likely origin is earlier European 'translations' of acupuncture texts.[118] This idea appears to originate with the French authors Albert Chamfrault and Nguyen Van Nghi, whose writings during the 1960s were among the few books available in a Western language.[119] These authors appear to have promoted a novel model whereby *yuan qi* is associated with the extraordinary vessels.[120] Chamfrault and Van Nghi cite Chapter 62 of the *Ling Shu* as justification,[121] although none of the versions of the *Ling Shu* we consulted had any such reference.[122] Neither does Soulie de Morant's immense, and then-available, French-language compilation of Chinese acupuncture literature.[123] This supports Peter Eckman's conclusion that this idea may originally be of Vietnamese origin.[124] Put simply, an idea that is at best an Asian or European variant has come to stand for the entire tradition because there are too few scholarly safeguards protecting the transmission of that tradition.

What is most important here is that facts in Traditional East Asian Medicine (TEAM) do not exist outside of context and, if transmitted without that context, they are easily altered by readers' expectations. Because the force of those expectations has not been routinely restrained by referencing and translation disciplines, ideas in acupuncture have become more idiosyncratic than they actually are. For example, the extraordinary vessel model just discussed was assimilated by many clinicians and writers who used Chamfrault and Van Nghi as sources – clearly evidencing the danger of one-and-only textbooks and secondary sources. Only one of the authors cited who assert an association between the extraordinary vessels and the *jing qi*, *yuan qi*, and/or kidneys claims to have translated Chinese, and he cites no sources for those statements.[125] Thus, an understanding of the extraordinary vessels that is less founded in the source literature than the ideas it has replaced becomes 'standard.'

Again, the most important issue is, why? This idiosyncratic understanding has influenced practitioners, because its authors became popular in the West and the education system has yet to provide a sufficient means of peer review. For example, there has never been any sinological review of the facts demanded of students on licensing examinations. Furthermore, there is literally no way to challenge those ideas. This is very important because, as Paul Unschuld has noted, there is a strong tendency among Westerners to accept whatever notion best fits Western needs.[126] Because this idea fits best the behavior of energy in Western thought — linear, point-to-point, circuit-like relations — it appears natural, and thus true to Western minds. Because it satisfies the Western craving for integrated knowledge, it is easily accepted. Because theories of *qi* are assumed to describe the universe as Western theories do, the metaphoric nature of *qi* is forgotten. Because Western thought assumes singular truths, an idea that East Asian clinicians might take as a school of thought, or a model appropriate to a particular treatment system, becomes a 'truth,' variance from which is 'wrong.' As we will see in Chapter 3, Eastern minds are not so exclusionary.

Fortunately, a new generation of scholars and researchers has begun to address these problems by making more Asian-centered views available. Kevin and Marnae Ergil, Volker Scheid, Nigel Wiseman, and others have established well-founded doctoral level investigations that give us greater access to the Asian roots of tradition. Marnae Ergil's research allows Westerners to see TCM in its native Chinese context — for example, how students are selected and trained in China — information that is critical not only to the successful Western adaptation of Chinese approaches, but also to understanding the role of the written materials that Westerners decide to translate and teach. Kevin Ergil is exploring the challenge to medical hegemony that acupuncture is said to make. Many claim that acupuncture is a fully developed model, 'an alternative medicine.' Yet, the way in which Westerners practice acupuncture actually undermines that claim. Ergil cites examples of how the biomedical model dominates traditional ideas. He quotes the example of a patient whose TCM diagnosis is 'blood stasis and uterine fibroids.' The latter is a purely biomedical diagnosis that has entirely replaced long-standing traditional concepts.[127] Similarly, Manfred Porkert studied 2000 case histories at the Beijing College of Traditional Chinese Medicine, and found that every diagnosis was of biomedical origin.[128]

In both East and West, the dominant culture of biomedicine often completely overrides traditional interpretations. Simplification of translation methodology further encourages the replacement of Asian ideas by biomedical terms. This is particularly true of those traditional ideas that do not fit Western expectations.[129] Thus diagnostic competence subtly shifts from acupuncturists to physicians, a shift that is anything but trivial, because it reinforces the dominant cultural bias, and thus deeply challenges acupuncturists' claims of independence.

Kevin Ergil is also exploring the strategic representations acupuncturists make when trying to clinically validate traditional practices. These efforts rely heavily on labels that are meant to impart authenticity by implying a coherent body of knowledge with a long, continuous practice.[130] Effective iteration over millennia is offered as proof of clinical validity (the 'test of time') and is assumed to be an effective substitute for conventional Western validity testing. However, as we have seen throughout the history of Chinese medicine, there has never been one right way of practice or a static continuity. It would be more accurate, but perhaps overly dramatic, to say that no system of practice has ever been older than its most longevous master–apprentice line. The means of reporting and validating claims of clinical success are thus far from firmly established, something we will explore in detail later in the text.

Paul Unschuld's research shows us how Westerners have chosen acupuncture and pharmacotherapeutics from the variety of traditional techniques to represent all of Chinese medicine because it is these ideas that most closely resemble our own. Nigel Wiseman shows how the words popularly chosen to translate Chinese medicine hide qualities of the Chinese art that do not fit the expectations of readers. Writers such as Dan Benksy, Charles Chace, and Andy Ellis are giving voice to Chinese clinicians, historic and modern, through reliably translated texts and accounts of traditional medicine. Marnae Ergil and Bob Flaws have pioneered Chinese-language training for future clinicians and educators.

It is fair to say that there is progress on many fronts, and that the integration of acupuncture in the West would never have occurred without the enthusiastic pursuit of its original proponents. However, until there is a workable way to label ideas attributed to tradition and personal experience, students and clinicians will have no means to judge the source of purported facts. Until disinterested scholars have a reasonable chance of affecting curricula and licensing examinations, the predominance of popular interpretation will burden the development of acupuncture. Without an effective peer system, there is no possible check on commercial trends. Early, simplistic, and sometimes misleading attempts to authenticate acupuncture today leave it vulnerable not only to the attack of skeptics, but also the internal conflicts fueled by competing interpretations and personal rivalry, despite its vast gains in public and professional acceptance. Until the more secure and workable methods of transmission, education, and clinical validation are achieved, the continued acculturation of acupuncture cannot be assumed.

THE NUMBERS GAME
China[131]

Western medicine is dominant in the People's Republic of China. Recent estimates put the number of health-care workers trained in acupuncture at more than a million. Although the number who currently practice acupuncture is unclear, we do know that most are trained in traditional medicine, *zhong yi*, typically herbal pharmaceutics and acupuncture. How many practice acupuncture or herbal medicine alone or in combination is unknown but more than 300 000 traditional doctors have graduated from China's 24 medical colleges, where they received 5 years of training in basic biomedical sciences, acupuncture, and herbal medicine. More than 30 000 assistant traditional doctors have graduated from 3-year programs that offer the same subjects in less detail. There are many Chinese biomedical physicians who have attended abbreviated acupuncture courses, and more than 2000 physicians have graduated from both a traditional and a Western medical program. By the early 1980s over 1 million Barefoot Doctors had been trained in 6-month to 2-year programs. Today, these famous worker-practitioners are paramedics who learn essential herbal medicine, Western medicine, and acupuncture techniques in Western-style programs. An unknown number of people have begun private acupuncture practice since it was again permitted during recent economic liberalizations. The training of these practitioners is unknown.

Herbal medicine is far more popular in China than is acupuncture, which retains its traditional lesser prestige. Thus the number of practicing acupuncturists is probably lower than the training statistics suggest. Acupuncture services are part of China's socialized medical system, but increasing numbers of patients now pay out-of-pocket as China's private sector grows. It thus is unclear what percentage of the population receives acupuncture treatment.

Taiwan[132]

Biomedicine is also the dominant medicine in Taiwan; however, traditional medicines survive and flourish. There are an estimated 7500 Chinese medical doctors, about 10% of whom practice acupuncture extensively. There are some 2000 biomedical physicians trained in acupuncture and actually practicing. Although insurance coverage for acupuncture is common, the percentage of the population that uses acupuncture is unknown.

Japan[133]

Although Western medicine is by far the dominant medicine, Japan's variation of herbal medicine (*Kampo*) and acupuncture are comparatively popular and thriving. Current estimates are that over 60 000 national licensees use some combination of acupuncture, moxibustion, and massage, each of which is separately licensed after completion of 3-to-4-year training programs. About 40% of these acupuncturists are blind. In the early 1980s there were about 6000 physicians practicing acupuncture. There are probably more today. The training of these physicians is variable and unknown. Acupuncturists do not prescribe herbal medicine, only physicians or pharmacists are so permitted by law. Health insurance only pays for acupuncture when it is performed at the referral of a physician from an independent clinic, or is for treatment of one of the six approved indications. Thus most acupuncture is a discretionary expense. Recent estimates suggest that at least 2% of the Japanese population uses acupuncture, this use being concentrated in the larger cities.

The USA[134]

Like most Western countries, biomedicine is by far the most popular medicine. However, recent studies suggest that over one-third of the US population is using an 'unconventional medicine.' These same studies estimate that the proportion of the population using acupuncture is 1% or less. There are an estimated 11 000 acupuncturists in the USA, approximately 3000 of whom are biomedical physicians. Current estimates are that the numbers will increase to 21 000 by 2005 and 40 000 by 2015. Specifically trained graduates complete 2- to 3-year programs, in which acupuncture may be taught in combination with Chinese herbal medicine. The scope of acupuncture education in the USA varies, with some schools integrating herbal medicine, massage, homeopathy, or other natural therapies. Current estimates are that by the year 2001 these schools will be graduating 2000 students per year. Physicians' interest is increasing and physicians can practice in many states without formal training; however, more and more physicians are training in postgraduate nonresidential programs. Over half the states have some form of licensure, with variable degrees of autonomy, scopes of practice and requirements for practice. There are also an unknown number of drug detox specialists who are trained in an acupuncture protocol, and who, working under trained acupuncturists, administer acupuncture as part of drug treatment in centers throughout the USA. There are also an unknown number of dentists, veterinarians, and chiropractors who practice acupuncture, after training programs of variable content and length. Some states have extensive insurance reimbursement available for acupuncture; most do not. Most acupuncture is paid for by patients. Recent estimates put the number of treatments per year at at least 12 million.

The UK[135]

The numbers of practitioners and the extent of their training is unclear, largely because of what is called Common Law. This allows therapies like acupuncture to be practiced without any specific training. However, it is estimated that there are over 2000 practitioners in the UK. An unknown number of these are physicians. Recently, the British government has allowed acupuncture to be covered by the National Health Service, if it is supervised by a general practitioner as part of their practice. It is thought, however, that most acupuncture is paid for out-of-pocket. As in the USA, many acupuncturists combine acupuncture with other therapies such as Chinese herbal medicine, massage, and homeopathy. Recent estimates put the proportion of the population using acupuncture at around 1%, although it is thought to be increasing.

France[136]

Generally the practice of acupuncture is a subspecialty of biomedicine. Only physicians are legally permitted to practice acupuncture.

Although there are over 10 000 physicians trained in acupuncture, there is a considerable but unknown number of nonphysician practitioners, many of whom are Vietnamese. Many physicians combine other therapies with acupuncture and biomedicine. Recent estimates place the proportion of the population using acupuncture at over 20%, probably because it is an insurance-reimbursable medical specialty.

Germany[137]

An estimated 20 000 to 30 000 physicians and 2000 *heil-praktikers*, or natural therapists, practice acupuncture. Natural or traditional therapies are very popular in Germany, with more herbs consumed by Germans than most of Europe combined. It seems that acupuncture is relatively popular among the general population. Certainly it is more widely used in Germany than in the USA and UK, and probably as much as in France. Many acupuncturists combine acupuncture with other therapies, especially homeopathy and phytotherapy (an herbal medicine based on higher potency extractions).

Utilization worldwide

In a recent Canadian survey it was estimated that less than 1% of Canadians use acupuncture.[138] In European countries, especially those where laws restrict acupuncture practice to physicians, the percentage of use is routinely higher. Recent estimates suggest 3% in Denmark, 6% in Belgium, and 2% in the Netherlands.[139] The Netherlands is an interesting and perhaps representative case. Although only physicians and physiotherapists were allowed to practice acupuncture legally (there were 2000 such practitioners) they were actually a minority. Recent studies estimated that there were over 5000 nonphysician, nonphysiotherapist acupuncturists working in the Netherlands.[140] These 'underground' practitioners were not only tolerated, but their numbers were great enough to force legislative change. It is possible that the same phenomenon may be found in other European countries.

Table 2.1 Pan-European utilization of acupuncture

No. of organizations	Countries
1	Egypt, Hungary, Iceland, Poland, Sweden, Switzerland, Turkey
2	Austria, Denmark, Netherlands, Portugal, Slovenia
3	Czech Republic, Norway
4	France, Greece
5	Belgium, Bulgaria, Spain
8	Ireland
9	Finland
10	Germany
17	Italy
19	UK

Alfio Bangrazi of the Istituto Paracelso in Italy compiled a list of 109 organizations throughout 24 European and Middle Eastern countries that promote or are involved in acupuncture. Although not a formal survey and now slightly dated, this compilation suggests widespread use of acupuncture in Western and Eastern Europe.[141] Table 2.3 shows the number of organizations in these 24 countries. Although this cannot be assumed to be authoritative, it is nonetheless usefully indicative.

It makes sense that the number of acupuncture treatments is greatest in less industrial countries, where it is has been used historically, where it is inexpensive, and where it benefits from political and economic support. However, among industrialized countries it is relatively more popular where its practice is dominated by Western physicians, making it part of nations' mainstream health-delivery and medical-payment systems. In industrialized countries like the USA and the UK, and even Japan where acupuncture has a long history, it is largely excluded from mainstream medical finance, and is thus less widely used.

Acupuncture has significantly increased in popularity throughout the world since the 1970s, particularly since Richard Nixon's trip to China and James Reston's post-appendectomy articles. Western interest has increased the amount of attention that acupuncture receives in East Asia. The WHO reports that it has helped develop Chinese acupuncture programs that have already trained people from over 100 countries.[142] Practitioners can now be found in Korea, Vietnam, Malaysia, Sri Lanka, Pakistan, India, Russia, Romania, Hungary, Austria, Italy, Switzerland, Finland, Sweden, Norway, Eire, Spain, Portugal, Greece, Australia, New Zealand, South Africa, Nigeria, Ghana, Israel, Saudi Arabia, Ecuador, Brazil, Mexico, and on and on. With most of the national boundaries that it has crossed, it has changed and adapted to suit the needs of the peoples to whom it was presented.

Nineteen-hundred years from its first thorough elaboration, acupuncture is effectively a modern art. It is no longer anywhere primarily supported by the philosophical tenets from which it arose, even in its own lands. Although philosophical loyalties and divergent views still divide its practitioners, its most powerful political opponents and proponents are almost universally moved by economic and social demands. The worldview of its foundations, the principles on which its practices are derived, must now do service to the cultural demands of the 21st century. It is these aspects that we will explore in Chapter 3.

NOTES

1   Manaka Y, Itaya K, Birch S 1995 Chasing the dragon's tail. Paradigm Publications, Brookline, MA, p 11
2   Hillier SM, Jewell JA 1983 Health care and traditional Chinese medicine in China 1800–1982; Routledge & Kegan Paul, London, p 13.
3   Ibid. p 15

4   Unschuld PU 1985 Medicine in China: a history of ideas. University of California Press, Berkeley p 229
5   (a) See note 2, p 29 (b) For a very compelling and moving account of the period through the eyes of one family, see Chang J, 1992, Wild Swans, Flamingo, London
6   Ibid. p 39

7   See note 4, p 246
8   Ibid. p 245
9   Ibid.
10 See note 2, p 309
11 Ibid. p 56
12 Chace C, Zhang TL (trans) 1997 A Qin Bowei anthology, Paradigm Publications, Brookline, MA, p 4
13 See note 4, p 250
14 See note 2, p 60
15 Ibid. p 66
16 Ibid. p 83
17 Ibid. p 313
18 Unschuld, PU 1998 Chinese Medicine. Paradigm Publications, Brookline, MA, p 83
19 Rosenthal MM 1987 Health care in the People's Republic of China: moving toward modernization. Westview Press, Boulder, CO, p 172
20 Evans JR 1988 Medical education in China. In Bowers JZ, Hess JW, Sivin N (eds) Science and medicine in twentieth century China: research and education. Ann Arbor, Center for Chinese studies, University of Michigan, p 244
21 See note 2, p 315
22 See note 3, p 251
23 One of the most influential books in the transmission of the TCM system of acupuncture was: O'Connor J, Bensky D 1981 Acupuncture: a comprehensive text. Eastland Press, Seattle. This book is a translation of texts written in 1962 and 1974 by the Shanghai College of TCM (p. xv). It reflects the pioneering work of the College in the 1950s and 1960s. One of the more striking features of the acupuncture described in this text is a considerable increase in the recommended depth of needle insertion at the acupuncture points. To explore this issue systematically, Birch examined historical and modern acupuncture textbooks, including *Acupuncture: A Comprehensive Text*, to tabulate the depths of insertion in *cun*, or 'body inches.' Major acupuncture points in the following important historical acupuncture texts were noted: *Zhen Jiu Jia Yi Jing*, by Huang Fu-mi (282), *Tong Ren Shu Xue Zhen Jiu Tu Jing*, by Wang Wei-yi (1027), *Zhen Jiu Ji Sheng Jing*, by Wang Zhi-zhong (1220), *Zhen Jiu Ju Ying*, by Gao Wu (1529), and the *Zhen Jiu Da Cheng* by Yang Ji-zhou (1601). Based on the number of points recommended at each needle depth, Birch calculated the mean depth of insertion and median depth of insertion as indicators of relative depth. Table 2.1 lists the numbers of points at each recommended depth range given, the overall mean depth of insertion, and the median depth of insertion for these five historical sources (for points that were given a range of depth of insertion, the midpoint of that range is given in the table).
    Birch then tabulated the recommended depths of insertion for all the major acupuncture points in four modern Chinese textbooks on acupuncture: *Essentials of Chinese Acupuncture*, Anon. (1981), *Chinese Acupuncture and Moxibustion*, by Cheng (1987), *Acupuncture: A Comprehensive Text*, by O'Connor & Bensky (1981), and *Fundamentals of Chinese Acupuncture*, by Ellis, Wiseman & Boss (1988). In addition, he calculated the overall mean depths of insertion, and the median depths of insertion. Table 2.2 lists the numbers of points recommended in each text in the depth ranges given, the overall mean depths of insertion and the median depths of insertion for these four modern sources (for points that were given

a range of depth of insertion, the midpoint of that range is given in the table).
    All the modern texts recommend deeper needle insertions than the historical texts. Looking at the mean depth of insertion and median depth of insertion as general indicators, *Acupuncture: A Comprehensive Text* recommends needling more than twice as deeply as the historical texts. Clearly, the practice of acupuncture changed in China during the 1950s and 1960s, when the work that preceded the publication of these modern texts was done. Although any absolute measure of the *cun* will vary because it is a relative measure that varies between individuals and areas of the body, changes in the *cun* concept cannot account for these increases in insertion depth. A modern Chinese researcher has estimated that the *cun* is approximately 2.23 cm (Chen et al 1979), while classical scholars estimate that the *cun* was about 2.31 cm in antiquity (Harper 1982).
24 Felt. Interview of Tin Yao So. So, who was named the 'father of acupuncture in America,' has played a historic role in the acculturation of acupuncture in the USA. Both of the present authors studied with Tin Yao So, Birch formally. We also have access to written and video materials from which we can make statements from So's perspective. Thus, references to acupuncture before the Second World War and Chinese apprentice training are frequently referenced to Dr So.
25 See note 2, pp 320–321
26 (a) Felt. Interview of Ping Chang (b) For a disturbing but compelling account of the major events and their bizarre events and consequences of the Cultural Revolution see note 5(b)
27 See note 2, p 322
28 This is a complex issue. Although there is probably some degree of chauvinism on the part of Westerners, there is evidence that this is the case. See, for example: Unschuld PU 1985 The evaluation of acupuncture anesthesia must seek truth from facts (see note 4, p 160)
29 This development is discussed in: Shudo D 1990 Japanese classical acupuncture: introduction to meridian therapy. Eastland Press, Seattle, 5 ff
30 Soichiro Tobe. Personal communication
31 Kodo Fukushima. Personal communication
32 Anon 1986 *Shukan Bunshun*, Bunshun library June 26, 128 (in Japanese)
33 Felt. Interview of Yoshiharu Shibata, MD
34 Anon 1947 Serious news. *Ido no Nippon* 6(7): 44
35 Anon 1947 Demonstration by the blind. *Asahi Shinbun*, October (in Japanese)
36 Anon 1947 (in Japanese) Compensation for our efforts: status law is passed. *Ido no Nippon* 6(9): 46 (in Japanese)
37 Yanagiya S 1948 The future of acupuncture. *Ido no Nippon* 7(1): 50 (in Japanese)
38 Birch S 1989–1991 Acupuncture in Japan; an introductory survey. *Review*: Part 1, 6: 12–13, 1989; Part 2 7:16–20, 1990; Part 3, 8:21–26; Part 4, 9:28–31, 39–42, 1991
39 See note 38
40 These are the personal estimates of Yoshio Manaka and Kodo Fukushima
41 Yoshio Manaka. Personal communication
42 Soichiro Tobe. Personal communication
43 (a) Tsutani K, Shichido T, Sakuma K 1990. When acupuncture met biostatistics. Paper presented at the

Second World Conference of Acupuncture and Moxibustion, Paris.
(b) Shichido T 1996 Clinical evaluation of acupuncture and moxibustion. *Ido no Nippon* 623(8,7):94–102

44   Hiroshi Watanabe, Kiichiro Tsutani. Personal communication

45   World Health Organization 1980 Use of acupuncture in modern health care. *WHO Chronicle* 34:294–301

46   Song Jang-Heon 1985 The role of Korean oriental medicine. Korean Oriental Medical Association, Seoul

47   See note 46

48   Tiller WA 1972 Some physical network characteristics of acupuncture points and meridians. Proceedings of the Academy of Parapsychology and Medicine Symposium. Stanford University, Stanford, CT

49   See note 45

50   Levinson JM 1974 Traditional medicine in the Democratic Republic of North Vietnam. American Journal of Chinese Medicine 2(2):159–162

51   Kleinman A 1980 Patients and healers in the context of culture. University of California Press, Berkeley, p 12

52   Wiseman N. Personal communication

53   Felt RL Interviews with Bill Prensky

54   Felt RL Personal account

55   Wolpe PR 1985 The maintenance of professional authority: acupuncture and the American physician. Social Problems 32(5):409–424

56   See note 55

57   Felt RL. Interviews with Mercy College faculty

58   Felt RL. Interviews with Bill Prensky

59   Accreditation Commission for Acupuncture and Oriental Medicine 1997 Accredited and candidate programs (as of May 4, 1997), Acupuncture and oriental medicine accreditation. ACAOM, Washington DC

60   Based on presentations at the Workshop on Acupuncture, co-sponsored by the Office of Alternative Medicine and the FDA, April 1994, (see the special issue of Journal of Alternative and Complementary Medicine 2(1), 1996, and presentations at the Consensus Development Conference on Acupuncture at the National Institutes of Health, November 3–5, 1997

61   Mitchell B 1996 Educational and licensing requirements for acupuncturists. Journal of Alternative and Complementary Medicine 2(2):33–35

62   (a) Lytle CD 1993 An overview of acupuncture. US Department of Health and Human Services, Public Health Service, Food and Drug Administration, Center for Devices and Radiological Health.
(b) Helms JM 1993 Physicians and acupuncture in the 1990s: a report. The AAMA Review 5(1):1–6(c) Cooper RA, Land P, Dietrich CL 1998. Current and projected workforce of nonphysician clinicians. JAMA 280(9):788–794

63   See note 62(a)

64   (a) Eisenberg DM, Kessler RC, Foster C, Norlock FE, Calkins DR, Delbanco TL 1993 Unconventional medicine in the United States; prevalence, costs, and patterns of use. New England Journal of Medicine 328(4):246–252
(b) Eisenberg DM, Davis RB, Ettner SL, Appel S, Wilkey S, von Rompay M, Kessler RC. Trends in alternative medicine use in the United States 1990–1997: results of a follow-up national survey. JAMA 280(18):1569–1575

65   There are no central sources of treatment data from which solid conclusions can be drawn. These are assumptions based on commercial evidence. For example, the bulk of both USA and European advertising directed to practitioners via their periodicals is TCM-centric, as are new book releases and the products offered. Sales of Japanese acupuncture equipment, such as disposable needles are proportionally high but, because of trends in Western populations, TCM practitioners routinely purchase these devices.

66   Califano JA, Kleber HD 1992 Center on addiction and substance abuse. Annual report. Columbia University

67   Goldkamp JS, Weiland D 1993 Assessing the impact of Dade County's Felony Drug Court. National Institute of Justice, US Department of Justice, NCJ 145302

68   Finn P, Newlyn AK 1993 Miami's 'Drug Court', a different approach. National Institute of Justice, US Department of Justice, NCJ 142412

69   See note 67

70   See note 67

71   Presentation, Washington, DC, May 1994

72   Brumbaugh AG, 1993 Acupuncture: new perspectives in chemical dependency treatment. Journal of Substance Abuse Treatment 10:35–43

73   See note 62(a)

74   Alpert S. In: Birch S, Hammerschlag R (eds), Acupuncture efficacy. National Academy of Acupuncture and Oriental Medicine, New York

75   Anon 1998 Acupuncture: NIH consensus development panel on acupuncture. JAMA 280(17):1518–1524

76   Because of the unsettled economic and political status of acupuncture in the West, labels are often claims of 'belonging' to a particular view. Thus there is acrimonius debate concerning the use of 'lay' and 'non-physician' as labels for acupuncturists who do not have a physician's training, or the use of the title 'Doctor' to label acupuncturists or traditional Chinese herbalists with or without degress like the Oriental Medical Doctor (OMD) or Doctor of Oriental Medicine (DOM). We are using 'specifically trained' to label acupuncturists who do not hold standard Western academic or medical credentials because this label reflects patients' concern for their practitioners' relevant experience and training. This further directs attention to the long-term issue of acupuncture education rather than transient intra- and interprofessional tensions. We recognize that some physicians have a didactic and/or clinical training just as specific as specifically trained acupuncturists, and that this could justify refering to them in parallel as 'multiply trained.' However, that is not the case for all, and thus the label is inappropriate except for specific individuals. From the patient's perspective, what counts is experience in the system practiced. Thus, where a physician may be advantaged in the practice of a system with a biomedical basis, they would be disadvantaged relative to a specifically trained acupuncturist with greater experience with traditional skills.

77   Hill S. Personal communication

78   Kaptchuk TJ 1997 Foreword. In: Maciocia G 1997 Obstetrics and gynecology in Chinese medicine. Churchill Livingstone, Edinburgh

79   Shifrin K 1993 Setting standards for acupuncture training – a model for complementary medicine; Complementary Therapies in Medicine 1(2):91–95

80   The difference between a professional master's degree and an academic master's degree is one of accreditation standards and agencies. Typically, issues such as credits

for courses taken, transfer, and admission standards are determined within accrediting systems. For example, a person with a professional master's degree in acupuncture might receive 'life experience' credits from some academic institution, but probably would not be admitted to a doctoral program based on their professional degree.

81 Hill S. Personal communication

82 Stephen Dorrell clarifies the position on alternative and complementary therapies; Press Release, December 3, 1991

83 Anglo Dutch Institute for Oriental Medicine Magazine, Spring: 11 1997

84 Anon 1997 Integrated healthcare. A way forward for the next five years? The Foundation for Integrated Healthcare, London

85 O'Neill A 1994 Enemies within and without. LaTrobe University Press, Bundoora, Victoria

86 Bensoussan A, Myers S 1997 Towards a safer choice. University of Western Sydney, Macarthur, 23

87 MacLennan A, Wilson D, Taylor A 1996 Prevalence and cost of alternative medicine in Australia. Lancet 347:569–573

88 See note 64

89 See note 86, p 22

90 Hemken A, 1995 The Anglo-Dutch Institute for Oriental Medicine and the situation on alternative medicine in the Netherlands. European Journal of Oriental Medicine 1, 6:30–31

91 Stux G. Personal communication

92 Eckman P 1996 In the footsteps of the yellow emperor. Cypress Book Company, San Francisco

93 Bossy J 1993 History and present status of acupuncture in France. In: Abstracts of the Third World conference on acupuncture. World Federation of Acupuncture and Moxibustion Societies, Kyoto

94(a) See note 64
(b) Thomas KJ, Carr J, Westlake L et al 1991 Use of non-orthodox and conventional health care in Great Britain. British Medical Journal 302:207–210

95 Nogier PFM 1983 From auriculotherapy to auriculomedicine. Maisonneuve, Saint-Ruffine

96 For discussions of the differences, see:
(a) Kenyon JN 1983 Modern techniques of acupuncture, vols 1 and 2. Thorsons, Wellingborough.
(b) Tiller WA 1989 On the evolution and future development of electrodermal diagnostic instruments. In: Energy fields in medicine: a study of device technology based on acupuncture meridians and chi energy. Proceedings of a symposium sponsored by the John. E. Fetzer Foundation, pp 257–328

97 See examples in: Matsumoto K, Birch S 1986 Extraordinary Vessels. Paradigm Publications, Brookline, MA

98(a) Bragin E 1993 Present and future of traditional medicine in Russia. In: Abstracts of the Third World conference on acupuncture. World Federation of Acupuncture and Moxibustion Societies, Kyoto
(b) Praznikov VP 1993. The role of acupuncture in modern medicine. In: Abstracts of the Third World conference on acupuncture. World Federation of Acupuncture and Moxibustion Societies, Kyoto
(c) Rudenko M, Kabaruchin B 1993 The system of education in traditional Chinese medicine in Russia. Abstracts of the Third World conference on acupuncture. World Federation of Acupuncture and Moxibustion Societies, Kyoto

99 Stoyunovsky D 1981 Acupuncture reflexotherapy: handbook–atlas. Cartya Moldovenyaske, Kishinev (in Russian)

100 See note 98(b)

101 See note 98(a)

102 See note 98(b)

103 Ionescu-Tirgoviste C 1991 Acupuncture in Romania. Complementary Medicine Research 5(2):89–92

104 Paul helped found the Midwest Center of Oriental Medicine in Chicago, IL, and contributed to the development of programs at the New England School of Acupuncture in Boston, MA.

105 Unschuld PU 1998 Chinese medicine. Paradigm Publications, Brookline, MA p 87

106 The following are representative examples:
(a) 'The extraordinary vessels all derive their energy from the Kidneys and all contain the Essence which is stored in the Kidneys. They circulate the Essence around the body.' Maciocia G 1989 Foundations of Chinese medicine. Churchill Livingstone, Edinburgh, p 355
(b) '[Four of the extraordinary vessels] are interlinked for the production, circulation, discharge and regeneration of the Essence.' Maciocia G. 1997 Obstetrics and gynecology in Chinese medicine. Churchill Livingstone, Edinburgh p 24
(c) 'Jing circulates in the Jing Luo system, and in particular in the network of the eight Extraordinary Channels.' Ross J 1985 Zang Fu, 2nd edn. Churchill Livingstone, Edinburgh, p 67
Other references to this concept are:
(d) Pirog JE 1996 The practical application of meridian style acupuncture. Pacific View Press, Berkeley, p 158.
(e) Seem M 1992 American acupuncture comes of age: perspectives from the front lines. American Academy of Medical Acupuncture Review, 4(2):16–23
(f) Seem M 1993 A new American acupuncture. Blue Poppy Press, Boulder, CO, p 52

107(a) 'Yuan qi is most concentrated in the curious meridians [extraordinary vessels].' Helms JM 1995 Acupuncture Energetics. Medical Acupuncture Publishers, Berkeley, CA, pp 523–524
(b) 'The irregular vessels [extraordinary vessels] function on a deep, fundamental level, and this is in perfect accord with the traditional statement that they are the carriers of the yuan ch'i(sic) or ancestral energy.' Low R 1983 Secondary vessels. Thorsons, Wellingborough, pp 70, 147–164
(c) 'In addition, all the extraordinary vessels are in some way connected to the kidneys or to the kidney meridian, and by extension to the original qi.' See note 106(a), p 156

108 See note 106(b), pp 22–24, and note 106(d), pp 156–158

109 See: note 107(b), pp 70, 147; note 106(a), p 355; note 106(b) p 22: note 106(d) p 156

110 One of the clearest discussions of the diverse descriptions of the *qi jing ba mai* can be found in: Matsumoto K, Birch S 1986 Extraordinary vessels. Paradigm Publications, Brookline, MA, pp 4–137

111 See discussions in note 110, pp 4–6

112 When empirical observation and experience indicate that acupoints or naturally occurring medicines have unwelcome effects in particular circumstances or combinations these contraindications appear in the literature. Although there are variances in these contraindications over time, had treating the extraordinary vessels created a significant history of iatrogenic effects,

there would be obvious contraindications in books describing the use of their acupoints.

113   These texts are all discussed in Chapter 1 and in Appendix 2. They all made significant contributions to the theories and uses of the extraordinary vessels. The salient passages are translated by Matsumoto & Birch (see note 110)

114   See: note 106(a), p 355; note 106(b), pp 22–24; note 106(c), p67.

115   Direct translations of modern TCM textbooks from China make no mention of these associations. The relationships described are to the liver, kidney, and minor organs, and there is specific mention that the extraordinary vessels are so named because, unlike the regular channels, 'they have neither a continuous interlinking pattern of circulation, nor are they each associated with a specific organ.'

See: Wiseman N, Ellis A 1994 Fundamentals of Chinese medicine. Paradigm Publications, Brookline, MA, pp 40–43.

Yuan qi, original *qi,* is defined by Chinese sources as 'right *qi,*' which stands in opposition to any entity that may harm the body, and 'source *qi,*' which is the basic *qi* of the body. It is specifically noted as not appearing in the *Inner Canon. Yuan qi* is not uniquely associated with the kidney, but with a combination of the essential *qi* of the kidney, the *qi* of food via the spleen, and the *qi* of air through the lung. It is specifically stated as accessed via the source points of the regular channels.

See: Wiseman N, Feng Y 1998 A practical dictionary of Chinese medicine. Paradigm Publications, Brookline, MA, pp 421, 507, 548

116   See: note 106(d), p 158; note 106(e), p 52; note 107(a), pp 523–524; note 107(b), pp 147–164

117   Zand J 1997 Presentation at the Pacific Symposium, San Diego, November 6

118   Use of the term 'translation' typically asserts a more or less word-for-word version of a foreign-language source. However, in English-language acupuncture literature the label is freely applied to works that are loosely referenced and which contain undifferentiated quotation, paraphrasing, and original writing. The antiquity of Chinese medicine's generative literature also contributes to discrepancies in interpretation. Because these ancient documents were recorded on perishable materials, they exist as archaeological fragments, references in other archaeological fragments, and quotations or attributions in later editions of those texts. Thus translations of these works require an assembly and verification process known as 'collation.' Because the contents have been assembled in different eras and reflect the assumptions of those that produced, commented upon, and sometimes edited those editions, the content of these texts is a complex issue. This is rarely noted, nor are the commentaries that accompany Asian editions typically available.

119   See note 92, p 163.

120   Chamfrault A 1969 Van Nghi N 1969 L'energetique humaine en medicine Chinoise. Imprimerie de la Charente, Angouleme, p 241

An English-language exposition of this model appears in Yves Requena's work. Requena is a direct student of Van Nghi and played an important role in the early years of the transmission of acupuncture. He references the model directly to Chamfrualt. See: Requena Y 1986

Terrains and pathology in acupuncture, vol 1, Correlations with diathetic medicine. Paradigm Publications, Brookline, MA, p 14

121   See note 120

122   We looked at:
(a) Kitasato kenkyujo huzoku toyoigaku sogokenkyujo rinsho koten kenkyuhan: 1982 *Reisu Rinsho Sakuinshu,* the *Lingshu* Clinical Index. Kokusho Kankokai, Tokyo,
(b) Anon 1988 *Ling Shu Jing.* Chung Hwa Book Company, Taipei
(c) *Huang Di Nei Jing Ling Shu Yi Jie.* 2nd edn. Chinese Republic Publishing Company, Taipei, 1978

Note, however, that because Chinese literature is so extensive (the vast majority of the literature has never been translated into any Western language), there is no physical evidence for much of what is reputed to be in these early, seminal texts, only fragments of which survive. Thus it is impossible to make definitive statements. It is the continual presence of an idea in a broad range of the surrounding and following commentary and related literature that is the most reliable evidence of authenticity. Although the references here are necessary, the best evidence for the idiosyncrasity of this idea is its isolation in the writings of European and European-influenced American authors.

123   Soulie de Morant notes that *yuan qi* is 'mostly used in the sense of vitality, strength and resistance,' a definition that accords with Chinese sources. Soulie de Morant G 1994 Chinese acupuncture. Paradigm Publications, Brookline, MA, p 46

124   See note 92, p 163

125   See: note 106(a), p 355; note 106(b), pp 22–24

126   Unschuld PU 1992 Epistemological issues and changing legitimation: traditional Chinese medicine in the twentieth century. In: Leslie C, Young A (eds). Paths to Asian medical Knowledge, University of California Press, Berkeley

127   Ergil KV 1990 A challenge to medical hegemony? Epistemological issues informing the practice of TCM in the United States. Paper presented at the Third International Congress on Traditional Asian Medicine, Bombay

128   Porkert M, The difficult task of blending Chinese and Western science: the case of modern interpretations of traditional Chinese medicine. Quoted in Sivin N 1987 Traditional medicine in contemporary China. Center for Chinese Studies, University of Michigan, Ann Arbor, MI, p 28

129   See: Wiseman N 1990 Introduction. In: Wiseman N, Boss K A glossary of Chinese medicine and acupuncture points. Paradigm Publications, Brookline, MA

130   Ergil KV 1992 Strategic representations: 'oriental' medicine at large. Paper presented at American Anthropological Association Annual Meeting

131   This section is based on: (a) Evans JR 1988 In: Bowers JE, Hess JW, Sivin N (eds) Science and medicine in twentieth-century China: research and education. The Center for Chinese Studies, University of Michigan, Ann Arbor, MI.
(b) Hillier SM, Jewell JA 1983 Health care and traditional Chinese medicine in China 1800–1982. Routledge & Kegan Paul, London
(c) Rosenthal MM 1987 Health care in the People's Republic of China: moving toward modernization. Westview Press, Boulder, CO

132   This section is based on Nigel Wiseman's interviews with his colleagues at the Journal of Chinese Medicine and the China Medical College (Taichung, ROC)

133   This section is based on:
(a) Birch, Acupuncture in Japan (see note 38),
(b) Sonoda K 1988 Health and illness in changing Japanese society. University of Tokyo Press, Tokyo

134   This section is based on presentations at the Workshop on Acupuncture sponsored by the Office of Alternative Medicine and the FDA (see the special issue of Journal of Alternative and Complementary Medicine 2(1), 1996 and presentations at the Consensus Development Conference on Acupuncture at the National Institutes of Health, November 3–5, 1997

135   Based on:
(a) Birch, Acupuncture in Japan (see note 38)
(b) Fulder SJ, Munro RE 1985 Complementary medicine in the United Kingdom: patients, practitioners, and consultations. Lancet 542–545
(c) Thomas KJ et al (see note 94(b))
(d) note 62(c)
(e) note 64(a and b)
(f) Cooper RA, Henderson T, Dietrich CL 1998 Roles of nonphysician clinicians as autonomous providers of health care. JAMA 280(9):795–802
(g) Wetzel MS, Eisenberg DM, Kaptchuk TJ 1998 Courses involving complementary and alternative medicine at US medical schools. JAMA 280(9):784–787

136   Based on:
(a) Bossy J 1993 History and present status of acupuncture in France. Abstracts of the Third World Conference on Acupuncture. World Federation of Acupuncture and Moxibustion Societies, Kyoto
(b) Bouchayer F 1990 Alternative medicines: a general approach to the French situation. Complementary Medicine Research 4(2):4–8

137   Based on:
(a) Aldridge D 1990 Pluralism of medical practice in West Germany. Complementary Medicine Research 4(2): 14–15
(b) Heise TE 1986 Historical development of traditional Chinese medicine in West Germany. Journal of Traditional Chinese Medicine 6(3):227–230
(c) Stux G. Personal communication

138   Anon 1991 One in five Canadians is using alternative therapies, survey finds. Canadian Medical Association Journal 144(4):469

139(a) Rasmussen NK, Morgall JM 1990 The use of alternative treatment in the Danish adult population. Complementary Medicine Research 4(2):16–22
(b) Sermeus G 1990 Alternative health care in Belgium. Complementary Medicine Research 4(2):9–13
(c) Uddin J 1993 Acupuncture, Europe and the law. European Journal of Oriental Medicine 1(1):53–55

140   Hemken A, Personal communication.

141   Bangrazi A, Tsutani K 1998 Global communication on acupuncture (10) Directory of Societies in the field of Acupuncture. Journal of the Japan Society of Acupuncture 48(2): 176–185

142   World Health Organization 1985 The role of traditional medicine in primary health care. WHO, Geneva WPR/RC36/Technical Discussions/s

3

The theoretical basis of acupuncture: fundamental concepts and explanatory models

In the first two chapters we have reviewed the long history of acupuncture. Because so many societies have found it useful, and the social, political, and medical needs of Asian nations have not been static, it has already undergone several acculturations. Even before biomedicine began rapidly to circle the globe from its origin in Western Europe, acupuncture was growing outward to meet it from vaguely seen origins in India and China. Each culture that has absorbed acupuncture has influenced its development. Each culture has contributed its own technical and theoretical achievements. Because acupuncture is a human skill, a process for observing and thinking, it has become multifaceted, reflecting the talents, needs, and expectations of each society it has served.

All this makes providing any absolute but general definition of acupuncture unwise. With so many diverse environments for its development and with so many languages for its discussion, it has been explained in many different ways. Because it has adapted to the philosophical foundations of several societies, there are contradictions between one writer's ideas and another's. There are many traditional explanatory models and, recently, a growing number of scientific models. So how are we to contend with this diversity? Is it possible to create a picture of acupuncture that excludes no major system or style? Is it possible to resolve the contradictions among various systems?

Of course, we intend to try. First, however, we should note the limits to success. Like the elephant examined by blind men in the famous fable, acupuncture's intellectual foundation is not so much indecipherable as huge. Just as sightlessness in this fable is a symbol for the intellectual blindness of judgements based on an individual's personal experience, theories about acupuncture have tended to focus only on what is relevant or interesting to whomever seeks the explanation. Just as each of the blind persons imagined that they had examined the whole elephant, investigators tend to feel that they have finished when their own needs are met, they have satisfied the prejudices of their culture, or have reached the limit of their vision.

There is a diversity of ideas and opinions about acupuncture that results from this process, a process that has occurred on the same temporal and intellectual scale as the deepest expressions of being human — mythology, philosophy, and religion. On the one hand, when traditional thinkers discussed what happened when a physician inserted an acupuncture needle, they talked about *qi*, an idea that is so deeply rooted in Asian thought that it cannot be entirely separated from ideas of consciousness or being. On the other hand, Chinese physicians also understood disease in ways that were not very different than our own. Long before Chinese traditional medicines adapted to the medicine of the West, Chinese physicians understood that tuberculosis was carried from the ill to the well by an unseen entity that they named for the spores they saw in nature, just as we speak of 'germs.' Chinese physicians listed these unseen 'worms' alongside phlegm, food, wind, cold, fatigue, and fear as causes of disease.[1] They also knew that smallpox lesions contained a factor that could protect others, and they used that knowledge to create a very early form of immunization.[2]

It is also important to understand that modern biases have blinded some who have examined this particular elephant. Among scientists and physicians, both in the West and East, these biases have led to some fascinating contradictions. All of acupuncture has been dismissed because there are acupoints that seem to be associated with nervous system structures, but acupoints have also been dismissed because they cannot be related to nerves. Modern popular writers who find acupuncture an answer to a cultural demand for holistic health care tend to ignore features of Chinese traditional thought that do not fit their view.[3] Not only did Asian physicians and scholars understand and apply biomedical principles, at times they thought about medicine just as we do today. The famous physician-scholar Xu Da-Chun compared the use of medicine to the attack of an army on an invading enemy, a metaphor that is exactly like those used to explain antibiotics. Indeed, these metaphors are found in many of the most significant theories of Chinese medicine.[4]

Finally, we cannot ignore the obvious — nothing travels for nearly 2000 years without acquiring a considerable layer of dust, strains, pains, and quite a few bruises. Both the critics who dismiss entire traditional concepts with diminutive labels like 'metaphysical manipulation' and the admirers who see only modern answers in this ancient art are concentrating on too small a picture. There is no possibility that acupuncture is flawless. But neither is there any chance that it contains nothing of value.

Certainly, given the analytic bent of the West, what we now call 'acupuncture' as a whole will, when fully acculturated, belong to a variety of different disciplines. So, to do our job fairly we must not only consider the limited descriptions of our own experience, but also a library full of theories and explanations, past and present, in languages and cultural biases as various as humanity. Just as the fable of the elephant teaches the impossibility of completely understanding something through inherently limited observation, we must recognize the impossibility of stating a complete and final model of acupuncture from any single perspective. However, having begun with an historical and cultural perspective, we can add to this a working knowledge of clinical and scientific matters. Then, we can sketch a reasonable outline of the theoretical bases of acupuncture. At least we can achieve one that captures most of the salient points.

To develop a more comprehensive model we will also need to consider the evidence that has begun to emerge from modern research. Since the majority of books on acupuncture apply some traditional description, this is where we will begin. However, later, in an effort to incorporate current scientific views, we will explore more recent views of acupuncture, attempting to find the common ground in both approaches.

THE QI PARADIGM

The most basic traditional concepts, those first described many centuries ago and still in use today, focus on the idea of *qi* and describe a model of how acupuncture works that we have chosen to call the 'qi paradigm.' As noted earlier, we chose the word 'paradigm' because the idea of *qi* is closer to a model than it is to a fixed entity. In the *qi* model all the ideas central to the traditional explanations of acupuncture and its traditional practice — *yin-yang*, five phases, channels, and acupoints — depend on some characteristic of *qi*. All the most basic ideas of health, disease, pathology, and therapy derive from observations of *qi*. Almost everything we describe in the following chapters – the techniques and processes, terms, methods of diagnosis and patient assessment, and the many treatment strategies and techniques – has its conceptual roots in the idea of *qi*.

THE IDEA OF *QI*

Qi is an Asian speculation about the nature of being that has been believable to so many people through so many generations that it is impossible to conceive of Asian culture without *qi*. It is very old; it has been used continuously from the first Chinese writing to modern times (Box 3.1). Indeed, the term *qi* is still routinely used in modern Asia. A modern general Chinese-English dictionary where ancient definitions have been reduced or eliminated still describes a very broad range of meanings for the Chinese character transliterated as *qi*:[5] (1) gas; (2) air; (3) breath; (4) smell, odor; (5) weather; (6) airs, manner; (7) spirit, morale; (8) to make angry; (9) to get angry; (10) to bully, insult; (11) in Chinese medicine – vital energy, energy of life. Among

those uses are some that still reflect ancient roots. In Japanese, where '*qi*' is pronounced '*ki*,' the routine daily greeting equivalent to 'Hello, how are you?' is *Ogenki desu ka?* — How is your original *qi*?'

气　米　氣　气　気
(1)　(2)　(3)　(4)　(5)

Box 3.1 *Qi (ki)*

The earliest form of the character *qi* (in Japanese *ki*) (1) means 'curling vapors rising from the ground to form the clouds above.' With the incorporation of the idea that these vapors helped nourish the body, the character became associated with vapors that came from food. Since rice was the central crop, it symbolized all food. Thus the rice radical (2) was added to make the character (3). Recently, in China older Chinese characters were simplified and the modern character was returned to its initial form (4). Another form is now used in Japan (5).

Qi has been variously translated as 'vital force,' 'vital energy,' 'energy,' 'pneuma,' 'influences,' 'spirits,' 'subtle spirits,' 'configurational energy,' 'air,' 'breath,' and 'finest matter influences.' It is often incorrectly associated only with living things. In fact *qi* was considered the foundation of everything, both animate and inanimate.

The idea of *qi* is neither antique nor static. Scientific terms coined in the present era make good use of the generality of the character. *Qi ya* is barometric pressure, literally '*qi* pressure.' For a modern Chinese person, *dian qi* is electricity, literally 'lightning *qi*.' *Qi dao* is the bronchii, literally the '*qi* or breath way,' and the trachea is the '*qi* or breath pipe,' *qi guan*. Many of these extended meanings and modern uses of the term carry over to medical terms.[6] Like other characters that once represented concepts in Chinese medicine, *qi* has been used to translate modern Western ideas into Chinese. Yet, despite these new uses, *qi* continues to serve the purpose it has always served in the traditional medical context. It provides a way to describe qualities and relationships that, although common to many things, are not obvious to the naked senses.

Because *qi* is such a large idea, it is the subject of much debate. Like any idea that has a long history of use, its meaning has varied and evolved through the centuries. In this regard we can find parallels in Western tradition. For example, we need only look at Middle Eastern religious ideas to find the same diversity of interpretation. In fact, just as the faithful of most religions refer to specific passages that have been passed down from ancient times, Chinese medical writers refer to their body of ancient literature as a source of authority. In fact, it is the source of intergenerational definition in Chinese medicine.[7] Although this analogy is by no means exact, it is not unfair to say that the canonical works of Chinese traditional medicine, what are often called 'classics' or 'canons,' were to Chinese medical writers what ancient religious texts are to the faithful. Just as those texts are the source, not only of doctrine, but also of the ideas, images, and metaphors that permeate entire cultures, the Chinese medical classics are intimately linked to a cultural heritage. Even today, 1800 or more years after they are believed to have been written, these books are much more than out-of-date clinical manuals. They are expressions of ideas that form the core of Chinese culture.

Thus, the roots of the idea *qi* and many of the most important acupunctural concepts are not only at the very heart of Chinese culture, but are also similar to root ideas in any society. However, whereas most Indo-European languages use alphabets and compose words by stringing together letters that represent spoken sounds, Asian languages use symbols to stand for objects and ideas. Although there is rarely something that reflects a subject in the string of letters that form a Western word, Asian readers are sometimes presented with a visible symbol of the idea. This is particularly true of the older forms of the characters.

In recent times, the Chinese government has promoted 'simplified characters' to achieve greater literacy and to eliminate the social barriers inherent in traditional methods of education. However, looking at the original picture-like forms can often explain part, but not all, of its meaning and history. This approach emphasizes the linguistic roots of a character but not the technical, psychological, or social meanings acquired through time. Just as Western philosophers speak of how the meaning of a word lies in its use, the etymology of a Chinese character tells us something, but not everything, about the idea itself. Thus before we look at the various ideas *qi* represents, we can usefully examine its image. (See Box 3.1).

It is generally accepted that *qi* ((1) in Box 3.1), the modern character in its oldest form (4), is related to the concepts of vapor, breath, and smoke. The character evolved from images of the steam or vapors that rise from cooking rice (3). The internal portion of the character (2) is a picture of a sheaf of bound rice stalks. This image is accessible to everyone; just visualize rice cooking in a heavy pot. It smells wonderful. We cannot see a smell, we experience it. Even separated by age and distance we can imagine how significant the aroma of cooking rice must have been for an ancient Chinese for whom — like agrarian peoples everywhere — neither the next meal nor a good harvest was an iron-clad guarantee.

The relationship between a warm hearth, a full belly, and the human sense of well-being unites humankind because it is an experience almost everyone knows. In most cultures, the aromas of cooking and the image of the hearth fire are inseparable from our most cherished memories and thoughts. Artists from every era called upon these images to portray feelings that are common to all humankind. In the same way, the image of *qi* and its associations permeate many of the technical meanings of *qi* and the diverse cases in which it is applied.

THE LITERATURE OF *QI*

In the literature of ancient China before the medical classics were written, *qi* was used in a very broad cosmological sense to refer to that which arose at the beginning of things and from which all else derived. If God is the creative agent in Western cosmology, *qi* is the medium of creation in Eastern cosmology. Again, even these esoteric aspects of *qi* are something that Western cultures share or to which we can, with a little conceptual discipline, relate to with some success. Today, many Westerners are greatly intrigued when they are introduced to the *dao*, through translations of Lao Zi's world classic the *Dao De Jing* (*Tao Te Ching*). In that work, we find passages that describe the *dao* as the undifferentiated whole from which all else comes to being. Piecing together passages from translations of similar ancient texts, we discover that the *dao*, 'the one,' differentiates into two, *yin* and *yang*. From *yin* and *yang* all else emerges. Original *yin* and *yang* are typically represented as heaven and earth. In the line of reasoning that is fully developed in old texts like the *Yi Jing*, heaven and earth interact to create a third level — human beings (Fig. 3.1).

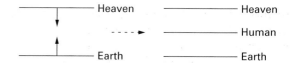

Figure 3.1 Interactions between heaven and Earth and the origin of humankind.

This human-centered view is central to understanding the ancient Chinese medical model. In both medicine and philosophy we find a line of reasoning that, to borrow a phrase, 'in the beginning,' there was the *tai yi* – the great one. In *tai yi* the original *qi* (*yuan qi*) began. The light *qi* rose upward to become heaven, the heavy *qi* bore down to become the earth. The *qi* of heaven and earth interacted to create the myriad things, including all life and human beings (Fig. 3.2).

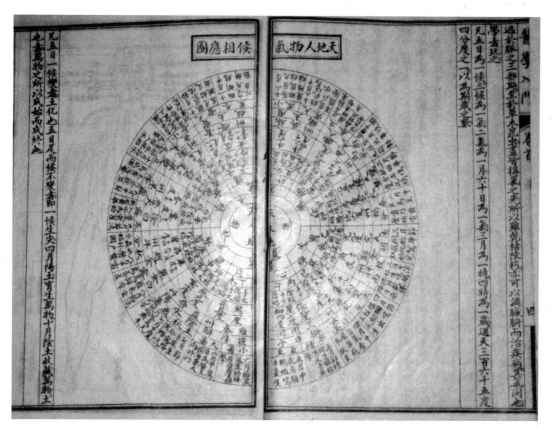

Figure 3.2 The relationship between Heaven, Earth, Humankind, the myriad things, weather and *Qi in The Gateway to Medicine* (1515 *Ming*). (Courtesy of Paradigm Publications.)

In an ancient song that was probably written before –400, human beings are elegantly described as being at the center of this interaction:

Heaven and earth have correct *qi*. Its form is flexible and fluid. In the lower parts, it is in earth's rivers and mountains. In the upper parts, it is in the heaven's sun and stars. In it human beings are said to be overwhelmingly and universally immersed.[8]

Some nonmedical authors took these ideas a step further and explicitly described the origin of human beings. Zhuang Zi (Chuang Tzu), another ancient daoist, wrote: 'The birth of the human being amounts to an accumulation of *qi*. When it has accumulated, birth takes place, and when it has dissipated, death takes place.'[9] Later, the philosopher-scientist Wang Cong would write: 'As water turns into ice, so *qi* crystallizes to form the human body.'[10]

In this perspective, *qi* refers to an undifferentiated whole that is the precursor of everything in nature, including human beings. Everything that is, is *qi*. Everything reflects *qi*. *Qi* is the medium by which one thing reflects another because it is the ocean of being from which all arises and returns.

We know that this view of a universal *qi* influenced the early medical writers. But to best understand the view of health and disease that underlies acupuncture and the qi paradigm we must examine the traditional Chinese views of the body and its relationship to nature. For example, traditional East Asian medicines today retain the ideas and terms for correct qi: upbearing and downbearing. Because moral tones are eschewed in Western science, many of the terms chosen to describe *qi* phenomena in English eliminate this element of 'correct.' Nonetheless, the image is an ideal of proper order within the human body. It is a qualitative concept of 'right,' not the statistical idea of 'normal.' The moral imperative 'should be' is far more strongly implied than is the sense of a quantitative measure.

QI IN NATURE

The Chinese observed nature and recorded the patterns of natural variation with a degree of skill and subtlety that led the world until the scientific revolution was well progressed. To support medical practices and theories the qi paradigm evolved specialized distinctions and differentiations. These developments occurred along two linked and parallel tracks. The first saw human beings as in an indivisible relationship with nature. The second looked inside the human being to subdivide and categorize bodily functions. The former is the root of concepts that explain how behavior, and ultimately health and disease, result from changes in nature. The latter results in descriptions of how the body works, and thus greatly influenced Chinese concepts of healing. Both were expressed in terms of *qi*. The concept of *qi* thus helps provide a unitary picture of nature that describes humans as both functional entities and, because *qi* is the universal stratum from which everything evolved, an inextricable part of all creation.

It is also a natural outcome of the idea of *qi* that everything in nature can be described in terms of *qi* (Table 3.1). If *qi* permeates all, everything will resonate and reflect all else. There is a *qi* of climate and weather, a *qi* of each season, a *qi* of plants, animals, and minerals. There is the *qi* of the earth, a *qi* of the sun and moon. There is a *qi* of the rarest jewel, a *qi* of the dung heap. All phenomena share qualities and relationships based in their common origin in *qi*.

It was also natural for these concepts of *qi* to evolve toward a point of view in which the macrocosm and microcosm were seen to be parallel and related. As things change 'out there,' corresponding things change 'in here.' However,

Table 3.1 *Qi* concepts in nature

Qi	Name
Tian qi	The *qi* of earlier heaven, referred to the general influences of heaven
Di qi	The *qi* of Earth, referred to the general influences of Earth
Da qi	The great *qi*, or cosmic *qi*, related to the breath
Ren qi	The *qi* of the human, which results from the interaction of *tian* and *di qi*
Yuan qi	The original *qi* from which all other forms of *qi* derive
Yi qi	The *qi* of meteorologic influence: cold, wind, damp, heat, dryness

things out there did not cause change, or vice versa; both were changing in reference to their foundation in *qi*. Thus, this concept of relatedness subtly differs from similar-sounding ideas that developed in the West. For example, where the 'as above, so below' maxim of Middle Eastern astrology depends on the idea that a cosmic energy impels human events through time and space, the Chinese universe was alive. Things resonated with *qi*, even when unlinked in time or space. Humans changed with the interminable cycle of the universe because they were living expressions of the *qi* that formed that universe, not because they were impelled by a separate and irresistible power. Humans, heaven, and earth breathed with one breath; that breath was *qi*.

Naturally, this was reflected in Chinese thought about medicine, and has been described as interlocking reactions. The late British sinologist Joseph Needham states it as follows:

…things behaved in particular ways not necessarily because of prior actions or impulsions of other things, but because their position in the ever-changing cyclical universe was such that they were endowed with intrinsic natures which made their behavior inevitable for them … They were thus parts in existential dependence upon the whole world-organism.[11]

In a general way this difference is like that between the Newtonian and Einsteinian ideas of gravity. In the former, gravity is something that objects possess; each attracts the other. In the latter it is the result of each object's effect on space and time itself. Thus, for example, in Chinese thought calendric cycles could predict the weather, epidemics, or human events, not because they impelled them, but because everything reflected *qi*.[12] There are passages from very old texts that describe how similar things resonate with one another, just as plucking a string on a musical instrument causes other strings to vibrate, or several strings to sound in harmony. Analogies such as these are very difficult for Westerners to appreciate, because we immediately think of sound waves, harmonics, and forms of energy, for a phenomenon that the Chinese would have conceived as a universal, qualitative relationship.

These analogies do offer us important clues for how to think about Chinese ideas of interaction, particularly those between humans and nature. It also helps us understand how Chinese medical thinkers were able to produce sophisticated systems of correspondence that could predict the course of an illness or the outcome of a therapeutic intervention without what seems to us the necessary concept of causation. Because human beings were seen to be in constant interaction with the universe, disease processes were described in terms of those interactions, a subject we will later explore in greater detail.

Another natural consequence of this perspective was that human actions were seen as affecting natural phenomena. This relationship is described in Chinese literature that concerned philosophy, religion, and social and ceremonial duties, as well as in medical texts. In addition to the expressions of *qi* founded on daoist images of life and nature, there were also images that derived from another of China's great philosophical movements, Confucianism. Like the daoist image of nature, the Confucian concepts of personal, familial, and social responsibilities were not one dimensional but two-way. The Confucian classic *The Great Learning* contains an elegant expression of this idea:

The ancients who wished to exemplify illustrious virtue throughout the world first ordered well their own states. Wishing to regulate well their states, they first regulated their families. Wishing to regulate their families, they first cultivated their own persons. Wishing to cultivate their persons, they first rectified their minds. Wishing to rectify their minds, they first sought for absolute sincerity in their thoughts. Wishing for absolute sincerity in their thoughts, they first extended their knowledge. This extension of knowledge lay in the investigation of things. Things being investigated, knowledge became complete. Their knowledge being complete, their thoughts became sincere. Their thoughts being sincere, their minds were then rectified. Their minds being rectified, their persons became cultivated. Their persons being cultivated, their families were regulated. Their families being regulated, their states were rightly governed. Their states being rightly governed, the world was at peace.[13]

Just as peace was interdependent with proper behavior, disharmony and illness resulted when people did not use their bodies, insights, and thoughts in the manner custom demanded. As we noted in our review of history, this link was an important step in the development of all Chinese thought, not just medicine. In practice, the view of the human body held by a Chinese physician came to be a reflection not only of the cosmos and nature, but also of humankind and its social and personal actions. What humans could do, 'rectify,' and 'regulate,' was what the cosmos did and, later in history, these same qualities would be attributed to medicinal substances and acupoints, often using exactly the same words. This is particularly clear in the names of acupuncture points, *xue* or 'holes.'

Chinese doctors did not label acupoints as we do in the West; they gave each a name. Some acupoint names were memory aids that helped students remember their location. Some were codes that hid one teacher's knowledge from another teacher's students. Yet, many acupoint names were images of the *qi* that permeated the universe. These *qi* moved in cycles that were timed by natural phenomena, enveloping the human body through the *jing-luo* network of 'channels.'[14] Early Western authors who wrote about acupuncture used the word 'meridian' for the horizontal, upward, and downward components of the *jing-luo* system, because they saw that network as analogous to the global meridians of longitude.[15] In the 1980s the influence of modern Chinese books in English made 'channel' the term more commonly used. 'Channel' is probably the word most used today. To the Chinese, however, *jing-luo* and *xue* did not represent the precise geometrical grid that words like 'meridian' and 'point' imply. Instead, they perceived a more natural landscape. As we saw, when acupuncture was becoming a systematized art, China was becoming an organized empire. Many terms, for example, 'depots' and 'palaces,' the terms for body organs, reflected the 'high technology' of a first-millennium Chinese economy based on the storage and transporation of essential goods. Thus words like 'conduit' may more aptly reflect the tenure of classical Chinese.

These channels were named for the major qualitative divisions of *qi*. The needle insertion points found on those channels expressed details of the human body and its relationship to the environment in terms of *qi*. There are acupoints named for *yin* and *yang*, and for aspects of *qi* and its collection or circulation.[16] For example, the acupoint *qi hai*, 'sea of *qi*,' was seen as a whole-body reservoir for *qi* and, always in close relation, breath.[17] Acupoints were also named for astronomic and meteorologic phenomena, and for the animals and objects of nature. So too were they named for human structures, human anatomy, and places of human activity, sometimes in meaningful juxtaposition. For example, *zang fu*, 'celestial treasury,' is the name of the acupoint where the *qi* of the lung gathered, just as taxes were collected for the treasury.[18]

However, as vast and complex as these relationships sometimes are, Chinese thinkers were also very skilled at observing individual behavior just as we do today. Thus there are many instances where the functions or parts of the body are explicitly likened to human behaviors. In the *Nan Jing*, there are very practical descriptions of what we might today call 'lifestyle issues' or aspects of 'environmental medicine'.

Grief and anxiety, thoughts and considerations harm the heart; a cold body and chilled drinks harm the lung; hate and anger let the influences flow contrary to their proper direction; they move upward but not downward. This harms the liver. Drinking and eating [without restraint], as well as weariness and exhaustion, harm the spleen. If one sits at a humid place for an extended period, or if one exerts one's strength and goes into water, that harms the kidneys.[19]

Unlike some similar relationships in Western thought, these were not heavenly punishments for proscribed behaviors, but practical observations of nature described in terms of the qi paradigm. When, for example, the channel related to the lung was less than ideally supplied with *qi*, there would be a hollowness, a vacuity of *qi* that left room for another *qi* to enter. This less than ideal defense of the body could allow an 'evil influence' or 'evil *qi*' (*xie qi*), cold in particular, to enter those channels and harm the lungs.[20] Demonological ideas that are persistent in Chinese thought from its beginnings are also reflected in these terms.

These correspondences were universal and always based in *qi*. The *qi* of plants, animals, and minerals was important to the understanding of pharmacotherapeutic actions of substances. In one image, Xu-Da Chun describes the results of misprescription of a drug with a hot quality as if the patient were being roasted in a fire, where his 'eyes turn red, and his stools are blocked, his tongue loses its moisture and his teeth dry out.'[21] The *qi* of the seasons was important in describing and classifying basic processes both in nature and in the body. For example, in Spring everything goes through a phase of growth and expansion. Thus all phases of growth and expansion, including physiological processes, share a correspondence to Spring. The *qi* of various celestial objects such as the sun and moon was important in describing the natural cycles of the environment and the human organism.

Although these images and associations help us understand *qi* conceptually, *qi* is not just an idea. It is a human experience. If *qi* were not an experience that could be shared, it would not have deeply affected Asian cultures. Thus we must also examine Asian peoples' experiences of *qi*.

THE EXPERIENCE OF *QI*

For many modern people, Asians and Westerners alike, *qi* is an idea understood intellectually, like grammar or a technical procedure. In traditional Asian cultures, and still in some schools of acupuncture today, *qi* is an experience – you are said to understand *qi* not because you can recite facts but because you can display human skills that reflect your ability to control *qi*. For example, when Felt trained with a Japanese teacher, mental concentration, physical skill, and stamina were considered the *sine qua non* of knowing *qi* because you cannot achieve concentration, skill, and stamina without developing your *qi*. Put simply, you cannot expect to influence another's *qi*, thus you cannot heal, until you can control your own. *Qi* was experiential, in his teacher's words: 'Practice without theory is stupid, theory without practice is dangerous.' But neither was *qi* only practical and physical; for example, fear, loss of self-control, and poor

memory were also signs of having failed to cultivate *qi*. Likewise, in certain acupuncture schools you are considered unqualified to practice until you can predictably change the *qi* of your patients as measured by, for example, a change in their pulse.

The experience of *qi* most familiar to Westerners is found in practicing one of the Asian martial arts. Among these, *qi gong* is both a martial art and part of China's medical tradition. Today arts like *qi gong*, *tai chi*, and *aikido* are practiced by thousands of people in Asia and the West. After years of repression in China, these arts are once again an active part of traditional medicine and research. *Qi gong* has already been adopted into some aspects of the French medical system.[22] In *qi gong* people learn both to feel and to increase their *qi* and, with great practice, to project it within and without their bodies.

In one *qi gong* story, American physician David Eisenberg describes his 1979 encounter with a *qi gong* master when Chinese law still forced such meetings to occur in secret. Although he had never tried such a demonstration, the master agreed to attempt moving without touching just the tassels on a large metal and glass lantern. After Dr Eisenberg determined that the tassels could not be moved by physical means, fanning or blowing, he waited as the master prepared himself:

Then it happened. Though he was three feet away, the tassels moved — all six of them. Slowly, the lantern began to move back and forth. I was speechless. Either I had been tricked or this was my first exposure to forces that Western science had not yet defined.[23]

Although stories like this one command our attention, the experience of *qi* is not reserved for the martial artist or the religious adept. From the domestic realm of cooking and working, to the love-making and child-rearing of family life, all experience is perfused with *qi*.

In the literature on acupuncture there is often talk of 'feeling the *qi*.' The theory of *qi* circulating in the channels is not put forward as an abstract model, but as something perceived, felt, experienced. Some acupuncturists are trained to feel the *qi*. As *qi* is universal, this refers to sensing a specific subset of *qi* that circulates through the body. In practice, a treatment should stimulate the *qi* to move. In part, this is described by practitioners as 'feeling the *qi*' or 'gathering the *qi*.' When treated with acupuncture you may also feel something moving. These sensations are sometimes called 'propagating sensations,' *de qi*, or 'the arrival of *qi*.'

Some people are very sensitive to *qi*. These *qi*-sensitive people experience a vibrating, tingling sensation that radiates from an acupoint to a particular body area, or even along an entire channel. However, most people experience the stimulated movement of *qi* as a rooting or tightening around an inserted acupuncture needle and, depending both on the needling technique and the patient's sensitivity, acupuncture may produce sensations that range from nothing at all to a dull, almost painful ache accompanied

by a feeling of heaviness. In forms of practice that use powerful stimuli, the sensation can be noxious, and truly painful. This is a defining quality of acupuncture practice, and we discuss the systematic study of these phenomena later in the text. Of course, *qi* is supposed to circulate constantly without our awareness, so these sensations are only one aspect of the circulating *qi*.

Observations of these kinds help support the *qi* circulation model, and probably played a role in its development. Such naked-sense observations are typical of the perceptual mode by which things are known in acupuncture, and it is entirely possible that these observations influenced the theories, models, and written descriptions of acupuncture. This possibility is supported by Birch's experience with senior blind acupuncturists in Japan (Box 3.2).

Box 3.2 Experiences studying with senior blind practitioners in Japan

Steve Birch has had the good fortune to study with experienced blind acupuncturists in Japan. He, his wife Junko Ida, and colleagues Martin Feldman and Joseph Kay had the honor of a private intensive seminar with the senior teachers of the Toyohari Association (literally the 'East Asian Needle Therapy Association'). Kodo Fukushima, Toshio Yanagishita, Akihiro Takai, and others each taught for one or two days. This was not only an incredible learning experience, but also an insight into the wonderful tactile sensitivity that blind practitioners have developed.

Many people think that blind acupuncturists would be heavily or even solely reliant on study through practice rather than book-learning. This impression is reinforced by the first line of the preface to Kodo Fukushima's book. It warns readers: 'if you are reading this book you are not needling.' Thus we were surprised when we visited a blind practitioner who had compiled a personal library of every major Chinese and Japanese classic, including all the major commentaries, in Japanese braille. In fact, we were astonished to learn how very much more information is available in Japanese braille than in English. We were equally astonished by the significant differences in clinical practice and techniques. Their sense of touch is very different. Although Birch has studied with other senior practitioners, the sense of a blind practitioner's touch is that the hands are more 'intelligent.' That is, blind practitioners feel and discriminate subtleties that are not ordinarily available. Just as the microscope opened an unseen world, their tactile abilities provide a new lens for viewing bodily phenomena.

In particular, by palpation of the radial arteries at the wrists they could describe in detail gradations of change that were to us a blur. It was as if our ruler had been recalibrated from the rough and ready milimeter scale to the finer gradations of a micrometer. For example, while Birch was practicing the location and needling of a point using a non-insertion needle technique, one blind teacher was feeling one radial artery, while Birch's colleagues were feeling other arteries. With each movement, as his fingers lightly searched for the point, the teacher would gauge the accuracy of his point location based on what he felt in the pulse. Simultaneously, the students would confirm the observation — each from a different pulse. The teacher could assess if Birch was too inferior, superior, proximal, or distal to the point.

When he located what is called the 'presently alive point,' Birch would hold his left hand at the point and introduce the needle slowly, towards the skin. As he did the teacher would report the condition of Birch's body. For example, the teacher noticed when he was tense in the knees. He knew the weight of his fingers at the point, his respiration, and his focus. He knew the relative depth of the needle, in a technique where 'relative depth' refers not to the depth of the needle in the flesh, but to the flow of *qi* perceived to flow at or just above the surface of the skin.

This description does not adequately capture the actual experience, but the system of detailed feedback is called the *Kozato hoshiki*, 'the Kozato study method,' after Katsuyuki Kozato, one of the founders of the *Toyohari* system. It enables advanced teachers to teach their students (especially their less sensitive, sighted and, therefore, handicapped students) how to practice this art.

Although it is common knowledge that blind people tend to have one or more of their other senses heightened, few societies have made so elegant a use of this phenomena as have the Japanese. For some this sensory compensation comes in the form of acute hearing, and in the West the skill of blind piano-tuners is well known. However, as we described earlier, since the end of the 19th century, the blind in Japan have been strongly encouraged to study massage and acupuncture, both of which focus on touch. These practitioners are further trained to develop their tactile senses. In fact, the blind acupuncture teachers in Japan have developed their touch to such a degree that they have discovered new diagnostic and therapeutic techniques. The detail with which they can describe what happens beneath their fingers, and the methods they have developed for teaching this sensitivity, surpass anything in traditional or modern acupuncture. Practicing with these modern masters, it is the sighted student who feels handicapped!

The experience of those who study with such masters highlights what has probably been a significant factor in the historical development of both the qi paradigm and acupuncture. Direct naked-sense observations were refined, studied, recorded, and catalogued. The Chinese achieved the intellectual heart of modern science without its measurement machinery – they confirmed their theories of life and nature through experience and repeated observation. To make their observations reliable they maintained both written records and created disciplines to train their senses. To insure reliable communications they developed methods of apprenticeship by which each generation supervised and confirmed the skills of those who followed. For example, their technical literature stored some thousands upon thousands of concepts because many ideas survived generation to generation as new ideas arose.[24] These concepts were able to archive a library of case histories, theories, methodologies, and other medical writings of some 10 000–12 000 volumes. Indeed, the role of observation and preservation of naked-sense information is so profound that the idea of *qi* is best thought of as rooted in human sensorial skills.

The Chinese have never lacked for logical prowess. Although they did not develop statistics, their process of organizing data did involve confirming observations, correlations, and questions. Because they were able to retain information over time, they recognized that some events occur simultaneously or synchronously with other events. Over time, these observations were systematized as patterns, and further links were discovered. Another early observation was that certain synchronous events shared specific qualities. Thus frameworks for organizing observations evolved and the qi paradigm developed refined theories of correspondence. As we saw in Chapter 1, in medicine these theories became 'the medicine of systematic correspondence.'

In the medicine of systematic correspondence, two doctrines are pervasive: the doctrine of *yin* and *yang*, and the doctrine of *wu xing* or five phases. These doctrines were used to organize, catalogue, and label vast amounts of sensory information. These general principles became intertwined. For example, because *qi* was used to describe all things in nature and the cycling of the seasons provided observations that were critical for an agrarian society, seasonal correspondences were highly evolved. Paul Unschuld describes how the ancient analysis of short- and long-term cycles of climatic phenomena developed as a set of interlocking concepts such as the 'stems and branches, and the 'five periods and six *qi*,' derived from astronomical observations.[25]

We know that during the spring, the inactivity and solitude of winter unravels as activity and growth increase throughout the whole environment. Suddenly, new plants, flowers, and blossoms rise everywhere. In summer, vegetation matures and reaches its lushest state, and nature reaches a peak of activity. In the fall, activity slows as seeds and fruit are produced, growth stops, and trees shed their leaves. Then, during the winter, we experience solitude and lack of activity, yet know that the growth of the coming spring is stored in the seeds and fruit of the autumn harvest. This pattern of activity can be drawn as a sinusoidal *qi* wave (Fig. 3.3).

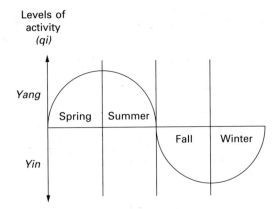

Levels of
activity
(qi)

Figure 3.3 Correspondence between season, qi level, and yin-yang.

The portion above the midline in Figure 3.3 represents the increased activity of spring and summer and is *yang* in nature. The portion below the midline represents the decreased activity levels of fall and winter and is *yin* in nature. Other parallels now become clear (Box 3.3). In the *yang* phase, the environment is lighter and hotter; in the *yin* seasonal phase it is darker and cooler. In the *yang* phase there is growth and expansion, which characterizes the surface and maleness (men in traditional Chinese culture ventured outward to farm or fight). In the *yin* phase, there is retreat in growth, and more storage or contraction, which characterizes the interior and femaleness (women in China's agrarian society mothered, and processed and prepared food). Following this line of reasoning, many aspects of the activity of nature, that is, the levels of *qi* in nature, were explained and catalogued in terms of yin and yang.[27] (Table 3.2).

This simple sinusoidal wave of annual *qi* activity also gives rise to the systematic use of the five phases (Fig. 3.4). Spring, with its rapid growth, increasing activity, expansion, and environmental warmth, relates to the phase of nature that is symbolized by wood; trees and vegetation being a universal symbol for growth. Summer, with the maximum activity of continued growth, maturity, expansion, and maximum heat, relates to the phase of fire. The declining levels of activity, slowing of growth, increasing coolness, and retreat to the seed state that occur in the

Box 3.3 *Yin-yang (yin-yo)*

陰　　陽　　坤　　乾

yin　　yang　　kun　　qian

Yin etymologically refers to the shaded side of a hill, and thus, by implication, coolness, darkness, less activity, and by analogy to these qualities, femaleness. *Yang* refers to the sunny side of a hill (literally a lizard basking on a sunny hill side), and thus heat, light, greater activity, and, by analogy, maleness. The polarity of *yin-yang* has been captured in Chinese thought as related images expressed through other characters that are polar in relation one to the other. One well-known image comes from the *Yi Jing. Kun* (earth) is *yin*, and *qian* (heaven) is *yang*. This complementary polarity of opposites was given high priority in the Chinese conception of natural order. For example, in basic cosmological speculations we find:[27]

> The myriad things emerge and are created in the Great One, [from] the transformations of *yin* and *yang*. (*Lu Shi Chun Qi*)

Here the image refers to:

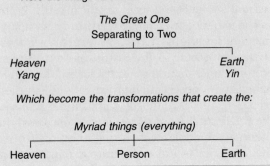

The Great One
Separating to Two

| Heaven | | Earth |
| Yang | | Yin |

Which become the transformations that create the:

Myriad things (everything)

| Heaven | Person | Earth |

Table 3.2 *Yin-yang* basic correspondences

Yin	Yang
Fall, winter	Spring, summer
Less *qi* activity	More *qi* activity
Storage of seeds	Growth of plants
Hibernation of animals	Growth and reproduction
Contraction	Expansion
Interior	Exterior
Dark	Light
Heavy	Lightweight
Cooler, cold, water/ice	Warmer, hot, fire
Night	Day
Moon (dark, cool)	Sun (light, warm)
Female	Male

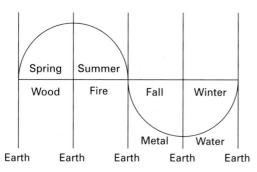

Figure 3.4 Correspondence between season, *qi* level, and the five phases.

fall are symbolized by the solidity of metal. (This image is clearer when you forget such cold metals of modern invention as steel and aluminum and imagine instead the softer, fall-colored surfaces of the ancient metals gold, copper, and bronze.) Winter, cold, and stillness, with minimal levels of activity, hibernation, dormant seeds, and maximum coldness were related to water — deep, still and cold, yet teeming with life beneath the surface as in frozen rivers and streams. Just as ice would melt in the spring, revealing the life of lakes and streams, so too would winter pass, revealing the innate fecundity beneath the surface. The fifth phase, earth, was initially described in relation to the four periods during the year where one season transitions to another — the balance points where the wave crosses the midline as it ascends or descends. Thus the earth phase is associated with the center, with transitions and transformations.[28]

To fit later systematizations of the five-phase model, the earth phase was seen in relation to 'long summer,' the period Americans call 'Indian summer,' the transition between the summer and fall, when the weather is often an ideal balance of seasonal qualities (Table 3.3, Box 3.4).

At this level of analysis, *yin-yang* and the five phases provide means of labeling or categorizing the levels of *qi* activity in nature. By extension through the recognition of qualitative relationships, the phases came to label the body and the aspects of nature that affect it. Because qualities of the heart and its function matched the qualities of the summer season and the phase of fire, the heart was known as the fire organ. As the only methods of observation employed the naked senses, the most important models in acupuncture deal in qualities that correspond

Table 3.3   The basic five-phase correspondences

	Wood	Fire	Earth	Metal	Water
Season	Spring	Summer	Long summer	Fall	Winter
Activity	Increasing	Maximum	Transitional	Decreasing	Minimal
Plants	Sprouting	Growth	Maturity	Seed production	Seed storage
Temperature	Warming	Hot	Transitional	Cooling	Cold
Light	Longer days	Longest days	Balanced	Shorter days	Shortest day

closely to nature. In explaining the qualitative relationships associated with the liver, the wood organ, Chinese expert Nigel Wiseman writes with truly poetic elegance:

Suppleness is the only defense of trees. Being immobile, they must bend to foil their major enemy, wind. Healthy plants are sufficiently supple to survive a wind. The wood of the body can also be blown by wind, especially internal wind. When a wind rises in the body, it can shake the sinews, causing convulsions (*chou feng*, literally 'wind tugging). In wind stroke it can — metaphorically — 'snap' the branches (limbs), so that they no longer move at all. One Chinese expression for hemiplegia is *pian ku*, hemilateral 'withering,' which describes the condition by analogy to the dry deadness of a broken branch. Wind is swift and changeable, and takes its victim by surprise. Wind-stroke, epilepsy, tetanus (*po shang feng*, literally 'wound wind') all share this characteristic. In the same way, a sudden fright can make the sinews jerk, so that liver disorders are sometimes characterized by a susceptibility to fright.[29]

Just as this interwoven natural analogy elucidates the major illness patterns associated with the liver, the phase of wood, all the essential components of the qi paradigm are natural relationships and qualities expressed through the concept of *qi*.

QI IN MEDICINE

If things and events in nature can be described in terms of *qi*, so too can the human body. But without multiple distinctions and subdivisions, it would have been difficult to explain how bodily systems function in health and illness. Thus each organ has its *qi*: the heart *qi*, the liver *qi*. Different tissues and body areas have different *qi*: the *qi* of the head or *qi* of the legs, for example. In the chest, *zhong qi* was associated with the heart and lungs. *Ying qi* was related to blood and circulation. If these *qi* were sufficient and free-flowing, there was health. Conversely, were there a vacuity, a less than ideal supply or quality, or a condition where the *qi* of one or more channels or organs was either replete or stagnant, there was illness. Some representative examples are given in Table 3.4.

Qi is not in essence a thing, an entity; it is a dynamic. It is associated with movement and process. An important component of the qi paradigm is the notion of constantly repeating cycles. In the qi paradigm everything is in constant flux and there are cycles that can be regularly observed in nature. *Qi*, for example, ebbed and flowed like a tide. A biorhythmic flow measured in 2-hour intervals was used to describe phases of relatively higher and lower activity of the *qi* in the channel system.[31] Longer periods were also associated with *qi*: the cycling of the seasons and calendric periods. As a dynamic concept *qi* is associated with virtually every change that occurs in nature. Wind is a kind of *qi*. In the spring the *qi* of nature expresses itself with growth and blooming. In the body, all physiologic functions are also a specific form of *qi*, a movement of *qi*, or a transformation of *qi*. For example, eating and assimilation involve the extraction of various *qi* from food, followed by the transformation and transportation of these *qi* to other parts of the body, where they circulate, express a specific function, or are transformed further. For example, the *qi* of food eventually transforms to blood.[32]

One of the ideas that best characterizes acupuncture theory is the idea that some forms of bodily *qi* cycle in specific patterns. There are said to be two primary forms of circulating *qi*: the *ying*, or nutritive *qi*, and the *wei*, or defense *qi*. The defense *qi* cycles across the body surface, providing an active defense against those environmental *qi* that have the potential to cause disease by disrupting the normal flow and function of bodily *qi* or *zheng qi*. In particular, the *qi* of various climatic phenomena — wind, cold, damp, heat, and dryness — can be disease vectors, or 'evils' that invade the body by overwhelming an insufficient *wei qi*[33] (Fig. 3.5). This *wei qi* model is a very interesting example of how ideas were absorbed and adapted into the qi paradigm from the earlier demonology that we noted in Chapter 1.

Nutritive *qi* circulates through bilateral channels on the limbs, torso, and head. It flows in continuous, connected upward–downward, inward–outward cycles. There were said to be

Table 3.4 Body-*qi* concepts[30]

Qi	Description
*Yuan qi**	Original *qi*, the *qi* one receives from one's parents, also called *xian tian zhi qi*, literally 'the *qi* of earlier heaven,' the congenital *qi* acquired at conception, or of which conception is a result
Hou tian zhi qi	Literally 'the *qi* of later heaven,' the acquired *qi* that one assimilates after birth from the cosmic and microcosmic *qi* environments
Yuan qi[1]	The source *qi*, a deep-lying *qi* that results from the blending of one's congenital and acquired *qi*
Zhen qi	*True qi*, a generic name for all normal physiological *qi*
Zheng qi	Right *qi*, a generic term for all *qi* that maintains health
Qing qi	Clear *qi*, a generic term for the purified *qi* from assimilation processes such as digestion
Zhuo qi	Turbid *qi*, a generic term for impure forms of *qi* from what one assimilates and then excretes
Ying qi	Construction *qi*, circulates in and nourishes the body and is partially related to the circulating blood
Wei qi	Defense *qi*, circulating in the body and attacking harmful influences that invade it
Xue qi	Blood *qi*, but as specifically related to the functional interaction of *qi* and blood as distinct from the physical fluid, but not exclusive of it
Shen qi	Literally 'spirit *qi*,' but also usually associated with the blood
Jing qi†	Essential *qi*, associated with *ying* and *wei qi* and the *qi* of reproduction
Jing qi†	Channel *qi*, which circulates in the channel system (see below)
Gu qi	Literally, 'grain *qi*, derived from digested food
Zhong qi	Center *qi*, of the chest, primarily a product of respiration and digestion and responsible for heart and lung function
Organ *qi*	Variously: heart *qi*, spleen *qi*, liver *qi*, lung *qi*, kidney *qi*, colon *qi*, small intestine *qi*, bladder *qi*, gallbladder *qi*, stomach *qi*, *san jiao qi*. The qualities of each organ are a reflection of its *qi*
Xie qi	Literally 'evil *qi*,' the dysfunctional *qi* that primarily results from the action of external, climate-related *qi* on the body's *qi* (e.g. wind-cold *qi*)

*Transcription methods such as the Pinyin system used here represent the sounds of Chinese, not the individual characters. These two *yuan qi* are different characters, but have the same sound (homophone). In more technical books where there is a greater use of Chinese, tone marks are used to uniquely represent many more Chinese characters. However, in the case of these particular homophones even the tones are the same.
†As above, the two *jing qi* are different characters but have the same sound.

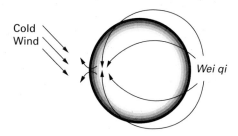

Figure 3.5 The *wei qi* model.

12 primary channels linked in a contiguous pattern. These 12 channels are categorized by a schema of arm-to-leg, arm-to-arm, and leg-to-leg pairings. We will discuss these and other categories in detail. As an example, Figure 3.6 illustrates the upward–downward, inward–outward cycles of one of these four channel sets.

Sets of channels are collectively referred to as the *jing-luo*, 'channels and network vessels.' Because there are no visible analogs for these channels, the *jing-luo* have been the center of a contentious debate that has lasted many years. Later we will review some scientific studies concerning the *jing-luo* system. However, what is most important about the idea of nutritive *qi* is not its presence as a measurable entity, but its use as an image for the regular and repeating patterns that Chinese medical thinkers observed. For example, where an insufficiency of defensive *qi* could lead to illness by allowing the invasion of an external *qi*, problems of the circulating nutritive *qi* were caused internally by obstruction. When nutritive *qi* ceased flowing freely, it was called 'obstructed *qi*.' If it flowed

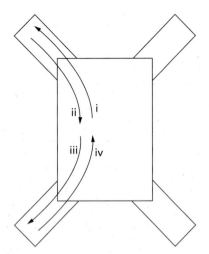

Figure 3.6 Part of the *ying qi* channel model. i + ii Arm–arm pair, iii + iv Leg–leg pair, i + iv Arm–leg pair (*yin*), ii + iii Arm–leg pair (*yang*), Circuit flows: i → ii → iii → iv...

in the wrong direction it was called 'counterflow *qi*.' If in a particular part of the body or channel, or in the whole system, there was a hollow quality to vitality or function, the resulting condition was a '*qi* vacuity.'

Each of these conditions was associated with specific clinical manifestations. If the *qi* of a specific organ was dysfunctional, there would be specific observable signs. For example, if the *qi* of the stomach is weak, digestive symptoms will manifest. If the *qi* of the kidneys is weak, elimination will be weak or will falter, and the lungs will suffer from an accumulation of water.

Qi is not limited to the physical realm. It also plays a role in the Chinese understanding of emotional or mental health, and social and spiritual life. In the West we compartmentalize the body and mind. The clear distinction Rene Descartes drew between mind and body continues to dominate medicine today.[34] If you have an abdominal pain, you will go to an internist once that pain exceeds your personal threshold of feeling normal. Yet, you are likely to offer that internist less information about your past and present mental life than you would share with an acquaintance over lunch. You will say where it hurts, you will discuss your symptoms and, if the internist is particu-

larly attentive, you might talk about how your life has been affected. Depending on your ethnic and familial background, you may notice direct relationships between your emotional state and your physical condition. On the other hand, if you are emotionally distraught or mentally disturbed, you will go to a priest, minister, rabbi, friend, or a psychologist or psychiatrist where, again depending on your background, you are likely to discuss physical signs only to the extent that they seem to have a bearing on your distress, or seem to result from it.

In acupuncture, mind and body are very much interconnected, because both mental and medical conditions are bound by *qi* (Box 3.5). This is clearly seen in the Chinese use of the same character, *xin*, to mean both 'heart' and 'mind.' Thus acupuncture literature catalogs many relationships between emotional states and the function of organs, and vice versa. In fact, these assumptions are so deeply ingrained in Asian culture that modern Chinese patients describe mental or emotional symptoms as physical signs. Illnesses that are recognized as emotional disorders in the West are experienced as physical discomfort in the East.[47] This happens to such an extent that minor psychiatric problems go unrecognized in China because patients report the secondary, physical complaints and not their anxiety, stress, or depression.

In the qi paradigm, both mind and body are expressions of *qi*. For example, rising *qi* can affect the liver, with an accompanying expression of anger. This too is a two-way relationship — the expression of anger can cause *qi* to rise and injure the liver. In fact, the condition may become chronic, in a degrading spiral where the liver problem causes *qi* to rise, predisposing further anger and irritability, predisposing further liver problems and, therefore, further rising *qi*. The liver problem, the rising *qi*, and the anger are simultaneous, synchronous events. Likewise, an obstruction of the circulating nutritive *qi* predisposes emotional states which simultaneously lead to further obstruction.[48]

Box 3.5 Psycho-spiritual dimensions in the traditional model

There are a number of terms used in traditional acupuncture books that seem to imply a psycho-spiritual dimension to the practice of acupuncture. Every traditional society has speculated on the origin of human life, usually in religious or spiritual terms, and the ancient Chinese were not an exception. As expected, these speculations can be found in both the early and later medical literature of China, Japan, and all of Asia.

In the context of acupuncture there are a few terms central to these implications:

神 *shen*, (1) translated as 'spirit'

(lightning 申 , altar 示)

精 *jing*, (2) translated as 'essence'

魂 *hun*, (3) translated as 'etheric soul'

(movement 云 , ghost 鬼)

魄 *po*, (4) translated as 'corporeal soul'

(white part 白)

These four concepts have been variously discussed and interpreted. The term *shen*, for example, has been translated as 'spirits,' 'spirit,' or 'mind.' Different authors have given it a religious-sounding meaning, a neutral meaning, or a pragmatic meaning. As we have seen in our earlier discussions of the history and development of acupuncture, it depends largely on the social, political, and individual context on how one interprets these terms.

For example, during the current era, the communist doctrine of materialism has directed Chinese post-Liberation interpretations toward secular, pragmatic, nonspiritual meanings. However, several working Western sinologists have been learned priests, and they have penned explanations that parallel the concepts of Christian faith. Other sinologists have emphasized social, political, linguistic, and clinical interpretations. That so many people can find so much of their own orientation in these terms is a testament to the extent to which the ancient Chinese were able to express the essential experiences of being human.

Today, psycho-spiritual interpretations are very popular in Western societies. Biomedicine, although powerful, can be frightening. Modern social trends are disturbing — in the USA, 48% of adults own guns, an estimated 250 000 children carry guns to school daily, and one in seven parents know a child who has been killed or wounded by a gun-wielding adult. The religious perspective is very deep in Western society, and America is the nation with the highest degree of religious following. For example, 69% of Americans believe in angels. Thus it is not surprising that people seek 'the wisdom of the ancients' in the words of those who created acupuncture and Oriental medicine. In addition, all healing can be seen to have a spiritual

impact, and acupuncture is not unique in this regard, although perhaps it is more explicitly part of the process. The following quotations from ancient medical and nonmedical texts may help you interpret these traditional Chinese ideas for yourself.

Shen is, etymologically, the image of lightning and an altar. This image is well known in the Judeo-Christian tradition, where, like the Chinese term, it signifies something wondrous or miraculous. *Jing* relates to the vital energies in living things, possibly those derived from food. It is seen as that which transforms to create the physical body. *Hun* refers to clouds, movement, and a ghost or wandering headless body. It implies what we would call 'soul' in the West. Thus it is associated with heaven (not to be confused with the Christian concept of heaven). On the other hand, *po* relates to the skeleton of the body, the white part, or what remains after death. It is associated with earth, as the skeleton returns to the earth after death.

> When the fetus begins to develop, it is [due to] the *po*. Then comes the *yang* part, called the *hun*. The *jing* of many things then give strength to these [the *po* and *hun*], and so they acquire the vitality, animation and good cheer of these *jing*. Thus, eventually there arises the *shen ming* [spirit and intelligence]. (*Zuo Chuan, c* –500)[35]

What do the words *hun* and *po* mean? *Hun* expresses the idea of continuous propagation, unresting flight; it is the *qi* of the lesser *yang*, working in people in an external direction and governing the nature [human nature-instincts]. *Po* expresses the idea of a continuous pressing urge on humankind; it is the *qi* of lesser yin, and works in people governing the emotions.

What do the words *jing* and *shen* mean? *Jing* is connected with the idea of quietness, it is the *qi* of emission and generation under the greater *yin*. It corresponds to the transforming power of water, which leads to pregnancy and life. *Shen*, on the other hand, is connected with the idea of 'blurred confusion,' it is the *qi* that is under greater *yang*. In general one may call it the origin of the changes and transformations in all the limbs [and organs] of the body (*Bai Hu Tong De Lun, c* 80)[36]

What are the *de* [virtue], *qi, jing* [essence], *shen* [spirit], *hun* [ethereal soul], and *po* [corporeal soul]? The heaven in one is *de*. The earth in one is *qi*. The *de* streams down and the *qi* reaches upward to it, subsequently there is life. Therefore the coming of life is called the *jing*. Both *jing* beat [meet] together, this is called the *shen*. Following *shen*, going and returning, this is called the *hun*. Paralleling *jing*, going out and coming in, this is called *po*. (*Ling Shu*, Ch. 8, *c* –200)[37]

Jing and *shen* are of the category of heaven. The skeleton and bones [the physical body] are of the category of earth. (*Lie Zi, c* –500 to –100)[38]

Heaven's *qi* becomes the *hun*. Earth's *qi* becomes the *po*. (*Huai Nan Zi, c* –120)[39]

Box 3.5 Psycho-spiritual dimensions in the traditional model *(cont'd)*

All living things have *qi*, they are born and then [later] they die. This is the common cycle of heaven and earth. This is nature. Death is when the primordial *qi* leaves the body and the *hun* disperses, returning to the root, returning to the beginning, returning to the cycle. (*Hou Han Shu, c* 25 to 220)[40]

Absolute *jing* has no form. The *jing* is tinier than [the concept of smallness]. Rough *jing* has form. No form means that it cannot be divided any further. (*Zhuang Zhou*)[41]

No form [*jing*] is the great ancestor of matter. The child [of no form – *jing*] is light. The grandchild [of no form – *jing*] is water. Everything is created from no form [*jing*]. (*Huai Nan Zi, c* –120)[42]

Form [the physical body] is the abode of life. *Qi is* the plenitude of life. *Shen* is the controller of life. (*Huai Nan Zi, c* –120)[43]

The *shen* transforms no form [the *jing*] to create living form. When the *shen* ceases to control the form — continuously transforming or activating the *jing* — the form returns to no form, [i.e.] death ensues. (*Huai Nan Zi* and *Lie Zi*)[44]

The *shen* is stored by the heart, the *jing* by the kidneys, the *hun* by the liver and the *po* by the lungs (*Nei Jing, c* –200)[45]

For further readings, see note 46.

Some examples of emotional/mental states and the related *qi–body* correlations are:

- Anger injures the liver and is the result of a liver *qi* problem.
- Excessive thinking or worry injures the spleen and is the result of a spleen *qi* problem.
- Fear injures the kidney and is the result of a kidney *qi* problem.
- Grief injures the lungs and is the result of a lung *qi* problem.
- Joy (meaning excessive expressiveness) injures the heart and is the result of a heart *qi* problem.
- *Qi* that rises and flows counter to its usual direction is associated with anger and damage to the liver.
- *Qi* that is disordered is associated with fright and damage to the heart.
- *Qi* that descends is associated with fear and damage to the kidneys.
- *Qi* that disappears (becomes dissipated) is associated with grief and tends to injure the lungs.
- *Qi* that is knotted (becomes stagnant) is associated with excessive thinking and injures the spleen.
- The will (*zhi*) and thoughts (*yi*) must be balanced to regulate the physiology of *qi*.

Some of the qi paradigm's traditional esoteric and complex mental, emotional, and physical relationships have been considerably de-empha-sized in modern China. As Chinese traditional medicines have adapted to the social, political, and economic challenges of the last 50 years, relationships that were in essence spiritual were expunged. Yet, as the following anecdote relates, for some the traditional orientation remains:

A group of respected Chinese traditional medical doctors came to Boston as part of a presentation on Chinese medicine. At the end of their presentation a member of the audience asked the esteemed practitioners how they treated patients with psychological problems. They talked among themselves for a while and then the translator answered 'We are sorry not to answer your question. But our Chinese colleagues cannot understand the difference between mind and body.'[49]

Since these physicians were accustomed to thinking of mental and physical events as integrated and in terms of *qi*, they had no frame of reference in which a problem could be solely psychological.

This is not to say that there is no room in the qi paradigm for expression of our inner life. Clearly it finds daily expression in all of Asia. Yoshio Manaka, for example, routinely spoke of the psychic interaction between people as a kind of *qi*. Most of us have had an experience where we thought of someone who then unexpectedly telephoned or walked into the room. Manaka described this as an example of people's *qi* interacting. The love that one feels for one's spouse, family, and friends is also seen as a manifestation of *qi*.[50]

In all aspects of life, the concept of *qi* permeates a broad range of both normal and pathological states. In fact, as Manaka also noted, of the some 50 000 characters that comprise the classical medical text *Huang Di Nei Jing Su Wen*, over 1100 are the character '*qi*.'[51] In that text and many others, *qi* is an ever-changing latticework of activities and movements that the Chinese described in both very general and very specific terms.

Smaller, seemingly discrete and localized forms of *qi* are inseparable parts of a whole. Each is an aspect of the undifferentiated or original *qi* from which everything derived. Thus the concept of *qi* refers to all things in nature, both animate and inanimate, and their relationships to one another. More than being a 'thing,' a state, an energy, or an abstract theory, *qi* describes perceptible relationships, it is the core of consistency in all phenomena.

IS *QI* REAL?

When Soulie de Morant first presented acupuncture to the West, he chose to describe *qi* as 'energy.' As he wrote, Henri Bergson's concept of an *elan vital* (human energy) was immensely popular in Europe. One can fairly imagine Paris nights when Bergson filled lecture halls as Soulie de Morant worked alone with his copious notes penning *Chinese Acupuncture*. In 'energy' Soulie de Morant found a popular and expressive notion to which he could associate *qi*.[52] This helped him persuade his often hostile audiences of physicians. He explicitly justified this idea by stating that the new and rapidly advancing science of neurology would eventually discover an aspect of the nervous system that would explain *qi*.[53] Thus he described *qi* to the physicians for whom he wrote as a working energy that could be less than necessary or 'insufficient,' or more than needed, 'excess,' exactly as early 20th century medicine described the economy of nervous impulses and biochemicals in the human body.

This strategy was clearly successful because 'energy' is today so closely associated with *qi* that it has come to stand for the whole of tradi-

tional East Asian medicine. When even consensus reports from the US National Institutes of Health bless the term 'energy medicine,' it is probably unwise for us to refuse a ride on that bandwagon.[54] In fact, a challenge to the *qi* = energy equation is often perceived as a challenge to acupuncture itself; it is thought to be the posture of an 'enemy.' However, as unwise at this may be, *qi* = energy is an equation that does not compute.

Neurology and biochemistry, for all their power, have not become the unique key to human function they once promised to be. Soulie de Morant's faith was unfulfilled and no neurological phenomenon has ever been equated with *qi*. Thus, as later writers borrowed 'energy' along with many of Soulie de Morant's words, they not only ignored his caution that he had chosen 'energy' 'for lack of a better word,' but also tended to ignore those aspects of acupuncture that did not conform to modern thinking about energy. Writers such as Felix Mann thus proposed that acupuncture was a neurological stimulus that 'sedated' nerves or 'tonified' the nervous system as did drugs. Again, ideas rooted in the *qi* concept were molded to the expectations of an audience, and layers of meaning that did not fit those expectations were lost. 'Sedate' means to settle, like silt at the bottom of a stream, where the Chinese term *xie* means 'to eliminate evils from the body.' In the context of acupuncture this refers to a needle stimulus intended to 'cause to flow' (the literal meaning of *xie*) accumulations of evil, stagnant *qi*, or blood. To sedate any of these would be to decrease flow, thus worsening the condition. In other words, the meaning has actually been reversed. 'Tonify,' an English neologism from the French '*tonification*,' implies bracing the entire organism like a tonic, something that is more a panacea than the specific supplementations of acupuncture.[55]

Thus, as the *qi* concept was scientized by emphasizing what seemed credible to Western writers, elements of acupuncture were lost. The Western idea of acupuncture was reduced to fit a culturally acceptable idea of *qi* and acupuncture's principles were squeezed into molds of words that fit early 20th century knowledge and expectations. What began as an analogy meant to explain and persuade became a bias: that to be 'real,' *qi* had to be an energy that science understood, something that could be measured and quantified just as the terms now used to talk about it implied. Later, we will discuss the consequences of these transformations for basic and clinical research.

Today, at one extreme, writers who are immersed in biomedical ideas still describe *qi* as nothing more than the impulse of nerves. These writers dismiss all other observations of *qi* as social or psychological phenomena. To them, *qi*-energy is real only to the extent that it is a measurable biological force. In their eyes, acupuncture — if it is not just an ancient recurring delusion — is a lucky combination of neurological pain control and the pyscho-immunological function of faith. Because they see acupuncture as a bag of tricks stumbled upon in Asia, they consider it burdened by a foreign, complex, and useless cultural debris, which it is useless to investigate.[56] This has often been the unspoken presumption beneath the 'scientific' study of acupuncture, acupoints, and channels.

At the other extreme, writers who are interested in promoting acupuncture as an alternative to the model of health and illness that dominates medicine today have revived 'vitalist' theories of body–mind interaction to explain *qi*. The energy of which these theorists speak is not the kinetic, working energy of a nerve impulse, but a mind–body, macrocosm–microcosm link. *Qi*-energy is seen to bind the parts and the whole like the impulsive force of Middle Eastern astrology.

There are also those who take a practical approach, emphasizing the fact that Asian *qi* techniques, such as acupuncture and *qi gong*, produce a feeling of increased energy or vitality. Many who practice massage have physically sensed a tingling, current-like exchange between giver and receiver. It is common for anyone, Easterner and Westerner alike, to experience sensations of uplift when practicing one of the Asian meditative or martial disciplines. Yet, as

scholar and experienced *qi gong* practitioner Ute Englehardt notes:

In my own and others' experiences, when practicing so-called *qi gong* exercises (which derive from life-nourishing techniques), one actually experiences an 'energy' that is parallel to the sensations described for *qi* ... However, at this point, there has not yet been found any valid proof in ancient texts to corroborate this theory of *qi* being the equivalent of 'energy.'[57]

Even if there were such proof, the question would remain whether these feelings of energy are *qi* or the body's response to its increase, the dynamic organization of known biological processes, or an as yet unknown phenomenon.

There are of course even much looser usages of '*qi*.' For some writers *qi* need not be described as a specific phenomenon or even be required to fit our modern understanding of nature. In fact, the idea of *qi* is sometimes described as matter and sometimes described as energy, and sometimes as both. Although many writers use the quantified language of science, speaking of *qi* excesses and deficiencies, they nonetheless propose that *qi* is not a measurable phenomenon. Instead, they explain *qi* by analogies to physics where, for example, light behaves like waves or particles depending on how it is observed. In effect, they say that *qi* has whatever properties it needs to explain what happens.

Ironically, the proponents of all these theories reflect the same assumption. They assume that *qi* and the modern model of nature are incompatible. Also, each chooses to retain or emphasize from Chinese thought only that which fits their particular argument. Vitalists reject the materialistic bias of the physical sciences. Scientists dismiss Chinese ideas that do not fit that model. Vitalists forget that the qi paradigm never excluded the material vectors in which biomedicine has specialized (and which are applied by thousands of Chinese daily). Scientists forget that they are demanding that *qi* fit a model of the universe that is itself outmoded (and which they reject for themselves). Not surprisingly, advocates of all sides can become somewhat strident. Scientists suggest dismissing all but empirical knowledge of acupuncture. Body–mind theorists see scientists as blinded by their own instruments. Scientists dismiss the work of vitalists as anecdotal; vitalists dismiss scientists and scholars who are not practitioners. This is the state from which the idea of paradigmatic walls arose. Tellingly, proponents of both approaches forget that *qi* was most often described neither as an abstraction nor as a physical fact, but as the response of a human observer.

Is there a resolution to this collision, some common ground? We believe so, but only by recognizing that it is the prejudice of the question that produces the clash. Since the Chinese model states that everything is *qi*, then *qi* is necessarily as real as anything else. In fact, the question, 'Is *qi* real?' is actually asked of only a very narrow aspect of *qi*, typically that which circulates in the channels. Because most Western researchers have been unaware of the scope of the concept, they have asked improper or inadequate questions, with the consequence that their research tells us little about acupuncture as it is actually practiced. This is discussed in greater detail later in the text. To resolve these problems we must look at the matter freshly, reconsidering the questions we ask.

In their work physicists do not ask whether a 'ripple in time' is real, they ask if the idea can predict something they can observe in the universe. Even a biologist seeking the electrical charge that activates a nerve refuses to ask what is real. Instead, he or she strives to discover whether a stimulus that is measured (current at an electrode) and a phenomenon (the reaction of a nerve) are more than randomly linked. Just as the most basic ideas of physics are not about 'stuff' that can be seen or held in your hand, *qi* is a construct, a way to explain what could not be observed directly with our human senses. It is, as we must not forget, an idea that arose among ancient Asian peoples to explain that which was beyond the range of their senses. The people who created the idea of *qi* could not see into the vast depths beneath the limits of their naked senses. However, this fact neither invalidates their ideas nor allows us to dismiss the down-to-earth patterns they recorded.

In fact, we could even think of *qi* as a theory. It does seem strange to discuss an idea that is ancient, vast, and various as if it were very modern and precise. Yet, *qi*, like a scientific theory, was used as a way to make statements about the universe that explain and predict what we observe. In other words, there is no reason we cannot ask about *qi* exactly what we ask about a ripple in time: Does the idea successfully predict something we can reliably observe? Thus the investigation of *qi* becomes a process of asking questions that not only fit traditional descriptions and practices, but also generates practical tests. *Qi* is a paradigm, a model, a framework within which all phenomena can be referenced. It parallels several 20th century developments in the way that scientists think about nature, and capture and describe the complexity of natural events. Thus, if we form our questions with help from these developments, we need not worry about paradigmatic walls.

It is now broadly recognized that things in nature interact constantly and are probably manifestations of some underlying substrate or matrix. As a matrix is that within which or from which something originates, takes form or develops, the concept matches the essential nature and utility of *qi*. In Western thought, systems theory and information theory provide this frame of reference (Box 3.6). This is how we have chosen to discuss *qi*. For example, to analyze the five phases from this perspective, Birch asked: *If everything about traditional five-phase theory were true, what could such a system do that fits our understanding of nature?* When this question was asked, an important discovery emerged.

If we assume that various cycles described by five-phase theory are an exchange of matter or energy, and then analyze the model mathematically, we find that it must be unstable. If what the five phases actually described was the transmission of energy, humankind and nature would fly apart. Energy would constantly build within the system. Thus, just as a flag shreds in the circling winds of a tornado, the idea that *qi* is energy shreds. However, if we assume instead that the five-phase model describes an exchange

---

Box 3.6   Systems theory and information theory: the basis for a conceptual bridge

Systems theory developed in the 1960s and 1970s as discoveries in science changed how we see the world. Essentially, these theories recognize that everything is composed of parts or systems that interact with one another, and that everything is part of even larger systems with which all smaller systems interact. In the realm of biology and medicine, these methods are used to develop a model of an organism — a human being — as the product of its various environments and interacting systems. 'The systems approach emphasizes basic principles of organization' where 'systems are integrated wholes whose properties cannot be reduced to those of smaller units.':[58]

celestial systems
↓
solar system
↓
terrestial eco-system
↓
close environment
↓
human being
↓
organ systems
↓
tissue systems
↓
cellular systems
↓
atomic systems
↓
subatomic systems

Information theory is also a product of the 1960s, and is related by conceptualizing the world that unites systems. Information can be generally thought of as 'a measure of order existing in a system.'[59] Information describes processes within or between organized systems:

...living systems exhibit multilevelled patterns of organization characterized by many intricate and nonlinear pathways along which signals of information and transaction propagate between all levels.[60]

The significance of these two models to acupuncture is considerable. One of the basic historical cosmological and philosophical theories of nature in China was the idea of three levels or systems that interacted with one another. This is exemplified by the central *Yi Jing* pictogram, the trigram:

_____ Heaven
_____ Person
_____ Earth

We can immediately see strong parallels to the latter 20th century systems model. The person interacts with, and is the product of the interaction between, heaven and Earth. Heaven and Earth, the traditional symbols for macrocosm and microcosm, are themselves composed of qualitative relationships. Recall too the Confucian model of how the larger environment, order in the state, is brought about by individual behaviors.

But the parallels do not stop here. In this cosmological model what underlies these three levels and interacts between them is *qi*. First there is the primordial *qi*; its heavy part sinks, becoming earth; its light part rises, becoming heaven. The person (humanity-life) is a product of the interaction between the *qi* of heaven and Earth. This strongly parallels the information model. Just as information propagates back and forth between all levels in the systems model, so too does *qi* propagate between the levels in the Chinese cosmological model. In fact, in this and many other contexts, you could replace the term *qi* with the term 'information,' without losing meaning.

The basic advantage of using systems theory and information theory is that it allows the use of a broadly accepted vocabulary that describes living systems without reduction and in a holistic or integrated manner. This is similar to the way in which the traditional qi paradigm describes the body. This not only helps us understand the traditional model, but also allows for the development of more relevant research models.

For those interested in reading more on systems theory and information theory, see note 61.

---

of information, the traditional system meets the most rigorous mathematical tests of stability. In short, the scientist–vitalist conflict can be resolved, at least in part, by thinking of *qi* as the information needed to maintain a complex system. The five phases of Chinese thought do not describe energy in an electrical circuit or the energy of a biochemical reaction, they describe the nature of the information exchanged.[62]

Because the media by which information can be exchanged are many (bioelectrical, biochem-

ical, biomagnetic, or any combination of these), neither the proposed identity of nerve impulses and channel *qi* nor a field-like body–mind are necessarily contradictory. Each of these ideas could be partial explanations. *Qi* in traditional use is a claim that there is a qualitatively similar relationship, not that there is a single absolute mechanism. Because information can be transmitted by biochemical or bioelectrical events that occur at energy levels far lower than those required for metabolic or neurological effects, we can rescue Soulie de Morant's hope of investigating all aspects of the qi paradigm and its systematic correspondences. Ironically, we must first surrender the comfort of the popular expression he chose.

In short, our inevitable Western search for the material or energetic basis of *qi* need not look for something that is strong enough to perform work. We can look instead for signals that stop, start, or moderate a process. In fact, the idea of *qi* as information matches the results of Paul Unschuld's sinological research showing that in classical Chinese thought the concept of *qi* most closely matches the idea of 'influences,' something that directs the course of the 'finest matter.'[63]

We propose that *qi* be thought of as a model of universal order and communication. It is an idea that supposes nature to be observably ordered. It proposes that natural patterns recognized by the senses and sensibilities of humans can usefully predict macro- and microcosmic events. As such, it is an expression of the faith in order that is shared by all science. We personally speculate that *qi* is one culturally determined way to talk about the permutations in some universal medium that none have as yet described with precision. In this regard, the closest parallel to *qi* in modern Western thought is a generative matrix in which all things interact with all other things through the exchange of information. Whether that matrix is 'real' (an actual fact of the physical universe) or 'logical' (a useful construct for ordering our observations) is both unclear and, to some extent, irrelevant. *Qi* labels what gives phenomena similar qualities, and establishes correspondences and relationships.

In the practice of acupuncture it is recognition of these relationships that counts. To understand acupuncture *qi* can be thought of as the observable results of the body's information-exchange mechanisms. The plural is important. Although a capitalized *Qi* can be proposed through the idea of a universal stratum, in the human body information exchange occurs by a variety of mechanisms. Thus the idea of a multidimensional array of communications paths that

are influenced by the physical and energetic universe gives us a very useful tool for thinking about our relationship to the environment. As we will see later in greater detail, temperature, punctures, pressures, and electrical stimuli of many different strengths and qualities are all capable of causing change in the human body. Thus, in its broadest sense, studying *qi* in acupuncture is the study of how stimuli can be used to moderate the natural phenomena from which humans seek relief.[64]

Regardless of how strange the qi paradigm may first appear to those trained in Western disciplines, it is an idea to be investigated, not a fraud to be debunked. Although no human activity is entirely free of charlatans, the idea of *qi* has been experienced and posited by so many that human courtesy (if not curiosity) demands that it be treated as genuinely motivated. We propose that investigating those culturally valid, precisely translated aspects of *qi* for which we can imagine useful tests should be the primary concern. Proving that any particular *qi* function is or is not a known phenomenon tells us nothing about any other *qi*. Thus, debunking efforts are useless. As we have discussed, it is typically Western writers who use the *qi* that was supposed to flow in the channels — described as energy — to stand for all *qi*. However, any culturally valid definition of *qi* actually ends with the gross physical senses. Imagine, for example, that a traditional idea like ancestral *qi* could be absolutely proven to be nothing more than an early observation of relationships that are now more usefully explained by genetics. Does this invalidate the host of clinical observations about acupoints that have beneficial effects for conditions described in terms of ancestral *qi*? No! It simply exchanges one explanatory model for another.

Qi is an entity known to a human observer. In what we feel, see, perceive, and sense, *qi* is a single word, but when we leave the realm of traditional thought and enter the realm of modern instrumentation we cannot assume it is a single entity or energy. The *qi* that allows a *qi gong* practitioner to move the tassels of a lantern may be a clever fraud, a faith effect, an energy

tists have yet to discover or, as
ch suggests, a human-generated
ae near-infrared range. However it
is n... ssarily the same entity that functions
in acupuncture. Proving that the *qi gong* master
wills metabolic heat to his hand, moving air
to flutter tassels, may disprove that *qi* is an
unknown energy, but it may tell us nothing
at all about the *de qi* produced by needling.
Indeed, it may be the case that different acupoints and acupunctural stimuli operate through
different mechanisms.

Thus, as a principle of investigation, we
suggest not only that *qi* be investigated based
only on culturally valid and adequately translated concepts, but also that it be investigated
as discrete functions. In the same way that
our knowledge of a primary concept such as
space–time is founded on the investigation of
many testable ideas, we must investigate *qi* from
the ground up. Just as some Western theories
have generated experiments that lead to new
and more useful theories, investigating the discrete aspects of the qi paradigm could produce
new, more useful perspectives. Although some
aspects of the *qi* paradigm may be replaced by
more modern conceptions, others may lead us
toward unexpected realizations and conclusions.

Finally, when we look at *qi* as the idea was
traditionally expressed, we find instance after
instance in which *qi* is a quality or a relationship.
Thus when we investigate *qi* we need to keep
in mind that the appropriate question may not
be 'What makes this happen?,' but 'Does this
happen reliably?' In other words, because so
much of what is discussed in traditional East
Asian medicines is pattern observed through
the human senses, the qi paradigm may be best
approached as problems of statistical reliability
or correlation.

It is important to realize that many things in
modern science are useful without being true
in any absolute sense. Underwriting statistics,
for example, tell us nothing about the causes of
death, only of their distribution in a given population. Similarly, ideas like *yin-yang* and the five
phases can be seen as tools rather than natural
laws. In fact, this is the attitude taken by

experienced Chinese clinicians, who will use
whichever traditional tool set works best for
a particular patient, without the slightest sense
of contradiction. Although it is obvious that a
five-phase concept like 'a lung vacuous constitution' is a less objectifiable idea than the presence of a specific bacillus, it is also true that
many useful biomedical syndromes are also
patterns that trained practitioners recognize
reliably. In short, if we are too intent on seeing
qi in terms of material or energy causes and
effects, we may miss its utility. Or, as in our
earlier example of the extraordinary vessels, the
Western conception of energy will so suppress
the Chinese metaphoric information, that clinical
options are lost.

THE CLINICAL EXPRESSIONS OF *QI*

Qi circulation: the *jing-luo* (channels)

As the qi paradigm developed there were many
facts and notions discovered that were similar
to medical discoveries made in the West.
However, the system of *jing-luo*, or channels,
is unique (Box 3.7). There is little in Western
biomedicine to match this system, and no clear
anatomical counterparts of the *jing-luo* have
ever been identified. The idea of *jing-luo* combines in a single–concept phenomena that were
seen as unrelated in the West. For example, the
observations of chronobiology (the idea that
human processes recur in calendric rhythms),
or biorhythms (the idea that psychological and
physical changes occur in regular patterns), are
both aspects of the *jing-luo* concept. The recognition that human physiology responds to the
environment is also intrinsic to the idea of *qi*
circulating in a channel system. Today, at the
frontiers of medicine, there are counterparts of
this ancient idea among those who see information processing as a distinct biological function.

There is a relatively fierce debate over the
physical existence of the channel system. We
will discuss this debate in Chapter 4. However,
whether or not the channels are a physically
founded entity, they are an important logical
component of acupuncture theory, because it is

Box 3.7 *Jing-luo (keiraku)*

經	经	絡	糸	
Jing	Jing (Simplified form)	luo	silk	Old form

Jing and the *luo* have various meanings. The radical common to both is the 'silk' radical. This gives both characters the connotation of threads in a woven fabric. Etymologically the *jing* refers to the vertical threads, the 'warp,' while the *luo* refers to the horizontal threads, the 'woof.' The term *jing* is variously translated as 'meridian,' 'channel,' 'conduit,' and 'sinartery.' The term *luo* is usually translated as the 'connecting' or 'network' channels or vessels. Just as together the terms *jing* and *luo* refer to the vertical and horizontal threads that are woven into a fabric, so too are the terms thought to refer to the *qi*-conducting fabric at the surface of the body. The primary function of the *jing-luo* is to distribute and circulate *qi*. The *luo* are the branches or divisions of the *jing*:[65]

> The channels (*jing*) are [located in] the lining [of the body]. The horizontal branch of the channel is the connecting channel (*luo*). The divergent [smaller] branches [of the *luo*] are the grandchild channels (*sun luo*). (*Su Wen*)

Here the analogy is to how the the *jing* (channels) divide to form the *luo* (connecting channels), which in turn divide to form the grandchild *luo*, just as large arteries divide to form smaller arteries, which further divide to form arterioles, then capillaries:[66]

> The channels are the routes by which blood and *qi* circulate, regulating *yin* and *yang*, keeping the bones and sinews moistened and the joints lubricated. (*Ling Shu*)

The *jing-luo* is the matrix, substrate, or medium of action of acupuncture. The traditional model posits that needles or other stimuli alter the flow of *qi* in the *jing-luo*, which in turn alters the body systems (organs, tissues).

on these channels that the *xue*, 'holes' or 'acupoints,' lie. Channel courses, interconnections, and branches have been elaborated since the idea of *qi* circulation was first clearly articulated in the *Nei Jing* (−200) and then more formally by the author of the *Nan Jing* (100). Channel and acupoint descriptions have been relatively stable since the era of the Bronze Statue (1027). The channels that students learn today are modern Chinese simplifications of those classical pathways.

There are a number of different channel systems in the body by which *qi* is said to circulate. The primary channels through which the *ying qi* circulates are the most commonly described and utilized channels. Each of these has a complement of acupoints. The other channel systems are used to varying degrees by different practitioners. Some are rarely used in modern practice. However, there are practitioners who specialize in even these rarely used systems. After the primary channels, the channel system most commonly employed in traditional East Asian medicine is the *qi jing mai*, or 'extraordinary vessels.' Two of these extraordinary vessels are particularly important in acupuncture because, like the primary channels, they have their own acupuncture points. The main channel types are listed in Table 3.5.[67] As the 12 *jing mai* are the most significant channels, the most thoroughly described and the most frequently used, we focus on these.

In acupuncture theory, channels are classified according to their 'yin-ness' or 'yang-ness,' according to their location on the upper or lower extremities, and according to whether they 'home' inside the body to a *zang* or *fu*.

Table 3.5 The main channel types

Name	Type	Number	Function
Jing mai	Regular channels	12	Circulate *ying qi*, have acupoints
Luo mai	Connecting channels	15	Alternative channels for *qi* circulation
Jing bie	Channel divergences	12	Alternative channels for *qi* circulation
Jing jin	Channel sinews	12	Associated with the body musculature, movement, bending, and stretching
Qi jing mai	Extraordinary vessels	8	*Qi* reservoirs, regulate *qi* distribution

These classifications were very practical, because all these qualities allow acupuncturists to select acupoints in treatment through their relation to clinical observations. Each channel has a surface trajectory (the lines you see traced on acupuncture charts). However, each channel also has an internal trajectory, by which it connects to at least two organs, in some cases more. In Chinese a channel is thus named by its *yin-yang* classification and its associated primary organ, i.e. the one to which the channel homes. Thus the stomach channel is more properly the *zu yang ming wei jing*, or 'leg yang brightness stomach channel.' These relationships are summarized in Table 3.6.[68]

The *yin* channels are generally thought to circulate *qi* in an upward direction, and the yang channels in a downward direction, but all channels pass through the lower abdominal center of the body. This is easier to visualize if you imagine someone standing with their arms raised over their head as in the *ying qi* circulation illustration (see Fig. 3.6). The *qi* is also thought to circulate in a continuous cycle. However, as with ocean tides, there is a minimum and maximum for each of the channels. This can be visualized by thinking of a wave with a higher peak and an opposite lower trough moving through the channels in the following order:[69]

lung ➡ large intestine ➡ stomach ➡ spleen ➡ heart ➡ small intestine ➡ bladder ➡ kidney ➡ pericardium ➡ *san jiao* ➡ gallbladder ➡ liver … (lung)

When an acupuncturist considers the use of the 12 primary channels, he or she generally thinks of the areas of the body that the channels traverse, their *yin-yang* characteristics, their five-phase characteristics, and the functions of the organs to which each channel homes. There are also sets of pathoconditions related to each channel. Treatment of one channel can affect many areas, associated organs, and interconnecting channels. *Ying qi* can be manipulated according to *yin-yang* and five-phase properties. For example, treatment of the large-intestine channel can affect the index finger, wrist, forearm, elbow, upper arm, shoulder, anterior portion of the neck, the jaw, mouth, teeth, and nose, because the channel traverses these areas. It can also affect the large intestine and lungs, and can be used to affect other channels, as indicated by the particular case.

Each channel also has a traditionally fixed number of acupoints located along its trajectory. These points have local effects – influences

Table 3.6 Classification of channels

Arm/leg	Yin/yang	Primary organ	Secondary organ
Arm	*Tai* (greater) *yin*	Lung	Large intestine
Arm	*Yang ming* (brightness)	Large intestine	Lung
Leg	Yang *ming* (brightness)	Stomach	Spleen
Leg	*Tai* (greater) *yin*	Spleen	Stomach
Arm	*Shao* (lesser) *yin*	Heart	Small intestine
Arm	*Tai* (greater) *yang*	Small intestine	Heart
Leg	*Tai* (greater) *yang*	Bladder	Kidney
Leg	*Shao* (lesser) *yin*	Kidney	Bladder
Arm	*Jue* (absolute) *yin*	Pericardium*	*San jiao*†
Arm	*Shao* (lesser) *yang*	*San jiao*	Pericardium
Leg	*Shao* (lesser) *yang*	Gallbladder	Liver
Leg	*Jue* (absolute) *yin*	Liver	Gallbladder

*Sometimes called the 'heart governor' or 'master of the heart,' *shou jue yin* is thought to have little relation to the actual heart envelope or pericardium.
†The *san jiao* is a complex concept with multiple interpretations; it is often translated as 'triple warmer,' 'three heater,' 'triple burner,' or, more interpretively, 'triple energizer.'

around the area of their location. Each also has distant effects — varying degrees of influence on locations traversed by the channel, related to the connected *zang* or *fu*, or a related channel. There are various classes of acupuncture points on each channel, and each class of acupoint has distinctive properties. The *xi* or 'cleft' points, for example, are traditionally employed for acute conditions. The five-phase or *shu* 'transporting' points are good for regulating *qi*, not only in the channel on which they are located, but also in channels associated through the relationships described by the five phases.[70] The number of points on each channel is given in Box 3.8. We have added the two most-used extraordinary vessels, the *ren mai* or 'controller vessel,' and the *du mai* or 'governing vessel.'

Box 3.8 The number of acupoints on each channel	
Lung	11
Spleen	21
Heart	9
Kidney	27
Pericardium	9
Liver	14
Ren mai	24
Large intestine	20
Stomach	45
Small intestine	19
Bladder	67
San jiao	23
Gallbladder	44
Du mai	28
Total	361

The pathways of all 14 channels and their acupoints are described below.[71] The illustrations show traditional and modern pictures of the large intestine, stomach, kidney, liver, *ren*, and *du* channels.

Lung channel. This channel starts inside the chest, in the lungs, surfaces in front of the shoulder, runs through the shoulder, down the upper arm, elbow, forearm, and wrist to end at the thumb. A branch runs from inside the chest to the large intestine.

Large intestine channel. This channel (Fig. 3.7) starts at the index finger, runs up through the wrist, forearm, elbow, upper arm, shoulder, up

the front of the neck, and through the mouth to end at the side of the nose. On the shoulder there is a branch that runs inside the body to the lungs and large intestine.

The stomach channel. This channel (Fig. 3.8) starts just below the eye, runs down the face to the jaw, upward to the temple and down the front of the neck to a line level with the nipple. From there, it descends down the chest and abdomen to the thigh, knee, shin, and ankle, ending on the second toe. At the clavicle there is a branch that runs inside the body to the stomach and spleen.

The spleen channel. This channel starts on the big toe, runs up the instep of the foot to the ankle, up the inside portion of the shin to the knee, thigh, groin, up the lateral aspects of the abdomen and chest to end below the armpit. On the abdomen a branch runs inside the body to the spleen, connecting to the stomach, and passing through the heart.

The heart channel. This channel starts inside the chest at the heart, surfaces near the armpit, runs downward through the upper arm, elbow, forearm, and wrist to end on the little finger. A branch runs from inside the chest to the small intestine.

The small intestine channel. This channel starts on the little finger, runs up the wrist, forearm, elbow, upper arm, back of the shoulder, and scapula to the back of the neck, where it rises to end on the face in front of the ear. At the shoulder a branch runs inside the body to the heart and small intestine.

The bladder channel. This channel starts at the inner corner of the eye, runs upward over the top of the head, and down the back of the head and neck. It traverses the back in two downward streams to the buttocks, continues down the back of the thigh, knee, and calf to the outer ankle, where it ends at the fifth toe. On the back a branch runs inside to the bladder and kidneys.

The kidney channel. This channel (Fig. 3.9) starts at the fifth toe, runs under the foot to the instep, to the inner ankle. It travels up the back of the calf to the knee and thigh, to reach the abdomen near the midline. From there it

(a)

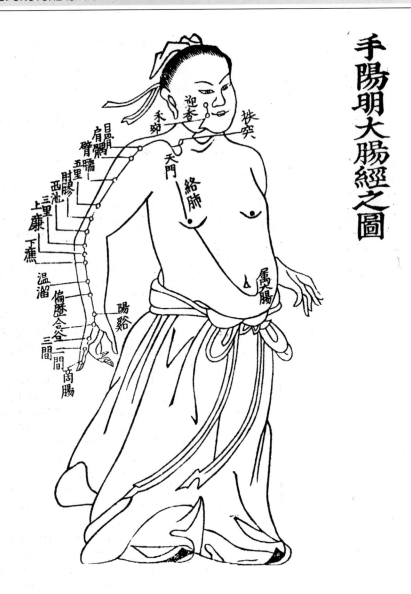

traverses the abdomen up to the chest, ending just below the clavicle on the edge of the sternum. On the abdomen a branch runs inside to the kidneys and bladder, also connecting to the heart.

The pericardium channel. This channel starts inside the chest at the *xin bao luo* (heart envelope), surfaces just above the breast, runs over the shoulder, down through the upper arm, elbow, forearm, and wrist to end on the middle finger. A branch runs from inside the chest to the *san jiao* (triple burner).

The *san jiao* channel. This channel starts on the fourth finger, runs over the back of the hand to the wrist, forearm, elbow, and upper arm to the back of the shoulder, across the shoulder to the side of the neck, to behind the ear. It ends at the outside edge of the eyebrow. A branch runs from the shoulder inside to the *xin bao luo* and *san jiao*.

The gallbladder channel. This channel starts at the outer corner of the eye, runs in front of the ear, zig-zagging backwards and forwards over the temple to the back of the neck. From

(b)

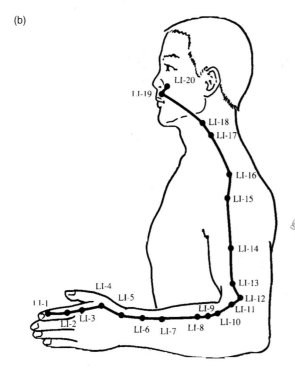

Figure 3.7 (a) Traditional and (b) modern (simplified) drawings of the large-intestine channel. (Courtesy of Paradigm Publications.)

there it proceeds down the back of the neck to the shoulders, to below the armpit, and down the side of the torso to the hip. Traveling from the hip down the side of the thigh, knee, calf, and outer ankle it ends on the fourth toe. A branch runs from the shoulder to the gallbladder and liver.

The liver channel. This channel (Fig. 3.10) starts on the big toe, runs up the top of the foot to the ankle, up the shin to the knee, and inside the thigh to the groin. It returns to the surface on the lateral aspects of the abdomen. A branch runs from the abdomen inside to the stomach, liver, gallbladder, and up through the lungs to the back of the nose and the crown of the head.

The *ren* channel. This channel (Fig. 3.11) starts in the lower abdomen and passes out to just in front of the anus below the genitals, runs upward along the midline to the abdomen, the midline of the abdomen through the navel, then the midline of the chest to the neck. It passes through the Adam's apple and over the chin to end just below the lower lip.

The *du mai* channel. This channel (Fig. 3.12) starts in the lower abdomen and passes out to just behind the anus, follows the spine upward on the midline to the back of the neck, over the midline of the skull from whence it descends down the nose to end at the frenulum of the upper lip, and where a branch passes to the kidneys.

There are also many points of intersection between these 14 channels. Each channel has connections to at least one acupoint on another channel, so that there are many 'intersection points' where two or more channels meet.[72] For example, *san yin jiao*, the sixth point on the spleen channel, intersects with the kidney and liver channels. Thus this acupoint can feature in the treatment of conditions related to the spleen, liver, and kidney channels. This is a great therapeutic advantage in treatments that must address complex problems or multiple symptoms.

The channels are also described as exhibiting a daily cycle of activity or maximum and minimum *qi*, sometimes vernacularly called the 'Chinese clock.' This information is used in both diagnosis and treatment. For example, a person who wakes around 2 a.m. every morning could be exhibiting signs of a liver-channel problem, because this is during the 2-hour period during which liver activity reaches its biorhythmic maximum. Likewise, when a person regularly presents a symptom in the afternoon around 2 p.m., it is possible to treat the small intestine channel with good results, because the small intestine channel is then at its biorhythmic maximum. By applying supplementing or draining techniques, using both the minimum and maximum of the channels, it is possible to create a range of therapeutic effects.

This cycle of maxima and minima, *zi-wu* or 'midday–midnight,' is presented in Box 3.9.[73] Different methods of diagnosis and treatment have evolved around each of these ideas. We will discuss aspects of diagnosis through *yin-yang* and five-phase phenomena in Chapters 6 and 7.

Symptoms related to these daily rhythms are certainly not the only channel-based manifestations. In Chinese medical thought a channel

(a)

足陽明胃經之圖

Box 3.9 The time of maximum activity in the daily cycle of channel activity	
11 p.m. – 1 a.m.	Gallbladder
1 a.m. – 3 a.m.	Liver
3 a.m. – 5 a.m.	Lung
5 a.m. – 7 a.m.	Large intestine
7 a.m. – 9 a.m.	Stomach
9 a.m. – 11 a.m.	Spleen
11 a.m. – 1 p.m.	Heart
1 p.m. – 3 p.m.	Small intestine
3–5 p.m.	Bladder
5–7 p.m.	Kidney
7–9 p.m.	Pericardium
9–11 p.m.	*San jiao*

can be vacuous (*xu*), void of *qi* relative to the overall flow in a particular individual. It can also be replete (*shi*), packed with *qi* relative to the overall flow. Typically, a repletion is not an excess of the channel *qi* but the presence of an invading evil.

The key to understanding these ideas is that in Chinese thought *yin* and *yang* are never quantitatively too little or too great; there is always balance. It is just that some balances do not support human life or comfort. *Xu*, vacuity, and *shi*, repletion, describe *qi* states that are relative

(b)

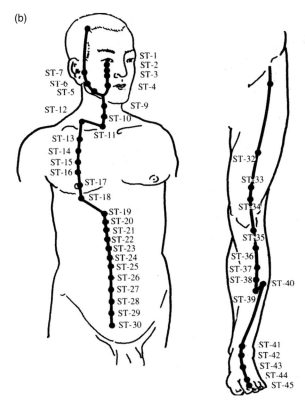

Figure 3.8 (a) Traditional and (b) modern (simplified) drawings of the stomach channel. (Courtesy of Paradigm Publications.)

to the individual, rather than comparisons with measurable norms and standards. There is little normative information used in Chinese medicine. Traditional Chinese physicians never meared the body's internal temperature, instead they noted the heat effused, palpably perceived on the patient's skin. Thus a given physically measured temperature that was cold for one person might be hot for another, depending upon the state of health and constitutional metabolism of the individual. Furthermore, the bedside orientation of traditional practitioners emphasized qualities, not comparisions. Thus, for example, heat was also differentiated by whether it was felt at the initial touch or after a time, and whether accompanied by dampness or dryness.

Furthermore, these concepts are frequently applied to phenomena Westerners have never

recognized as symptoms of disease. For example, the Chinese character for 'vacuity' expresses hypocrisy, unearned reputation, frailty, and strengthless flabbiness — the beer belly of a couch potato, not the powerful bulk of a sumo wrestler. Pathologically obese people who might be considered excessive in a material view are actually *xu*—vacuous—from the *qi* perspective. Clinically, a *qi* vacuity can manifest as a listless or spiritless demeanor, laziness, or sloppy mental habits. Gallbladder *xu* is not just the sum of the physical signs of gallbladder hypofunction because it also includes, for example, 'timid gallbladder,' a lack of courage.[74] There may also be physical signs that are subtle and thus easy to miss; these subtle distinctions are sometimes powerful clinical clues. For example, an aversion to drafts that is not really a physical chill or symptom, and is a recently noticed sensitivity, can give a clue to a treatment that will prevent a *shan han* — something that is sometimes just a 'cold.'[75]

Some practitioners, Yoshio Manaka being a particularly good example, focus their attention on the relative imbalance of a channel or series of channels, because their treatments center on producing systemic balance. Thus vacuity and repletion express constitutional qualities. These practitioners usually identify themselves as working toward 'root treatment.' In this perspective vacuity and repletion are visualized as deformations in the whole of the human — like a ball with a lump on one end and a matching depression at the other. For these practitioners, *xu* and *shi* are not symptom categories, excesses, or deficiencies, but an imbalance perceptible within the topological character of the body.

Traditionally, imbalance is the root of illness. Thus, when focusing on treating channels, the primary goal is to restore the normal flow of *qi*, a concept that implies a deep, essential balance of both mind and body. There are many, many treatment options, and the appropriate therapy might be indicated by the most subtle of a set of clues. For example, channel repletion need not evidence itself just as physical signs, but can be indicated by personality traits, tones of

(a)

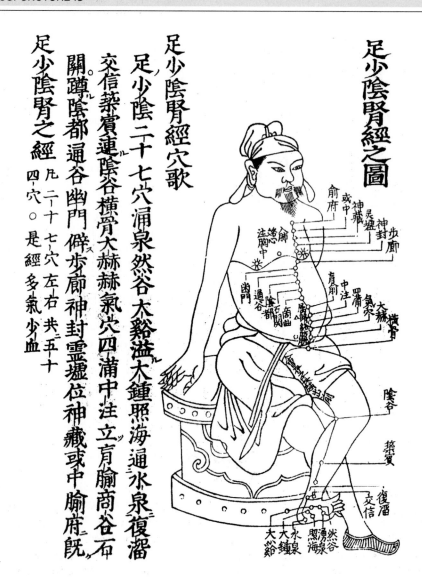

足少陰腎經之圖

足少陰腎經穴歌

足少陰二十七穴湧泉然谷太谿溢大鍾照海通水泉復溜交信蒸賓連陰谷橫骨大赫赫氣穴四滿中注立肓腧商谷石關蹲陰都通谷幽門僻步廊神封靈墟位神藏或中腧府畱

足少陰腎之經凡二十七穴左右共五十四穴。是經多氣少血

voice, ways of thinking, or a vacuity in another part of the body or in a different channel. It may be indicated by a distortion of the shape of one part of the body as compared to another.

A channel can also be stagnant, inhibited, a condition that occurs when it is difficult for the *qi* to flow properly. This condition can also arise for many different reasons. There may be trauma, bruising — actual physical stagnation — but there may also be a *qi* repletion or vacuity that distorts the relative balance between two or more channels, eliminating the differences in potential that create flow. For example, because *qi* and blood circulation are related, blood stagnation can lead to *qi* repletion in one area of the body and a *qi* vacuity in another. In some conditions the *qi* is thought of as being in 'counterflow;' that is, moving in a direction contrary to that required for good health. The viscera, bowels, and channels are also functionally interconnected, so organs can affect channels, and channels can affect organs to such an extent that they may be considered as practically inseparable.

(b)

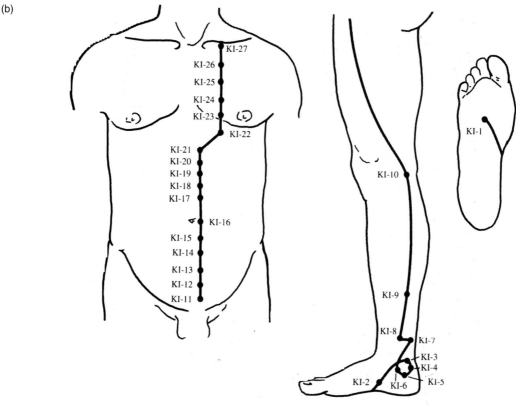

Figure 3.9 (a) Traditional and (b) modern (simplified) drawings of the kidney channel. (Courtesy of Paradigm Publications.)

Qi production and function: the *zang fu* system

The *qi* that circulates in the channels (*ying qi*), the *qi* that defends at the body surface (*wei qi*), and the numerous other *qi* are not related only because organs and channels are connected. Each *qi* has its own source of production and origin, and these sources are centered in the traditional Chinese notions of *zang* and *fu* (Box 3.10). The traditional literature clearly acknowledges that each *qi* must be produced somewhere and links these *qi* to many functions that are also described in the West as well as some that are uniquely Chinese. The traditional literature uses a vocabulary that often sounds strange to Western ears, but in many instances describes familiar features and events from a different perspective.

Some East–West differences are the result of the very early date at which Chinese medical theory and language formed. As we have seen, when the viscera, bowels, and channels were identified, China was an emerging state concerned with the development of its political and economic infrastructure — roads, canals, cities, and government storehouses. Thus, the *fu* organs are named by a character that has been translated as a 'grain collection center' or 'palace,' by analogy a place where blood and *qi* are produced. Similarly, the *zang* organs are labeled by a character that indicates their function as 'storage facilities' or 'depots,' where blood and *qi* are controlled or stored. Typically, however, modern clinicians refer to the organs that produce secretions, what are called 'clear fluids' in Chinese, as 'viscera.' The organs that handle the transportation and elimination of food and waste are known as 'bowels.'

(a)

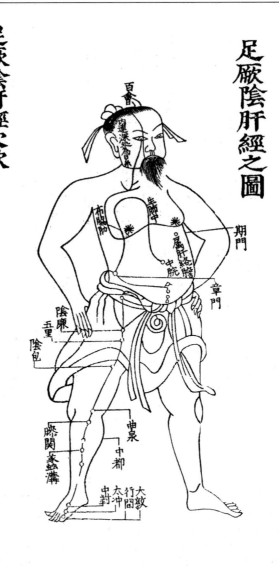

Box 3.10   *Zang-fu (zo-fu)*

臟   腑

zang   fu

The *zang*, the body's storage facilities, are variously called the 'depots,' 'viscera,' 'solid organs,' or 'yin organs,' and have the primary role of producing and storing vital substances, fluids, or *qi* in the body. They are the organs of primary significance, those to which attention is most commonly directed in diagnosis and treatment, because they perform the greatest number of functions. The *fu*, the body's grain collection centers, are variously called the 'palaces,' 'bowels,' 'hollow organs,' or 'yang organs.' Their primary role is transportation in the decomposition of food and the conveyance of waste.[76]

The so-called five viscera store essential *qi* and do not discharge waste. Thus they are full, but cannot be filled. The six bowels process and convey matter, and do not store. Thus they are filled, yet are not full. (*Su Wen*)

Although anatomical studies in ancient China were less sophisticated than those of today, the basic knowledge of the location, size, and function of the major organs was largely congruent with modern anatomical descriptions.

(b)

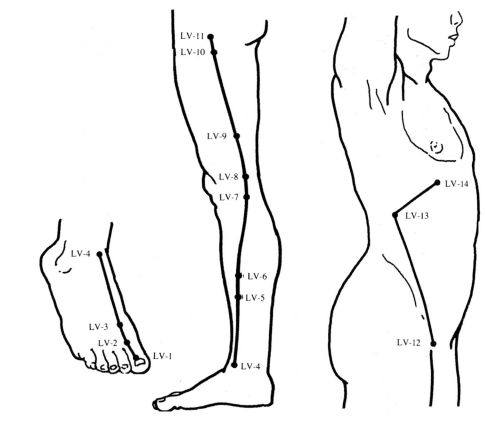

Figure 3.10 (a) Traditional and (b) modern (simplified) drawings of the liver channel. (Courtesy of Paradigm Publications.)

The Chinese did not limit themselves to descriptive names and analogies. The gross anatomy, placement, and relative sizes and weights of the different organs were also known. This anatomical knowledge depended on naked-sense observation, so it did not describe the microscopically fine detail accomplished by modern science. As we saw in our discussion of the modern history of acupuncture (see Ch. 1), Western anatomical knowledge quickly overwhelmed this indigenous perspective. However, the anatomical dissections undertaken were neither unimportant or trivial. It is recorded, for example, that it was by anatomical dissection that the correct depth of needle insertion was determined.[77] This implies a thorough examination of the visible blood vessels and anatomical structures that should not be needled if wounding is to be avoided. This

makes sense, because in acupuncture's generative eras, any infection was potentially serious.

Thus Chinese ideas of the production and transportation of *qi* probably began with the same observations with which Western anatomy and physiology began. For example, medical researchers in both cultures observed that ingested food was transformed in the stomach and passed along the digestive tract to be discharged as waste. However, rather than analyze the stomach wall, the glands, secretions, and intertwined biochemical reactions, as Western researchers would do hundreds of years later, the Chinese reasoned that the spleen and stomach absorbed the *qi* of the transforming food. This is another example of how Chinese thinkers perceive *qi* not as energy or matter but as the transformation within and relationship between events. What counted was the dynamic

(a)

coordination of digestion — how well it worked as a whole, not the molecule-by-molecule detail. For the acupuncturist, the spleen absorbs the vital essence of food, providing nurture for the body. Thus the spleen was titled the 'office of granaries,' an analogy to human government that expresses the function of governance over the 'qi of grain and water,' yet another example that reflects the state of Chinese cultural development during acupuncture's formative period.

From this basic observation and its logical extension, Chinese medical thought grew to complete the analogies between the functions of the organs and how nature could be seen to work. The spleen was like the earth — yellow-tan in color and central, the position it holds among the five phases. Therefore, like the earth the spleen must need water to be productive, but stagnation and rot will result if it is poorly drained. Just as the earth is the mother of all

(b)

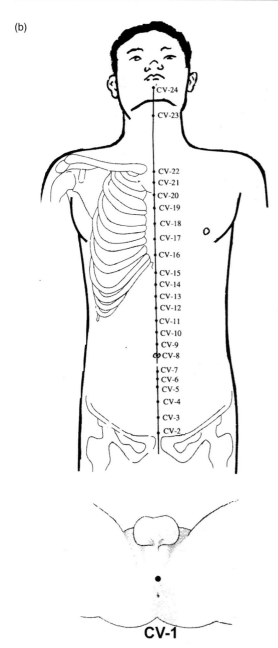

Figure 3.11 (a) Traditional and (b) modern (simplified) drawings of the *ren* channel. (Courtesy of Paradigm Publications.)

things, the *qi* provided by the spleen must be the root *qi* of the body, and thus life itself. Just as the spleen is the mother of our life and health, thought is the mother of our action and invention. Thus, the spleen was seen to govern thought.

In the same way, by the same logic, each of the *zang fu* were understood to be responsible for the production and expression of several *qi*.[78]

We cannot stress often enough that the very broad meaning of *qi* included any activity that occurred in an organized and consistent way, as we noted earlier in regard to the dynamic organization of food moving through the digestive tract. Chinese medical thinkers used the concept of *qi* to explain the same essential functions Western scientists would later describe. Thus, the *zang fu* system of organs described by the ancient Chinese has many similarities to our modern anatomophysiological knowledge. Both are rooted in observation of the same human body. Although clearly not based on the molecular science that characterizes modern biomedicine, or the physics of bioelectrical energies, and only marginally concerned with norms and measurements, Eastern and Western ideas of organ systems are often very similar. The following examples show clear similarities in the Eastern and Western ideas of the most essential functions:

- respiration – lungs
- blood circulation – heart
- digestion – stomach, small intestine, large intestine
- excretion – large intestine
- urine formation and excretion – kidneys, bladder.

These similarities are not restricted to generalities. The first and still one of most sophisticated Western attempts to relate Chinese and European physiological knowledge was that of Soulie de Morant. The associations he proposed between stimulation of the sympathetic nervous system and stimulation of the *san jiao* (triple burner) are listed in Table 3.7. This table summarizes some of his research on the characteristics of the triple burner. 'Greater' means increased function, 'lesser' means decreased function. As the table shows, the functions ascribed to the triple burner are largely those Western science ascribes to the sympathetic nervous system.[79] The table suggests that, even without identifying physical structures, and, in

(a)

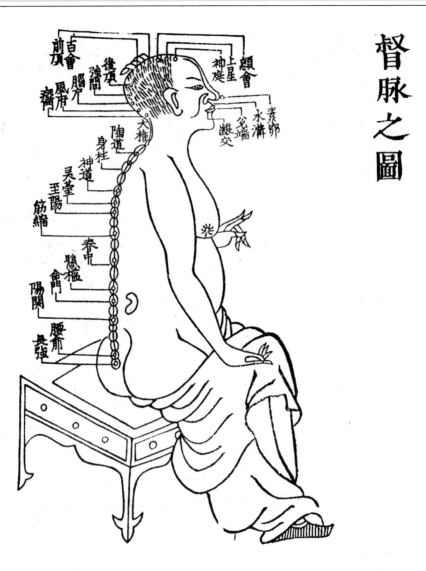

督脈之圖

fact, without even a concept of the nervous system, the Chinese observations of human function could nonetheless be detailed and accurate. Again, we can see that whether or not there is an actual entity that corresponds to the triple burner, the concept and the observations related to it are clinically useful.

In the traditional acupuncture literature each organ is also assigned functions that are clearly different from the modern biomedical perspective. Many of these are the result of the analogies to natural phenomena that the Chinese employed (for example, as we noted above, the presumed effect of the spleen on thought). Although focus-

ing on these often fascinating differences, it is important to keep the broad, essential similarities in mind and to remember that many of these functions carry cultural associations that are nearly 2000 years old. However, it is most important to remember that in acupuncture the only essential description of any organ is its relation to *qi*. *Qi* assimilation, production, storage, circulation, and function are the essentials of the *zang fu*, the channels, and every concept of human order and function. Even organ functions that are predominantly matters of blood production, storage, and transportation are matters of *qi*, because it is *qi* that animates the

(b)

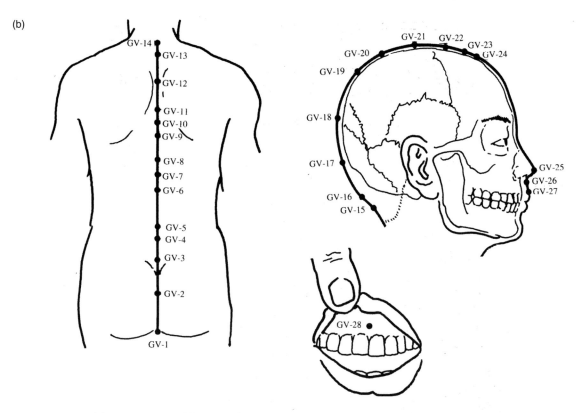

Figure 3.12 (a) Traditional and (b) modern (simplified) drawings of the *du* channel. (Courtesy of Paradigm Publications.)

Table 3.7 Associations between the sympathetic nervous system and the stimulation of the *san jiao* (Soulie de Morant[79])*

Function	Sympathetic effect	*San jiao* effect
Blood vessels in general	Greater	Greater
Coronary vessels	Lesser	Not known
Vessels of general application	Lesser	Not known
Heart: amplitude, rapidity	Greater	Greater
Bronchi	Lesser	Lesser
Lungs	Not known	Lesser
Smooth digestive muscles	Lesser	Lesser
Internal anal sphincter	Greater	Not known
Intestines	Lesser	Lesser
Pancreas	Not known	Lesser
Liver	Greater	Greater
Gallbladder	Lesser	Lesser
Spleen	Greater	Greater
Kidneys	Not known	Greater
Urinary bladder: expulsor muscle	Lesser	Lesser
Internal sphincter	Greater	Greater

*Greater, increased function; lesser, decreased function.

blood. As everything is *qi*, and everything that occurs in life is a manifestation of *qi*, every function imaginable is a permutation of *qi*. In fact, the two organ systems, the *zang* and the *fu*, are essentially described by their relation to *qi*.

The *zang* are *yin* organs and the *fu* are *yang* organs. The following names and characteristics of these two organ types are listed in Box 3.11.[80] Each organ also has functions beyond simple assimilation, production, and elimination. Because the qi paradigm is rooted in observations of nature, the movement and expression of *qi* and *qi* pathologies include both physical and mental states. Because everything was ultimately *qi*, emotional and mental states would not only alter *qi* but also alter the organs. This would manifest as a change in organ function. Thus organs were described with reference to human affects as much as the governance of *qi* circulation or the storage of blood. Even this was not a limit because the medium of *qi* was also seen as a spiritual link. Although spirit in Chinese thought is not the Western idea of an individual soul — something beneath, beyond, and dominant over the human realm — it is an expression of humans' relationship to the universe. This too is an essential reflection of *qi*.

Box 3.11 *Zang* and *fu* organs

Zang: *qi* production and storage	**Fu:** decompose food and convey waste
Fei (lung)	*Da chang* (large intestine)
Pi (spleen)	*Wei* (stomach)
Xin (heart)	*Xiao chang* (small intestine)
Shen (kidney)	*Pang guang* (bladder)
Xin bao luo (pericardium)	*San jiao* (triple burner)
Gan (liver)	*Dan* (gallbladder)
Interior	Exterior
'Solid' organs	'Hollow' organs'
Viscera	'Bowel'
'Palaces'	'Depots'

Basically, the organs were seen as having influence in the body, each one playing a role in *qi* production and having a special relationship to certain emotional, mental, and spiritual states. Each was also distinctly linked to specific tissues, particular channels, and specific environmental factors. In one traditional text these broad spheres of influence were likened to the 12 officials in a feudal government. In fact, the Chinese character used to describe this influence, *zhu* (governance), was actually borrowed from the vocabulary of imperial government. This is an analogy that is alive today in some modern systems of practice. In the People's Republic of China there has been a de-emphasis of all but the somatic aspects. For example, one text used to train traditional physicians in China's leading medical schools devotes only a single paragraph to the discussion of attitudes and emotions.[81] However, as discussed earlier, this change in emphasis reflects a change in social and economic priorities, not a proven lack of clinical utility.

In the following paragraphs, we briefly outline the main functions under the influence of each organ by using this extended analogy. In certain styles of practice, this knowledge is essential to diagnosis and the formulation of treatment plans.[82]

- The lungs hold the office of minister and chancellor; they govern respiratory function; they help regulate the flow of water in the body. They control the *qi* and govern the defensive exterior of the body, including the skin and hair. They are said to store the *po*, a 'corporeal soul,' that comes forth from the earth with life and returns to the earth with death.
- The large intestine is the organ responsible for transit; it governs transformation and conveyance of waste. It eliminates the turbid *qi* that remains from the digestive process.
- The stomach, with the spleen, is responsible for the storehouses and granaries; it governs ingestion and decomposition of digestate.
- The spleen governs movement and transformation of the digestate. The spleen was assigned overall control of digestion. Many scholars have concluded that what the ancient Chinese meant by *pi* included the pancreas and its important digestive functions. Thus some acupuncturists refer to either the pan-

creas only, or to the logical compound of 'spleen–pancreas.' The spleen governs the flesh and limbs, and is said to store the *yi*, 'thought.' Thus spleen condition has a strong relationship to mentation.

- The heart is the emperor, the supreme ruler. It governs the blood vessels and blood. It stores the *shen*, 'spirit' or clarity of consciousness. '*Shen*' is what breathes life into the body. There are many interesting discussions about 'spirit.' It is generally likened to a supreme ruler who governs the land and all its subjects, just as the rulers of ancient China were thought to provide for their peoples through communication with the supreme ancestor. In the body, *shen* is the most important manifestation of *qi* and must be properly nurtured and protected.
- The small intestine governs separation of the clear and turbid. It primarily extracts the clear *qi* that is to be assimilated and passes the turbid *qi* to the large intestine from whence it will be eliminated.
- The bladder is responsible for storage and elimination of fluid. It helps eliminate turbid *qi*.
- The kidneys are responsible for the creation of power. They govern water, which is a symbol for life itself. It governs the bones and creates the bone marrow. The brain is formed from the excess *qi* of the marrow. The kidneys are said to be the root of the body; they store the *jing*, or 'essence,' which is the prenatal foundation of the body. They are responsible for growth, development, and reproduction. They are said to store the *zhi*, 'will.'
- The pericardium is the outer casing of the heart, it serves primarily to protect the heart, the emperor, the *shen*. There have been numerous theories about the pericardium that give it various degrees of significance.
- The *san jiao* is responsible for the waterways and ditches. It has a significant role in regulating water metabolism, regulating and bringing about digestion. It serves to distribute *qi* globally in the body. Much has been said about the *san jiao* but little agreement has been reached. It is generally accepted as having a regulatory role for the organs of assimilation, circulation, and elimination.
- The gallbladder is responsible for what is just and exact. It primarily functions to support the liver. Audacious, strong-willed people were known to the Chinese as 'grand gallbladders,' and this organ was described by analogy to a general in feudal society, a tactical leader whose role was to defend and extend the state's territory.
- The liver is the commanding general, the strategist, responsible for decision-making. It governs the free coursing or flow of *qi* throughout the body; it stores the blood; it governs the sinews; it is said to store the *hun*, the 'soul,' which descends from heaven with life and returns to heaven at death.

The above are the primary organs and their functions. Among these, the most basic functions are those of *qi* assimilation, production, and circulation:

- Storage and dissemination of prenatal, essential *qi* – kidney
- Assimilation of *qi* from the environment – lung, spleen, stomach, small intestine, and large intestine
- Circulation of *qi* – lungs, liver, and *san jiao*
- Elimination of turbid *qi* (digestate and metabolic waste products) – large intestine and bladder.

Each of the organs is also described in terms of its *qi*-related functions, its blood-related functions, its *yin*-storing functions, and its yang-active functions. To continue the analogy of the spleen, its power to transform ingested food is a *yang* (active) function. Its governance of the flesh and limbs is a *qi*-related (circulating) function. In the case of the liver, the storage of blood is a *yin* (storing) function. The general circulation of *qi* by the liver is a *qi* function. Thus acupuncturists' diagnoses of organ problems go beyond identification of the troubled viscera or bowel, being instead an assessment of a specific dysfunction. In addition, the *yin-yang*, *qi*-, or blood-related problem is further diagnosed as fitting one of the same patterns of dysfunction used to categorize channel problems: vacuity or repletion, and stagnation. For example, a problem might be described as a 'depression of liver *qi.*' Each pattern indicates a general treatment plan that is individualized by the practitioner through point selection. However, in every case the primary goal of treatment is always restoration of *qi* circulation and organ function.

Again, even where entirely different-sounding vocabulary and concepts are used, these are often logical equivalents to biomedicine. The descriptions are very different because they are separated by hundreds of years and ideas of knowledge that are considerably different. However, the essential observations of the two medical systems are related, because in biological time hundreds of years are no more than a moment. And, although absolute one-to-one equivalences between patterns in acupuncture and biomedical diagnoses are probably not possible on any large scale because the methods of cognition are so different, the search for useful clinical correspondences is now a major research subject in China. There are appreciable differences in how medical problems were understood and resolved in the ancient East and the modern West; however, the human body is the same, many diseases are the same, and it is thus unwise to overstate either the similarities or differences.

Each system proceeded along different lines, guided by the attributes of its generative culture. The perspective of traditional East Asian medicines, and their development in advance of instruments that could operate beyond the range of the human senses, led to stressing observable relationships instead of the detail of organ biochemistry. In Western medicine, buoyed by the power of biochemical analysis, it was the biochemical organ functions that were stressed. Because the effects of acupoint stimulation are observed with the gross physical senses, patterns in acupuncture are based on those observations. Because the effects of drugs are understood as biochemical in nature, biomedical diagnoses concentrate on microscopic details. This makes neither system right nor wrong; what counts is their ability successfully to predict and control the outcome of therapy. In acupuncture, that control is achieved through the selection and stimulation of acupuncture points.

Acupoints

Many Westerners learn about acupoints through familiarity with the Asian martial arts, acupressure and shiatsu massage, or even a system where athletes use tennis balls to stimulate a series of acupoints to help them prevent and recover from injuries.[83] Most Westerners who approach these sources begin with the impression that each acupoint has a job, an effect — one for a headache, one for back pain, perhaps two or three for a complex problem. However, this is the case in only the narrowest sense. In traditional thought acupuncture points were an intimate part of the qi paradigm and were more than just switches for turning off symptoms. In a loose metaphoric sense, acupoints are like frets on a musical instrument, the finger positions by which the orchestration of human functions was kept harmonious.

In the acupuncture literature acupoints have locations, actions, and indications. Some have contraindications against particular stimuli, use in certain conditions, or needling depth. Locations were traditionally palpatory instructions. For example, according to the *Zhen Jiu Da Chang,* one of the must famous acupoints, *zu san li,* the thirty-sixth point of the stomach channel, is located 'three body inches below the knee, on the lateral end of the shinbone, in the fleshy part of the major sinew, at the point where it divides under pressure.'[84] (The *cun* or 'body inch' is a measure that is individual for each person.) Today, modern Chinese books use anatomical locations; for example, ST-36 is found 'roughly one inch lateral to the crest of the tibia.'[85] In some systems, acupoints do not have fixed locations. *Toyohari* practitioners use the textbook location as a starting point for feeling the 'currently live point.' This is determined by palpation, and may change as the patient's condition changes.

What points are thought to do also varies with the school of thought. In Traditional

Chinese Medicine (TCM), each acupoint is thought to have one or more 'functions,' as well as multiple 'actions and indications.' Functions are phrases that describe the point's role relative to TCM patterns. For example, an important and effective point like ST-36 has a dozen functions, one of which is to 'rectify the spleen and stomach.' This refers to its ability to harmonize digestive activity. Thus its indications refer to symptoms for which it may be applied (e.g. stomach pain, abdominal distension, and indigestion). The method of stimulation, needle or moxa instructions, and the sensation the patient should feel are also noted.[86] These too differ by system, and in systems where more subtle needling is applied the sensation referenced is that perceived by the acupuncturist, not the patient.

With the number of variables possible, lists of acupoint actions and indications can be extensive. Acupuncture points may be supplemented, drained, treated at particular hours of minimum or maximum activity, and needled with differing degrees of stimulation. Thus lists of effects for important points can go on for pages; Soulie de Morant's compilation for ST-36 mentions virtually every part of the body, every organ, and lists more than 100 signs and symptoms.[88] However, these lists are by no means as chaotic as this prose description may make them seem, because everything an acupoint can do is rooted in, and organized by, principles of correspondence.

Box 3.12   *Xue (ketsu)*

穴   氣穴   空穴

xue   qi xue   kong xue

The term *xue* is used alone or in conjunction with other terms to refer to the acupuncture points. However, etymologically the term refers not to a geometrical abstraction such as 'point,' but to a 'cave,' a 'hole,' a 'pit,' a real chamber below the earth. Some classical sources have suggested that the term refers to a grave because of its use in Chinese geomancy (*feng shui*) to refer to a gravesite in which it would be auspicious to bury someone. We use the vernacular word 'acupoint' in this book, but it is useful to remember that *xue* are really 'holes,' dynamic structures on the body surface that must be selected and located by appropriate means.

Commonly encountered terms are *xue* and *qi xue* (*qi* point/hole); these imply an association with the *qi* system. *Jing xue* (channel point/hole) implies an association with the channel system. *Kong xue* (hole, cave, or hollow) is a generic term referring to points/holes in general.

The acupuncture points were given names in the historical literature that have been largely replaced in English by the modern practice of numbering the points. For example, the ninth point on the lung channel is *tai yuan* (great abyss), in the West referred to as LU-9. The thirty-sixth point on the stomach channel is *zu san li* (leg three miles), referred to as ST-36. All the points have one or more names, which may or may not have clinical relevance but about which many have contributed interesting ideas and interpretations. Common referents in the classification of acupuncture points are given as follows.[87]

yin-yang, channels, *qi*, blood, organs

Yin gu	Yin valley	KI-10
Yang xi	Yang ravine	LI-5
San yin jiao	Three *yin* intersection	SP-6
Qi she	Qi above	ST-11
Xue hai	Blood ocean	SP-10
Xin shu	Heart *shu*	BL-15

Architectural, astronomic, geographic, meteorological associations

Jing men	Capital gate	GB-25
Xia xi	Pinched ravine	GB-43
Tian shu	Celestial pivot	ST-25
Feng chi	Wind pool	GB-20

Location and anatomy

Da du	Great metropolis	SP-2
Jian jing	Shoulder well	GB-21
Dan zhong	Chest center	CV-17

There are four major classes of acupuncture point. The first are those that lie on the channels, such as the examples above, of which there are said to be 670 (counting bilateral points twice). The second class are the 'extra' points; These points have identified properties and functions, but may not be on the pathways of the channels. Some of these points are only for use with needles, some only for use with moxa. There are a large number of these extra points. The third class is the *a shi* point, the pressure pain point, found with pressure. These may or may not be located on the channels. The fourth, more recent,

---

Box 3.12 *Xue (ketsu) (cont'd)*

class of points are the various microsystem points; these are special subsets of extra points relevant in specific microsystems, such as ear, hand, foot, periocular, perinasal, or scalp acupuncture. In the fourth system the whole body is reflected in one part of the body, and each major part of the body is a point within that region.

The main *xue* are those that lie on the channels. These *xue* can also be classified into major types. Each channel has one of the following classes of points: a five-phase (command) point (wood, fire, earth, metal, or water); a source point; a *luo* point; and a *xi* (cleft) point. Each channel also has a related 'back-*shu*' point and a related 'front-*mu*' point (reflex points located on the front and back of the body). There also may be intersection points between one or more channels. The following list classifies the 21 points of the spleen channel and associated points:

- *yin bai* (SP-1), wood, *jing*-well point
- *da du* (SP-2), fire, *ying*-spring point
- *tai bai* (SP-3), earth, stream *shu*, and source point
- *gong sun* (SP-4), connecting *luo* point and master point of *chong mai*
- *shang qiu* (SP-5), metal, *jing*-river point
- *san yin jiao* (SP-6), intersection point with liver, kidney channels, and *chong mai*
- *lou gu* (SP-7)
- *di ji* (SP-8), cleft-*xi* point
- *yin ling quan* (SP-9), water, uniting *he*-sea point
- *xue hai* (SP-10), as 'sea of blood' affects blood
- *ji men* (SP-11)

- *chong men* (SP-12)
- *fu she* (SP-13), intersection point with *yin wei mai*
- *fu jie* (SP-14)
- *da heng* (SP-15), intersection point with *yin wei mai*
- *fu ai* (SP-16) intersection point with *yin wei mai*
- *shi dou* (SP-17)
- *tian xi* (SP-18)
- *xiong xiang* (SP-19)
- *zhou rong* (SP-20)
- *da bao* (SP-21), great *luo* of the spleen
  Associated points:
- *zhang men* (LR-13), front *mu* point of the spleen
- *pi shu* (BL-20), back-*shu* point of the spleen
- *zhong ji* (CV-3), intersection point of spleen channel
- *guan yuan* (CV-4), intersection point of spleen channel
- *xia wan* (CV-10), intersection point of spleen channel
- *zhong wan* (CV-12), intersection point of spleen channel
- *qi men* (LR-14), intersection point of spleen channel
- *ri yue* (GB-24), intersection point of spleen channel.

Each acupuncture point is thought to have a number of properties associated with it. These properties can be thought of in relation to: the channel on which it lies, channels that intersect, local effects, the class or characteristic associated with that point (e.g. *luo point*, or fire point), and empirically observed actions of the point (i.e. stops bleeding, relieves pain in the inquinal region). Treatments are composed by selecting points that match or counter the observed problem.

The theories of systematic correspondence: *yin-yang* and the five phases

How can medical knowledge that is centered on qualities and relationships rather than specific disease states allow acupuncturists to help their patients? In the same way any medicine can. At the most basic level, all medicine is a link between what we observe and what we want. Like an engineer's theoretical 'black box,' we can visualize medical systems as machines into which we pour information and from which clinical instructions issue. How then do we examine the inner workings of the black box of acupuncture?

We have seen how observations of nature led to theories and how those theories led to the evolution of a medicine of systematic correspondence. So far though, we have only looked

at the theories of systematic correspondence in relation to major cycles and a limited number of common, corresponding phenomena. To understand how acupuncturists treat illnesses we need to explore correspondences that are pertinent to the details of human function, and thus to the decisions of clinical practice. Furthermore, we will need to understand how these phenomena promote health or illness. In other words, we need to learn what *yin-yang* and the five phases can tell us about things that have 'gone out of balance,' as well as how they help formulate treatments that encourage that balance.

We already know much about how observations are treated in the black box of acupuncture. We saw, for example, how the cycle of a year and its corresponding seasonal cycles were correlated to the general theories of *yin-yang* and the five phases. We saw how seasonal cycles and their corresponding fluctuations of activity — qi-activity levels — influenced the elaboration of these theories. We have seen that, not only by ordering the phases of qi but also by relating them to other phenomena in nature — the tables of basic yin-yang and five-phase correspondences — the qi paradigm allows us to understand one phenomenon in relation to another. For example, we can predict that fire signs will predominate in a fire season, that someone whose kidneys have been damaged by cold will manifest symptoms (or what Unschuld appropriately calls 'pathoconditions,' because they are not in all cases symptoms) that reflect the qualities of cold — depth, slowness, absence of warmth. We can also look for signs of cold through the entire sphere of influence associated with the kidneys. Thus, for example, we might look for pathoconditions related to the bones of the body.[89]

Because we know that the theories of yin-yang and the five phases can be applied to all phenomena, we know that the first thing that happens inside our imaginary black box is the classification of clinical observations according to whether they are relatively more yin or yang, whether they have qualities reflected by the symbols of wood, fire, earth, metal, or water, or whether they fit one of the extended jing luo, zang, or fu analogies. In effect, the processes in the black box are in an ordering exactly like what has happened, step by step, idea by idea, throughout the history of Chinese medicine. Just as the general theory of qi acquired multiple distinctions of qi types, Chinese physiology and pathophysiology acquired multiple distinctions through generations of experience in treating illness. Thus the first step for the acupuncturist is to recognize those specific aspects of qi that he or she can understand in terms of yin-yang and the five phases.

In terms of how the body was categorized, we have already seen how the obvious structures, systems, and functions, for example, the zang-fu were understood. We have also considered the most basic logical systems such as the jing luo. In addition, there are all the various body surfaces, tissues, and their products: sense organs, body fluids, colors, odors, and tastes. In acupuncture extensive lists of bodily phenomena and structures are related to both classification systems. In fact, we now need to extend that list because all of the body's external environment, especially those aspects of the environment that can relate to pathological conditions, must also be considered. This includes seasonal factors, time of year, time of day, climate, available foods, behavior, inherited constitution, and living and work habits.

In the traditional and modern acupuncture literature, practically everything has been classified in one or more of these systems. However, classification is not enough. Even if everything is related, and everything is classified according to relationships, we still cannot entirely understand the workings of our imaginary black box. To understand how the acupuncturist selects from this near-infinite number of possibilities we must also know the logic by which this information is processed. In modern terms, we not only need to know the inputs, but also to understand the algorithms, the software, by which that information is applied.

For Westerners, that logic is easy to understand because it is familiar. In East Asia, as in the West, medicine is 'allopathic,' that is, it treats a condition through its opposite. Unlike European homeopathy, which developed according to the law of similars, the idea that like treats like, Chinese medicine and acupuncture developed according to the idea that opposites cure. Literally thousands of statements, many from the earliest times, set out the essential strategy: 'If it is hot, cool it'; 'If it is replete, drain it.' Although Chinese medical logic also involves a kill-the-invader approach identical to that of biomedical drugs such as antibiotics, the clinical perspective stresses treatments that restore the body's desired functions. Thus the illness is not the invader but the weakness that allowed the invasion to succeed. The effects of acupuncture points are described not as curing a particular disease (although this does occur in modern literature), but as increasing or decreasing qi flow, or removing blockages (disinhibition) from one or more of the major or minor channels.

In sum, the black box we have imagined is principally a picture-producing machine. Information that is ordered by *yin-yang* and the five phases is used to form a picture of a particular individual based on detailed images of human function. Organ functions, channel conditions, and relationships describe an intercommunicating network of influences that are analyzed for breaks in communication. These breaks are seen as repletions, vacuities, or stagnations. *Yin-yang* and five-phase logic is applied to determine how these conditions may best be improved. In choosing their interventions, acupuncturists select from a repertoire of acupoint capabilities described in exactly the same language of images.

For example, in one system, when a patient is diagnosed with a damp condition, an acupoint such as *yin ling quan*, the ninth point on the spleen channel, will be stimulated because it is thought to eliminate dampness. In another system, a patient presenting a lung vacuity pattern will be treated at the *tai yuan* point, the ninth point on the lung channel. That point is chosen because it is the supplementation point of the lung channel, and will thus increase *qi* flow in that channel. Regardless of the system used, the logic and language of point and technique selection is the counterbalance of the problem identified.

Pragmatic considerations limit how any classification system is applied in practice. No acupuncturist can consider or acquire practical expertise with every system. In acupuncture what determines which correspondences are used most is a system of training, what is sometimes called a 'school of thought.' In Asia, schools of thought are not always based solely on adherence to a particular doctrine, being based also on particular approaches to learning physical skills. It is a philosophy of practice, or a problem-solving strategy coupled with a repertoire of techniques. Acupuncture, not unlike a sport or martial art, requires the development of physical skills, some of which are not easy to acquire. Just as knowledge of color theory, shade, and human anatomy cannot lead to a beautiful painting if an artist lacks skill with a brush, acupuncture cannot be practiced with knowledge alone.

When traditional medicine was standardized after the Second World War, the traditional training that was replaced involved literally thousands of small schools. These were often no more than an experienced practitioner and a few apprentices who learned as they worked. Interaction between schools was limited, because masters competed for apprentices, there being few other ways for the masters to increase their income in such a labor-intensive art. We have already noted how acupoint names were sometimes used to help keep a master's knowledge secret. However, even the more generally shared literature contributed to clinical and theoretical variance. For example, the traditional 'songs' (long rhyming lists) by which information about acupoint capabilities was made easily memorizable for illiterate apprentices lacked all the technical detail necessary for application. Thus, these too did nothing to discourage variation. Individual differences and circumstances, teachers of varying skills, economic competition for apprentices and patients, and the limits of the literature all contributed to a very uneven standard among traditional practitioners.

Given the needs after the Second World War, the remedy applied in all of Asia was standardization. Standardization elimininated many correspondence sets and rationalized those common to most systems of training. Worldwide it is these sometimes simplified correspondence sets that modern acupuncture students learn. Like modern, simplified versions of the channel system, these correspondence sets are summaries of the most broadly shared information. However, the apprentice system has not died out. It is still alive in styles of acupuncture that depend upon physical skills that are difficult to learn. It permits directed, intensive training, as well as student–teacher comparisons that build confidence. This is not surprising — both sport in the West and the martial arts in the East recognize the value of mental and personal focus in the development of complex physical skills. For example, in addition to their daily training, acupuncturists in the Toyohari school may eschew coffee, take exercise or meditative periods, or observe a fairly rigorous lifestyle, the aim of these disciplines being to increase the physical sensitivity that is their principal diagnostic tool. Today many Japanese practitioners still credit their best-developed skills not to the formal training by which they passed their examinations, but to their often lengthy study with a master acupuncturist. In China too individual masters who were once required to conform or retire during the period of standardization are now once again valued for their skill and practical experience.

Another way of looking at this is to say that, throughout history the place of acupuncture in Asian societies has encouraged the development of a variety of maps: navigation systems that organize information about a patient so that a therapy can be selected. Some of these maps – the now standardized curricula – were general knowledge, but even after traditional doctors in China were legally required to surrender their private knowledge, small schools survived outside of official sanction, and rivalry and irregular quality were never entirely eliminated. In Japan, the standardization imposed by government-controlled examinations had a similar effect. The same process can be seen in the West. Thus, more or less in all of the world, acupuncture is now a relatively more standard body of knowledge. However, within this standard there are still many different, practical approaches to gathering and assessing information and many different repertoires of hands-on skills.

Some of these differing approaches came to the West at various times and some have survived here. These systems share the use of the basic correspondences and techniques. Some Western schools concentrate on unique or ethnically derived approaches, and others specialize in particular diagnostic or therapeutic techniques. Of course, there is still rivalry among systems, and rivalry for students. Schools of practice still contend with one another over the value of diagnostic or therapeutic technique. However, it should not be forgotten that although this diversity has been a source of irregular quality, history has also shown it to be an adaptive advantage. Acupuncture and all Chinese traditional medicines have benefited by absorbing the creativity of individuals. In fact, as we saw in our review of Chinese history, less popular individual systems have sometimes succeeded when the popular orthodoxy failed.

Because acupuncture relies almost entirely on naked-sense observation and hands-on techniques, clinical success depends not only on the body of knowledge, or a particular strategy, but also on human skills. The senses of sight, sound, touch, and smell provide the basis of clinical judgment and must be carefully developed to successfully treat patients. This is perhaps an even greater difference from modern biomedicine than is theoretical perspective. In biomedicine the instrumentation of both diagnosis and treatment constantly increases in range. Indeed, with exceptions such as surgical skill, biomedical practitioners' naked-sense observations have become largely limited to reading instrument panels and print-outs. In traditional medicine the practitioner's physical and sensory self is his or her diagnostic and therapeutic instrument. Great practitioners are often those who have elevated sensory skills, such as radial pulse palpation and visual inspection.

This too has had a strong influence on what aspects of the total theoretical model are used in clinical practice. In short, the dependence on, and especially the refinement of, naked-sense methods that characterize acupuncture has tended to limit the phenomena that are taken into clinical account. Thus, for our descriptive purposes, there is a relatively short list of phenomena classified by the *yin-yang* and five-phase frameworks that are relevant to clinical practice.[90]

Each of the correspondences in Tables 3.8 and 3.9 is a naked-sense observation, some of which offer interesting insights into Chinese thought. 'Sinew' includes those bodily structures responsible for locomotion, such as muscles, tendons, and ligaments. In Chinese, *jin* has a meaning much like the word 'nerve' had in Western languages before modern biology specified

Table 3.8 Somatic yin-yang correspondences

	Yin	Yang
Topography	Interior	Exterior
	Anterior	Posterior
	Inferior	Superior
	Right	Left
Organs	*Zang*	*Fu*
	Lung	Large intestine
	Spleen	Stomach
	Heart	Small intestine
	Kidney	Bladder
	Pericardium	*San jiao*
	Liver	Gallbladder
Channels	Arm *tai yin*	Arm *yang ming*
	Leg *tai yin*	Leg *yang ming*
	Arm *shao yin*	Arm *tai yang*
	Leg *shao yin*	Leg *tai yang*
	Arm *jue yin*	Arm *shao yang*
	Leg *jue yin*	Leg *shao yang*
Temperature	Cool/cold	Warm/hot
Activity	Hyperactivity	Hyperactivity
	Vacuity	Repletion
	Weakness	Strength
	Quiet voice	Loud voice
	Withdrawn	Outgoing

nervous-system structures in great detail. Sinew, like *jin*, is a compound of structures (tendons, muscle, ligament, and nerve) and function (movement, bending, and stretching). It is what the human observer notes, not a presumed cause or mechanism. 'Affect' is interesting because it shows the need to be sensitive to Chinese medical writers' distinctions rather than our own. Preoccupation is not an 'emotion,' the vernacular term often used in English. A practitioner who looks only for what we experience as emotional will miss signs that are in reality, habitual mental patterns. 'Taxation' brings governmental taxes to mind, because the Chinese word comes from the idea of 'taking a toll,' paying a consequence. The medical idea is identical, each *lao* incurs a human toll. Humans are taxed by too much sitting, just as their bank accounts are taxed by a loss of resources. The five taxations are sometimes translated as 'injurious labors,' which is an interesting expression of a modern prejudice, because three of the five are actually inactive states.

Table 3.9 Somato-psychic five-phase correspondences

	Wood	Fire	Earth	Metal	Water
Zang	Liver	Heart, pericardium	Spleen	Lung	Kidney
Fu	Gallbladder	Small intestine, san jiao	Stomach	Large intestine	Bladder
Channels	Leg *jue yin*, leg *shao yang*	Arm *shao yin*, arm *jue yin*, arm *tai yang*, arm *shao yang*	Leg *tai yin*, leg *yang ming*	Arm *tai yin*, arm *yang ming*	Leg *shao yin*, leg *tai yang*
Tissues	Sinews, nails	Blood vessels, blood	Flesh, lips	Skin, body hair	Bones, head hair
Sense organs	Eyes	Tongue	Mouth	Nose	Ears
Colors	Blue, green	Red	Yellow	White	Blue, black
Tastes	Sour	Bitter	Sweet	Spicy	Salty
Odors	Greasy	Scorched	Sweet	Raw	Flesh, rancid
Tones	Shouting	Laughing	Singing	Weeping	Groaning
Body fluids	Tears	Sweat	Saliva	Runny nose	Semen
Affect	Anger	Joy	Preoccupation	Sorrow	Fear
Climate	Wind	Heat	Damp	Dryness	Cold
Taxation	Walking	Watching	Sitting	Lying down	Standing
Foods	Wheat, chicken, plum	Millet, flour, apricot, sheep	Millet, cow, date	Rice plant, horse, peach	Bean, chestnut, pig

In these central clinical correspondences we see again the principal features of our illustrative black box, the analogies behind the correspondences. Since wood relates to spring, the phase of growth and expansion, it is natural for wood to correlate to the sinews, those structures responsible for locomotion. Too much walking can thus be injurious to sinew and its governing sphere, the liver. As the fire phase relates to heat and maximal levels of activity, it is natural for fire to correspond to the most active organ in the body, the heart, and thus to blood and all the vessels. As water relates to minimal levels of activity, the coldest time of the year and the storage of seeds for the future, water is the controlling image for those organs most responsible for water functions, the kidneys and bladder, and the reproductive organs responsible for the seed of humans.

We can also see in these lists why no school of thought uses every correspondence. The range of each is so large that each school tends to target phenomena with which its practitioners can gain skill. This selection of correspondence sets in each school is often based on social and cultural factors. In the West, this has led to labeling each style of practice by its ethnic origins (e.g. Korean Acupuncture). This is natural from the point view of an importer. However, that viewpoint contributes little to our understanding, which would be better based on more practical considerations. For example, as we saw in Chapter 1, in China, Confucian influence was pervasive. Verbal interrogation rather than palpation became the dominant method of gathering information because touch between humans and displays of the human body were strongly discouraged. Thus correspondence sets that could be applied by asking questions came to the fore.

In Japan, where Confucian influences were less powerful and acupuncture became a traditional employment for the blind, palpation rather than interrogation was emphasized. A well-known modern Japanese acupuncture book is called *Diagnosis Without Asking Questions*. Palpation methods dominate the information-gathering process, as do correspondences more readily accessed by observation. This reflects a bias opposite to that found among Chinese practitioners. This, in turn, led to its own process of independent development. For example, palpation led to an awareness of the body and its structure. This naturally inspired comparisons, for example, of the length of one leg to the other. Thus, ideas that depended on observation of bodily topography arose in Japan, and Japanese clinicians developed diagnostic techniques based on, for example, comparisons of the body's left and right sides.

In addition, various political philosophies and religious beliefs affected how correspondence sets were utilized. In China, during the 1960s and 1970s the system of five phases was minimized because it did not fit the Marxist perspective or serve China's need for thousands of quickly trained clinicians (there was hardly time to train the physical skills of acupuncture, much less a subtle sensitivity to, for example, color or odor). During the same period in England, the nation that spawned Marxist thinking, the five-phase system found philosophical acceptance in that society's need for a more holistic view of human life. Ironically, that social need was in many ways a response to late 20th century industrialization, just as Marxism was a response to an earlier stage of the same process. Whereas many practitioners trained in England frequently question patients about their feelings about themselves and others, a Chinese practitioner trained during the same period is more likely to inquire after physical functions such as digestion and elimination. In fact, Japanese acupuncturists' matter-of-fact talk about matters of 'the bathroom' often surprises European and American practitioners.

Economic factors also play a role. Because English-speaking practitioners have, until recently, been largely isolated from biomedical institutions such as hospitals, their work tends to center on conditions treated on an outpatient basis. On the other hand, because many Chinese practitioners have trained and worked in hospitals, they have acquired a larger repertoire of treatments for acute conditions. In Japan, where medical insurance covers all of biomedicine, but only a few conditions when treated by acupuncture, acupuncturists have specialized in the treatment of chronic, recidivistic disease for which biomedicine offers less desirable outcomes or where the drugs commonly used involve dangerous or unpleasant side-effects.

Because social circumstances vary, clinical methods, practices, and education also provide a variable influence over which correspondences are used. The correspondences that involve techniques that are harder to learn tend to fit one education system better than another. For example, the *Nan Jing Classic of Difficult Issues* recommends subtle needle techniques that are difficult to learn without an apprenticeship. One must learn from someone who uses them successfully, not from books or lectures. As we saw earlier, this mode of education has been largely replaced in China by a classroom approach designed to resolve China's public-health problems. Consequently, those needle techniques necessary to support the five-phase model are rarely seen. In Japan, where apprenticeship is still common, the five-phase correspondence models are more common, and there is intense competition among graduating acupuncturists for apprenticeships with recognized masters.

These practical considerations also have a feedback effect on theory. The five-phase model has historically been used in association with a diagnostic and therapeutic focus on the *jing luo* (channels) and thus upon the complex of intellectual and physical skills this focus requires. This orientation has influenced practice in Japan, the UK, and the USA. On the other hand, approaches that focus on the *zang fu* were strongly influenced by the practice of herbal medicine, which was absorbed into the medicine of systematic correspondences at a much later date. It focuses on *yin-yang* because *yin-yang* correspondences such as hot–cold and surface–interior better fit the evil *qi* penetration model articulated during the Song-Jin-Yuan when naturally occurring drugs were first absorbed into the medicine of systematic correspondence. Furthermore, just as the ideas of *qi*

and channels reflect the sensations associated with acupuncture, hot–cold and interior–exterior, better describe the sensations felt after ingesting medicinals. Chinese herbalism's long history of empirical practice provided herbalism with a wealth of refined observations. Thus the sets of correspondences that are utilized change the clinical perspective, the clinical perspective changes the theoretical view and, coupled with historical and clinical factors, the theoretical view changes the course of clinical investigation, changing the correspondence sets.

In Chapters 6 and 7 we will explore the diagnostic methods, approaches, and processes of several schools of thought. Here, Tables 3.8 and 3.9 outline different correspondence sets in common use. It is important to remember that each and all of these have a common root in the qi paradigm. For the sake of description, we have concentrated on three commonly used sets of correspondence logic. First, the *ba gang bian zheng* system, the TCM model employed in the acupuncture of modern China. TCM primarily uses *yin-yang* and *zang fu* data. Next, there is the *yin-yang* balancing approach, which is sometimes called 'classical acupuncture.' It is perhaps better thought of as the acupuncture practiced by a set of schools that concentrate upon the practical refinement of traditional principles. There are many systems in this category, but they are all channel based. They also tend to think of acupuncture as it was expressed in the foremost clinical classics; for example, books such as the late Ming dynasty compilation *Da Cheng*. This system is exemplified in the West by Europeans such as Soulie de Morant. In Asia, Yoshio Manaka was an outstanding practitioner. Finally, there is the *keiraku chiryo* system of traditional acupuncture that developed in Japan. It is largely a five-phase system that has had both direct and indirect effects on Western acupuncture. The Toyohari and Traditional Acupuncture schools are good examples of this approach.

The *ba gang bian zheng* system. The *ba gang bian zheng*, or eight-parameter pattern, identification method primarily focuses on the *zang fu*, and within the *zang fu*, the liver, spleen, kidney, heart, and lung. It utilizes clinical signs and symptoms that are categorized as shown in Box 3.13.[91] The system uses techniques that focus on organ functions and dysfunctions. Treatment foci and treatment principles are used to select acupoints meant to counter these imbalances. The principles are direct: if hot, cool it; if cold, heat it; if replete, drain it. If the problem is external, the TCM practitioner will focus on external aspects. Although, as we discussed earlier, five-phase correspondences are implicit to the extended analogies on which the system is based, they are not explicitly invoked during diagnosis and treatment. In particular, the five-phase cycles or interactions are rarely, if ever, explicitly used. The five-phase logic inherent in the historical development of *zang fu* functions is thus the only presence those correspondences have in this system.

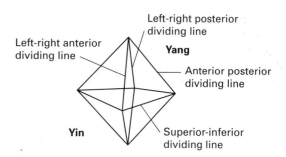

Figure 3.13   Structural octahedral body symmetry.

Box 3.14   Yin-yang balancing system: classification by body structure

Yin	Yang
Inferior	Superior
Anterior	Posterior
Right	Left

Box 3.13   Categorization of clinical signs and symptom in the *ba gang bian zheng* system

Yin	Yang
Cold	Hot
Internal	External
Vacuity	Repletion
Blood	*Qi*

The yin-yang balancing system.   *Yin-yang* balancing systems focus on the channels and ideas of interrelationship. This is the *sine qua non* of the approach. This orientation continues in systems derived from these traditional approaches. For example, the treatment philosophy developed by Yoshio Manaka focuses on the channels, but sees them as inseparable from the physical structure or topography of the body. Thus it classifies them according to structural polarities (Box 3.14).[92] The system focuses on a structurally based equilibration of *qi* distribution as defined by these topographic polarities (Fig. 3.13). The techniques used thus focus on regulating distribution and circulation of the *qi*. Five-phase theory and correspondences are used to help achieve this goal, as they represent another *qi* regulatory system.

The *keiraku chiryo* system.   The *keiraku chiryo* channel therapy or system focuses primarily on the channels, especially problems of vacuity and repletion. It is strongly rooted in information organized according to the five-phase system. In the simplest terms, the primary diagnoses are: lung vacuity, spleen vacuity, liver vacuity, and kidney vacuity. These four patterns combine phase and channel theory and serve as a springboard for therapy. Treatments target an equilibration of circulation and distribution of *qi* among the 12 channels, and an overall balance of the five phases.[93]

Each of these different systems of practice is rooted in the same traditional theories, whether the focus is on the *zang fu*, the channels, *yin-yang*, the five phases, or the general distribution and circulation of *qi*. Behind each are a series of stated and unstated assumptions. For example, a focus on equilibrating *qi* distribution is assumed to improve organ function. Likewise, a focus on five-phase channel balancing will also improve organ function, and the *zang fu* practitioner assumes that a focus on restoring normal organ function will restore normal *qi* circulation. These assumptions all exemplify the regulatory nature of *qi*, and thus the regulatory strategies provided by *yin-yang* and the five phases. Change in one part of the system initiates change and balance throughout the whole.

The general philosophical frameworks from which the theories of *yin-yang* and the five phases arose assumed a general unity in nature. Everything is implicitly connected with everything else, and a change in one part implicitly produces changes in other parts, some more directly than others. Symbolically, heaven is necessarily tied to earth, the blood is a reflection of the *qi*, interior relates to exterior, hot to cold, *yin* to *yang*. Nature was seen as a system of antagonistic–syntagonistic relationships. All things were not simply pairs of opposites, but opposites in complementary relation. The wood phase is implicitly tied to the phases of fire, earth, metal, and water; a change in any will potentially change any or all.

On the broadest level, the *yin-yang* and five-phase models describe basic rules that are assumed to operate globally to maintain an ordered balance in nature and humans. In modern terms, they are algorithms that form the operating system which controls the behavior and interaction of the human program. It is not that they do all the work (perform all the functions for which a computer may be used), rather it is that they govern the relationship between all the programs that the system may operate. These rules govern not only global interactions, but all the subsets of global interaction. In acupuncture, these subsets are each of the systems of correspondence. In mathematical terms, the body, and on a larger scale, nature, is a complex dynamic system. Thus *yin-yang* and the five phases are rules that describe the probable order within an infinity of possible behaviors.

Interactions, regulation, and balance

Yin–yang

So far we have looked at the theories of *yin-yang* in one dimension, as a vertical plane of contiguous relationships, as a wave, as sets of correspondences. However, these theories also apply on a horizontal plane; that is, as a series of interdependent qualities and relationships. In fact, it is these relationships that allow acupuncturists to predict therapeutic effects. In terms of *yin* and *yang*, the following generalizations can be made.[94]

First, *yin* and *yang* are interdependent. This principle is what is graphically epitomized in the famous *taiji* symbol of the *dao* (Fig. 3.14), but is general in East Asian thought rather than specific to daoism. Here *yin* and *yang* define each other. *Yin* cannot exist without *yang*. We cannot understand hot without cold. This is a very general human observation. For example, when we teach children the idea of 'hot' we often compare a safe source of heat to something cooler to the touch.

Furthermore, nothing is purely *yin* and nothing is purely *yang*. The seeds of one are always contained in the other. This is the significance of the opposite-colored dots in each half of the *taiji* symbol. Another way to think of this is to imagine *yin* and *yang* as polarities in a continuous cycle. Again, this is a universal human observation of interdependence. In nature there are continuous transformations between two extremes, neither of which is ever absolute. This is evident in the passage of day into night. The extreme of darkness and coolness continuously transforms into the extreme of lightness and heat, only to transform again to night. Even at the heat of high noon, there is dark (e.g. shade beneath a tree). Even at midnight, there is the light of the stars. Because everything ultimately follows these cycles of transformation, Chinese medical books refer to transformations between the two extremes or poles as 'the interdependence of *yin* and *yang*.'

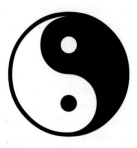

Figure 3.14 *Taiji*: the traditional *yin-yang* symbol.

Just as importantly, *yin* and *yang* balance each other. As each always contains the seed of the other, it is impossible for one to change without the other also changing. As opposites of one another, continuous interconnectedness manifests as balance. All the *yin* functions, surfaces, areas, and parts of the body are continuously balanced by all the *yang* functions, surfaces, areas, and parts of the body. A relative balance of all of these is health. If the *yin* functions of an organ are relatively balanced by the *yang* functions of that organ, there is a healthy condition. If the flow of the *yin* channels is relatively balanced to the flow of the yang channels, this too is a state of health. If the total strength and quality of *qi* in the lower half of the body is relatively the same as the strength and quality of *qi* in the upper half of the body, that too is healthy.

Pathology results when imbalances between *yin* and *yang* occur. If someone has poor breathing habits, a stressful lifestyle, and spends too much time thinking, a relative *qi* imbalance between the upper and lower halves of the body will ensue. From this many different conditions can develop. In Chinese this is called 'repletion above with vacuity below.' According to the principle of *yin-yang*, the body is always striving to maintain a normal state through natural counterbalances. It is these effects that are described by *yin-yang* correspondences. In other words, the body is always balanced, whether or not we like the means it employs to achieve that balance. When someone's physical or mental habits are so extreme that they cannot be counterbalanced comfortably, the body's operating system will initiate more violent measures. This is recognized in the West by the macabre slogan that 'cancer cures smoking.' Eating one meal that is too hot and too spicy for your digestive system may lead to nothing more than counterflow *qi*, the hot belching we Westerners call 'indigestion.' However, a drug so powerful or a habit so constant that it overwhelms the body's balancing ability produces a condition known as the 'separation of *yin* and *yang*.' When *yin* and *yang* separate, the precondition for life ceases and we die.

Acupuncturists are trained to recognize b problems and to utilize treatment methods help restore a normal state. Implicit in this id is the notion that the acupuncturist takes advantage of natural opportunities to restore balance. This is the therapeutic function of *yin-yang* logic, to help us recognize opportunities to restore balance. For example, in both of the above cases the acupuncturist would supplement the lower half while draining the upper half of the body. The practitioner would select points and techniques to strengthen the *yin* aspect on the lower half and to drain the *yang* aspect on the upper half. But the quality of the treatment chosen would also be in balance, a balance regulated by the quality of the condition treated. For simple counterflow *qi* the treatment would be fairly mild. For drug poisoning, it would involve the induction of vomiting or purging, powerful stimuli to drive the poison outward so that the body's restorative processes could successfully function.

The counterbalancing properties of *yin* and *yang* are frequently shown as a series of boxes (Fig. 3.15). As one increases, the other declines, like the two arms of a pivot scale. This is another good illustration of how Western biases affect our understanding because this view of complementary antagonism expresses only the primary theoretical aspect of *yin-yang*. It satisfies our desire for clear, precise statements, but it does so by hiding the clinical applications. Furthermore, it is often further interpreted as 'good [*yang*] and bad [*yin*].' Because *yang* qualities (activity, maleness, heat) touch certain chauvinisms prevalent in Western societies and characteristics we fear less as disease (fever, aggressivity, hyperfunction), *yin* with its more fearsome connotations of vulnerability to attack too often becomes 'too *yin*,' an absolute idea that does not fit *yin-yang*.

In the clinic the diversity of phenomena is so great and the manifestations of *yin-yang* interaction so various that the clinician must observe and interpret an entire complex of major and minor correspondences, all interacting simultaneously. When teaching, Dr Manaka often used a large, complex mobile to illustrate the multi-

N.B

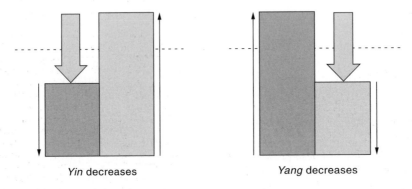

Equilibrium of *yin* and *yang*

Yin decreases   *Yang* decreases

Figure 3.15 Primary theoretical *yin-yang* balance.

dimensionality of clinical reality (Fig. 3.16). There are always many adjustments made by the body to counter a particular imbalance, just as can be seen in such a mobile.[95] *Yin* and *yang* are never absolutely excessive or deficient, there is always balance. It is only that some of these balance mechanisms are 'too much for comfort.' What the skillful practitioner seeks is the place upon the mobile where intervention can restore a healthy balance with the least force.

Clinically, this basic rule of counterbalance is applied in many ways. If the *yin* liver functions are weak, the *yang* functions can become replete and inappropriately active relative to the *yin* functions. This relativity is individual. For example, any liver function measured by Western biochemical means might be normal in one person, or even the same person at a different age. But, the identical measurement would be pathological for someone else. In fact, this is explicitly recognized in biomedicine because ideas of excess and deficiency are stated as ranges around a norm (standard deviations). In acupuncture,

however, these patterns are given clinical substance by constitutional systems, methods of generally categorizing types of relative balance.

Whichever categorization system is applied, in the case of a liver *yin* vacuity, the treatment would be aimed at strengthening the *yin* functions, termed 'supplementing liver *yin*.' However, in a more profound case where this would be inadequate to counterbalance the *yang* functions, the latter could also be made less replete by 'draining liver *yang*.' Here the image in Chinese is one of the *yang* aspect bursting forth, expressed as, for example, an overwhelming of the functions of the stomach and spleen.

If the lung channel is vacuous, that is, if there is a hollowness of the quality and force of qi, then the related *yang* channels, particularly the coupled large intestine channel, will be replete or stagnant. If you think of the lung–large intestine *yin-yang* pair as a three-dimensional figure, such as a ball, then one side is depressed, and the other is raised; the ball is out-of-round. In such a case, treatment

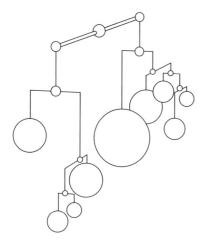

Figure 3.16 Clinical *yin-yang* balance.

might be aimed at strengthening the flow of *qi* in the lung channel (supplementing the lung channel). However, if this were insufficient to reduce the *qi* in the large intestine channel, the acupuncturist would choose points to drain the large intestine channel. With the right clues, the adept practitioner would look for the condition responsible for both the lung channel vacuity and the large intestine repletion, and eliminate both by treating the common source. (See Box 3.15).

When engineers praise a solution as precise, they call it 'elegant.' It does exactly what it must do, with the absolute minimum of steps. This same elegance is also a goal in acupuncture, which is why 'one point for one symptom' acupuncturists have often been ridiculed. In one of the most famous texts, the *Yi Xue Rumen* (1575), it is said:

A single puncture can make hundreds of illnesses disappear. Make at the maximum four punctures. Those who riddle the whole body with needles are detestable.[97]

The one-needle cure is an ideal (because it is by no means a daily reality); however, practitioners who achieve more elegant treatments tend to consider the whole human. They look for clues in a complex and dynamic system. Rather than seeing *yin-yang* as one dimensional, only supplementing the vacuous, or draining the replete, they perceive *yin-yang* and the five

phases as multidimensional feedback loops, like the complex mobile.

Five phases

Five-phase theory, for example, can be thought of as describing interaction between phases on more than one plane. As we discussed earlier, it is logically very similar to the *yin-yang* model, except that it is a little more complex, with five interacting components. Traditionally the five phases were described as interacting along four different pathways. The *sheng*, or 'engendering' cycle, and the *ko*, or 'restraining cycle,' are the

---

Box 3.15 *Yin-yang* relativity

While composing the example of relativity between lung channel vacuity and large intestine channel repletion, an interesting article appeared in *The Boston Globe*.[96] In this article the surprising result of a long-term Finnish study was detailed. The study of 29 000 male smokers in Finland was meant to show whether daily doses of beta-carotene and vitamin E prevented lung cancer in heavy smokers. The largest surprise to researchers was that the study contradicted previous research, showing that the two vitamins did not have a beneficial effect on the incidence of lung cancer. They also reported that those who took the vitamins had lower incidences of both prostate cancer (30% lower) and colorectal cancer (16% lower).

Traditional Chinese *yin-yang* logic provides a different view of lung cancer. Seeing smoking as a hot, dry stimulus, a Chinese physician would expect the lungs, which must be kept moist, warm, and free-flowing, to become replete or stagnant (lung cancer). In other words, people living in a cold, damp climate (Finland) will seek to warm and dry their lungs. Those who warm and dry their lungs with a hot, dry stimulus that is powerful enough to overwhelm the body's more comfortable balances (heavy smoking) risk the deadly balance of this disease (lung cancer). However, because the colon and the bladder (prostate) are most harmed by vacuity and cold, and the upward and outward dynamic stimulated by smoking keeps *qi* from stagnating in the lower body, those with the 'lung cancer balance' are less likely to exhibit diseases of lower body repletion and stagnation (such as colorectal and prostrate cancer). The Chinese physician would look for problems of cold and vacuity in the lower body, as indicated by the *yin-yang* adage 'hot above, cold below,' then ask what it might be about these vitamins, or the constitutions of the groups tested, that would affect lower-body repletion and stagnation.

most important. The counter-cycle pathways, and the counter-engendering and the counter-restraining cycles are of secondary significance. However, taken as a whole, these four paths yield a model of interactions where each phase is always in relation to all other phases.

The engendering cycle is stated as follows:[98] wood engenders (is the mother of) fire; fire engenders earth; earth engenders metal; metal engenders water; water engenders wood. By these principles, if there is an increase in wood, wood will then increase fire. If there is an increase in earth, earth will increase metal. This is represented diagrammatically as shown in Figure 3.17. Since each phase has a corresponding organ and channel, these principles can be used to strengthen weakness in the organs and, especially, the channels:

wood → fire → earth → metal → water
liver → heart/ → spleen → lung → kidney
    pericardium
gallbladder → small → stomach → large → bladder
      intestine/   intestine
      san jiao

The restraining cycle is stated as follows:[99] wood restrains earth; earth restrains water; water restrains fire; fire restrains metal; metal restrains wood; wood restrains earth. By these principles if there is an increase in earth, water is reduced; if there is an increase in wood, earth is reduced. Metaphorically this cycle is described by the following: metal restrains

wood – the bronze axe cuts down the tree; wood restrains earth – the growing roots of the tree displace the soil; earth restrains water – earth is used to bank up and dam water; water restrains fire – water puts out the fire; fire restrains metal – the heat of fire melts the metal. This cycle is represented diagrammatically as shown in Figure 3.18. These interactions occur between the organs and, especially, the channels:[100]

wood → earth → water → fire → metal
liver → spleen → kidney → heart/ → lung
               pericardium
gallbladder → stomach → bladder → small → large
                     intestine/ intestine
                     san jiao

The engendering and restraining cycles are usually shown in a single diagram (Fig. 3.19).

The counter-engendering and counter-restraining cycles are precisely the reverse of the above cycles. They are important to an understanding of the dynamics of the whole model, but are not as often used clinically. Most five-phase treatments focus on the engendering and restraining cycles. In our sample problem of vacuity in the metal phase, specifically, a lung-channel vacuity, an experienced practitioner would look for pathoconditions that correspond with spleen function. Finding these, he or she would strengthen the earth phase via the spleen channel. This takes advantage of the engendering cycle. Any action that increases earth will engen-

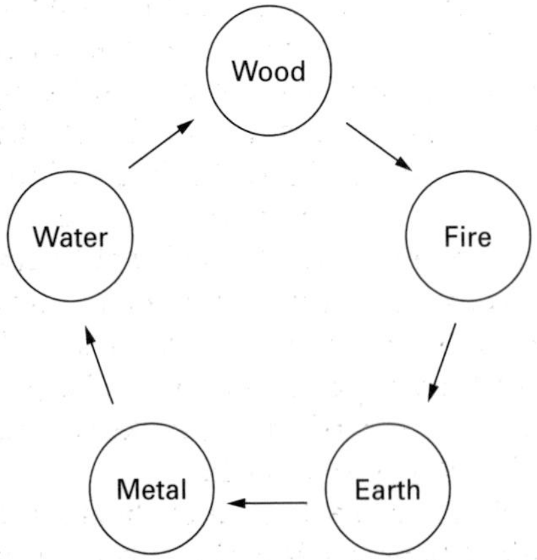

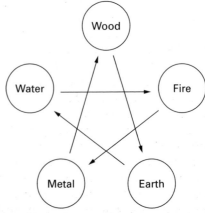

Figure 3.17 The engendering cycle of the five phases.

Figure 3.18 The restraining cycle of the five phases.

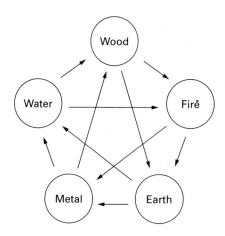

Figure 3.19 Composite diagram of the five phases.

der metal. Thus strengthening the spleen channel will strengthen the lung channel. This principle is the most basic approach to the practice of acupuncture using the five-phase model.

However, there are other approaches. In a vacuity condition of the lung channel, the heart or pericardium channels could also be drained to improve the condition. This takes advantage of the restraining cycle, specifically, the action of fire restraining metal. In this cycle, if fire increases, metal decreases. Any deliberate therapeutic action that reduces fire will tend to increase metal, by taking advantage of the natural action of fire on metal. This is also another important feature in clinical practice. The same condition can be treated in different ways, depending on the accompanying signs. It is the overall pattern that is most important, not any one part of the diagnosis. The most elegant treatment is thus the choice that addresses the broadest set of clinical observations.

As we will see in Chapters 6 and 7, these principles are not followed by all schools of thought, and the clinical techniques necessary to utilize these principles are used by some and not others. As with the *yin-yang* model, the five-phase model can be seen as describing rules of interaction where positive and negative feedback loops are used to maintain a stable state. Each school has developed from different backgrounds to deal with different clinical and historical circumstances. And, while they do

differ, and each has advantages and disadvantages, all represent some aspect of the many-faceted ability of acupuncture.

Traditional models and their clinical consequences

As we move on to examine diagnosis and treatment in clinical practice, please keep the essentials in mind – it is easy to get captured in the myriad details. The simplest description of what is portrayed by the *yin-yang* and five-phase models is to say that they are algorithms; that is, they are procedures for discovering how any given bodily event fits amidst the interactive systems that regulate the human body. As a famous acupuncturist (who we will not name) once said, 'Acupuncture is not God.' In other words, *yin-yang* and the five phases are not 'Truth' with a capital 'T.' They describe patterns that produce complex but predictable behaviors. *Yin* and *yang* are like the Mandelbrot set, a simple equation iterated over and over to generate a complex picture.

Like everything in nature, the body is unified by the idea of *qi*. *Qi* described what was predictable in the traditional Chinese view – the orderly manifestations of an indivisible whole. *Qi* explains the immaterial basis of repeatable observations operating beyond the realm of the human senses. As systems of medical practice evolved, it was necessary to subdivide and classify these *qi* so that they could be learned and used. Thus the most useful models of *qi* are splintered into numerous subsets. Because different subsets appealed to different people at different times, different schools of thought developed. Because different schools of thought needed to contend with different economic, social, and political trends, different techniques and clinical refinements developed. Because it takes not only time but also access to a skillful teacher and many patients to learn the practical clinical expressions of correspondences, schools of thought tended to specialize.

Thus what appears to be a confusing array of minuscule differences is really a long history of effective adaptation. Some degree of specialization appears to be necessary to the evolution of any medical practice. However, the root principles of acupuncture are more constant than is often assumed. As we have just seen, the various concepts of *yin-yang*, five phases, and *zang-fu* retain much of their original unitary nature, even if it is not always explicitly stated.

It is also important to remember that the general theories of *yin-yang* and the five phases describe both horizontal interactions (regulatory mechanisms within the body) as well as the vertical sets of correspondences (qualitative relationships between things and events) that may have no direct interaction in the sense-perceived world of temporal and spatial proximity. As we will see in Chapter 7, because everything is described according to these schemes, there is always a starting point for treatment.

In Chapter 6, as we explore the concept of health and the nature of disease, or imbalance, we will see that there are many different diagnostic patterns and methods of information gathering. Many of the systems we will explore use the principles outlined in this chapter. However, we will also describe approaches that consider only direct, empirical evidence, and those where devices replace what were traditionally human skills. Thus, it will be important to keep two more principles in mind.

First, traditional systems vary from modern systems in the assumption that treatment of any part of a whole takes advantage of interactions that affect the whole. You will see that this is particularly the case for treatment systems that deliberately take advantage of *yin-yang* and five-phase relationships, not just their correspondences. However, this is also implicit in other approaches to therapy, even when it is less explicitly stated. For example, practitioners who focus on the organs usually assume they are affecting the related channels.

Secondly, even though diagnosis of a pathology by biomedical means does occur in acupuncture, and so-called 'formula acupuncture' is not uncommon, traditional clinicians still assume that the whole can be realized through inspection of any of the parts. Practically, some systems are more straightforward, but all share this quality. A classic example is pulse palpation, but the same is true for abdominal palpation, visual observation, tongue inspection, and systematic questioning. Each of these systems focuses on particular information to acquire knowledge applicable to the whole body.

In sum, acupuncture is a widespread, philosophically varied practice that has done an unimaginably great service to humankind. We doubt that its service to our species has as yet been completely explored or applied. However, although it may have many wonderful new applications, those on which we will continue to concentrate are those that reflect the traditional world view from which it sprang. Thus far, that focus has been upon traditionally based acupuncture. Before examining the details of clinical practice in Chapters 6 and 7, it is important to examine acupuncture from the perspectives of modern science. As acupuncture has been assimilated and acculturated in the West, and as science has been assimilated and acculturated in the East, new models and new perspectives on acupuncture have developed. We will examine these in the next two chapters.

In Chapter 4 we introduce and explore evolving modern explanatory models of acupuncture, the investigative processes, and the questions asked. In addition, we will discuss some of the methodologies and technologies used in these investigations. In Chapter 5 we examine how to determine the conditions for which acupuncture is effective, and thus those conditions for which medical providers should consider referrals to an acupuncturist. The questions, issues, and methods of clinical trials are discussed in detail. The scientific investigation of acupuncture is critical to the future developments of acupuncture everywhere in the world, not only because this affects its future acculturation, but also because it is already an essential component of the continuing evolution and adaptation of acupuncture.

NOTES

1   Unschuld PU 1990 Forgotten traditions of ancient Chinese medicine. Paradigm Publications, Brookline, MA, pp 118, 200

2   See note 1, pp 339–340

3   See note 1, p 33

4   See note 1, pp 183–185

5   Beijing Foreign Languages Institute 1980 The Sino Chinese–English dictionary. Sino, New York, p 291

6   Wiseman N, Boss K 1990 Glossary of Chinese medicine and acupuncture points. Paradigm Publications Brookline, MA, pp xxviii–xxvix

7   Wiseman N, Feng Y 1998 Compilers' preface. In: A practical dictionary of traditional Chinese medicine. Paradigm Publications, Brookline, MA, p v

8   Wen Tian Xiang quoted in: Manaka Y, Itaya K, Birch S 1995 Chasing the dragon's tail. Paradigm Publications, Brookline, MA, p 5

9   Zhuang Zi quoted in: Needham J 1956 Science and civilisation in China. Cambridge University Press, Cambridge, vol II, p 76

10   Wang Cong quoted in: Matsumoto K, Birch S 1988 Hara diagnosis: reflections on the sea. Paradigm Publications, Brookline, MA, p 114

11   See note 9, p 281

12   Unschuld PU 1998 Chinese medicine. Paradigm Publications, Brookline, MA, p 40

13   Fung, Yu-lan 1952 A history of Chinese philosophy. Princeton University Press, Princeton, NJ, vol 1, p 362

14   Ellis A, Wiseman N, Boss K 1989 Grasping the wind. Paradigm Publications, Brookline, MA, pp 1–8

15   Soulie de Morant G 1994 Chinese acupuncture. Paradigm Publications, Brookline, MA, p 24

16   See note 14, pp 5–6

17   See note 14, p 309

18   See note 14, p 23

19   Unschuld PU 1986 Medicine in China: Nan Ching the classic of difficult issues. University of California Press, Berkeley, p 457

20   See: *xie qi* in: Wiseman N, Feng Y 1998 A practical dictionary of Chinese medicine. Paradigm Publications, Brookline, MA, pp 180–181

21   See note 1, p 216

22   Requena Y. Personal communication

23   Eisenberg D, Wright TL 1987 Encounters with qi. Penguin, New York, p 139

24   Wiseman N. Personal communication

25   Unschuld PU 1997 Chinesische Medizin; CH Beck, Munich, pp 45–63 passim

26   See note 10, p 71

27   The *yin-yang* and five-phase data are abstracted from: Wiseman N, Ellis A 1995 Fundamentals of Chinese medicine, rev edn. Paradigm Publications, Brookline, MA, p 15

28   Abstracted from: Ellis A, Wiseman N, Boss K 1991 Fundamentals of Chinese acupuncture, rev edn. Paradigm Publications, Brookline, MA, p 16

29   See note 6, pp xii–xiii

30   Abstracted from: Wiseman N 1998 A practical dictionary of Chinese medicine. Paradigm Publications, Brookline, MA

31   See: note 28, p 38; note 8, p 66 Manaka, Itaya, Birch

32   Abstracted from: Wiseman & Ellis (note 27, ch 2 passim)

33   Abstracted from: Wiseman & Ellis (note 27, ch 10 passim)

34   Foss L, Rothenberg K 1987 The second medical revolution. Shambhala, Boston, MA

35   Needham J, Lu GD 1974 Science and civilisation in China. Cambridge University Press, Cambridge, vol V, part 2, p 86

36   See note 35, p 87

37   See note 10, p 35

38   See note 10, p 110

39   See note 10, p 20

40   See note 10, p 84

41   See note 10, p 89

42   See note 10, p 90

43   See note 10, p 10

44   Paraphrased from note 10, p 91

45   See note 10, chs 3, 5, 6

46   (a) See note 10 ch 3
    (b) European Journal of Oriental Medicine 1(1), 1994

47   Wiseman N, Ellis A 1985 Fundamentals of Chinese medicine. Paradigm Publications, Brookline, MA, p xxii

48   See the discussion in note 10, ch 3

49   Mann H. Personal communication

50   Manaka Y. Personal communication

51   See note 8, p 5

52   George Soulie de Morant stated '… the name *qi* which we translate, for lack of a better word, as "energy." His descriptions of *qi* as energy are broader and more sophisticated than many of those that apply his choice of term. See note 15, p 46

53   See note 15, p 6

54   Anon 1998 Acupuncture. NIH consensus development panel on acupuncture. JAMA 280(17):1518–1524

55   See note 6, p xxxiii

56   Ulett G 1992 Beyond *yin* and *yang*; H Green, St Louis, MI

57   Englehardt U 1986 Translating and interpreting the *Fu-Ch'i Ching-i Lun*; experiences gained from editing a T'ang dynasty Taoist medical treatise. In: Unschuld PU (ed) Approaches to traditional Chinese medical literature. Kluwer, Dordrecht, p 130

58   Capra F 1982 The turning point. Bantam, New York, p 266

59   Cunningham A 1986 Information and health in the many levels of man: toward a more comprehensive theory of health and disease. Advances 3(1): 32–45

60   See note 58, p 282

61   (a) Foss L, Rothenberg K 1987 The second medical revolution. Shambhala, Boston
    (b) For a more technical model of information theory, see: Schffeniels E 1976 Anti-chance. Pergammon, New York
    (c) For discussions of the relevance of these theories in the Chinese model, see note 58
    (d) For more discussions of the relevance of these models in acupuncture, see note 8

62   For a description of the mathematical models summarized here, see note 8, pp 391–411. For one of the speculative models, see note 8, pp 391–397

63   Unschuld PU 1985 Medicine in China: a history of ideas. University of California Press, Berkeley, pp 67–68

64   See note 8, pp 17–37

65   See note 10, p 141

66   Wiseman N, Ellis A 1985 Fundamentals of Chinese medicine. Paradigm Publications, Brookline, MA, p 38

67   See: note 8, p 49; note 28, p 32

68   See: note 8, p 56 ff; note 28, pp 33–35

69   See: note 8, p 56; note 28, p 38

70   See note 28, pp 56–70

71   See note 28, pp 31–38

72   See note 28, pp 440–442

73   See note 28, p 45

74   The primary symptoms of gallbladder vacuity are: 'signs of anxiety and indecision, clouded vision, tinnitus and poor hearing, "timid gallbladder" (lack of courage) and suceptiblity to fright.' See: Wiseman N, Feng Y 1998 Compilers' preface. In: A practical dictionary of traditional Chinese medicine. Paradigm Publications, Brookline MA, p 236

75   See note 74, p 78

76   See note 66, p 66

77   See note 10, pp 134–135

78   See note 6, p xi

79   Soulie de Morant G 1994 Chinese acupuncture. Paradigm Publications, Brookline, MA, p 269

80   See note 28, pp 51–75

81   Sivin N 1987 Traditional medicine in contemporary China. Center for Chinese studies, University of Michigan, Ann Arbor, MI, p 287

82   See note 28, p 51

83   See: Coseo M 1992 The acupressure warmup. Paradigm Publications, Brookline, MA

84   See note 28, pp 132–133

85   See note 28, pp 132–133

86   See note 28, pp 132–133

87   Taken from Ellis, Wiseman & Boss (see note 14)

88   See note 79, pp 376–378

89   For a discussion see: note 27, pp 177–181

90   See note 27 pp 5–16 passim

91   See note 27, pp 127–144 passim

92   See note 8, pp 41–47

93   Yanagishita T, What is qi. Toyohari Seminars, Boston, MA May 1995

94   For a discussion see: note 27, pp 1–16, passim

95   See note 8, p 41

96   Boston Globe, April 13, 1994, V246, N103

97   See note 79, p 170

98   For a discussion see: note 27, pp 7–14 passim

99   See note 27, pp 7–14 passim

100   See note 27, pp 7–14 passim

4

How does acupuncture work?

This is a fascinating question that traditional Asians never asked. There was no need to ask because they already had an answer. *Qi* was that answer and it was sufficient for generations. In the West this is a critical question. Without an answer rooted in our own ways of thinking, acupuncture probably cannot be fully adopted. The mounting evidence that it does work has kept it from the ranks of outlaw medicines. Already, fewer and fewer people use the words 'acupuncture' and 'quack' in the same sentence. Regardless, nothing that science labels as 'merely empirical,' or 'unproven,' receives the social investment required for adoption by today's mainstream health-care systems.

The reason why scientific judgements are critical is that the majority of medical research, education, and development is funded by patient fees, government funds, and those who hope their investments in medical research will result in profitable products, typically pharmaceuticals or devices. Put bluntly, aquiring funding is the first and critical component of scientific investigation. Decisions about who will receive that funding are made by researchers from institutions steeped in the Western scientific tradition. Their decisions are based on working agreements among professional scientists conditioned by social, political, and commercial goals. When some majority trend is apparent, the people who have contributed to the development of that trend become the academic juries and government panels that decide what research will be funded. Research funding is the practical expression of professional consensus at any given time.

Although far fewer Western practices than most non-scientists believe have been put through state-of-the-art research scrutiny, new medical approaches are still required to face this trial. The first step in that trial is to engage the interest of enough professional scientists to acquire the necessary resources. One significant aspect of acquiring that interest is answering the question 'How?' (Box 4.1). Although that answer does not always need to be complete and totally seamless, it must be sufficient to satisfy the general criteria of the established science professions. To succeed in this attempt, acupuncture must overcome several considerable problems, not the least of which is the problem of *qi*.

THE PROBLEM OF *QI*

Today, for the most part, those who receive acupuncture treatment, as well as most of those who provide it, do not ask 'How did this work?' They are content with the fact that it did. The notion that acupuncture affects 'energy' is all the rationale most patients and practitioners need. Energy is for them what *qi* was for generations of Asians, a culturally credible answer that ends their inquiry. But is *any* energy *qi* and will that assumption satisfy the need for an engaging research rationale for acupuncture?

Although it is clearly possible that some phenomena labeled *qi* in traditional Chinese and Japanese texts are in fact forms of energy, perhaps even forms of energy physics has yet to define, as far as anyone yet knows *qi* is not energy at all. When people use the word 'energy' to translate *qi*, they are not translating a Chinese idea but using a familiar word to resolve Western fears concerning medicine and technology. It is easier to accept the idea of *qi* if it is replaced by the positive associations of the word 'energy.' In Paul Unschuld's words:

> By explaining disease in terms of energetic disturbances, Chinese medicine gains plausibility, but a plausibility that arises out of conceptual adaptation to Western fears, not out of the historical reality of Chinese thinking.[3]

It is fair to repeat the fact that, when any deep-seated Asian concept is understood as a familiar Western notion, it is probably misunderstood. But it is also fair to note that the idea of energy has become popular because it reflects human experience. Acupuncture makes you feel better, stronger, more positive. Therefore, by analogy, it provides energy, just as food or the company of good friends makes us feel more energetic.

In science, however, unlike *qi* in the traditional East or meaningful expressions in English, energy needs to be a measurable entity. Before acupuncture can achieve scientific acceptance, its functions must be explained. Energy alone is too narrow a research strategy. Thus, if we wish acupuncture

---

Box 4.1 Paradigmatic walls?

Skepticism about acupuncture is rooted in Western cultural predispositions about what can and cannot be true. Whether or not these examples evidence truly paradigmatic walls, they do show that it is doubtful acupuncture will win scientific acceptance by showing only that it is an effective medical intervention. It must also have a demonstrable physiological explanation of how it works. Otherwise the evidence simply disappears against the background expectations of what can and cannot be true. This requirement for scientific acceptance rarely surfaces in the scientific literature, because scientific writing formats leave so little room for the direct expression of individual opinion. However, it does at times nonetheless emerge. For example, in a review of homeopathic literature, a Dutch team analysed clinical trials of homeopathy. They found objective evidence that its effects were not attributable to placebo alone. However, despite their own conclusion, the authors paradoxically rejected homeopathy because current explanations of how it works were 'too fantastic to believe.[1]

After the US National Institutes of Health review panel concluded that acupuncture had evidenced success in clinical trials, a report on that meeting published in the *Journal of the American Medical Association* quoted Dr Fred Levit, who is described as 'knowledgeable about acupuncture,' as asserting that acupuncture 'works by suggestion.'[2] Despite any obvious participation in acupuncture research, his quote is given the prestige of publication, despite the fact that suggestion was accounted for by the controls of the clinical trials reported. In other words, the editors of this pervasive biomedical journal simply did not believe the evidence.

to survive its inevitable scientific trial, we need to understand how the Chinese conceived (and still conceive) of *qi*, and we need to know how those qualities relate to the problem of describing the function of acupuncture. To do so we must examine how *qi* is perceived in traditional East Asian medicines. Before we can hypothesize what *qi* is, or measure what we propose it to be, we must first look to what it has always been thought to do. Otherwise we cannot conceive of valid theories and tests.

There are thousands of descriptions of *qi*. As linguist Nigel Wiseman describes, to the Chinese, *qi* refers to anything that is perceptible but intangible.[4] It is used in Chinese to refer to anything we understand to be present but cannot actually perceive with our senses. In other words, *qi* is everything that plays a role without revealing itself to the naked human senses. Sinologist Nathan Sivin states that, in Chinese, *qi* is sometimes that which animates change in the material world. He also notes that in Chinese it is also used to describe the material in which change occurs.[5] Smell is intangible but perceptible; it does something to your nose. It was naturally called a *qi*. That *qi* is not merely a primitive expression for air-borne molecules or olfactory receptors. It is not even the idea of an odor; rather, it is the entire complex of the natural stimulus and the human response.

In Chinese, waste passing through the intestines is referred to as *zhuo qi*, or 'turbid *qi*.' It is in complementary opposition to the *qing qi*, or 'clear *qi*,' which the *pi* (spleen) is said to produce from food.[6] Although clear *qi* is reasonably seen as an analog of nutrients in modern biology, it is neither those nutrients nor any specific energy or process used in their production. It is a symbol for the observable sum of human metabolism. The Chinese observation recognizes that eating and excreting are intrinsically linked to life, and that the quality of someone's appetite, stool, urine, and other digestive functions are indicative of their state of health. This is the assumption behind the idea that appetite, stool, urine, and nutritional state tell us something about people's *qi*. The assertion of the Chinese expression is not that *qi* is one

energy that separates into two component energies. Instead, it asserts that there is a perceptible link between human health and digestive function. For the sake of definition, we can think of turbid *qi* as the movement of waste through the intestines, or we can think of clear *qi* as an energy that drives metabolism, but to the Chinese both were just *qi*.

All ideas of *qi* are the results of observation with the unaided human senses. *Qi* is thus as various as the human capacity for observation. As noted earlier, *qi* is felt to emanate from people, landscapes, even moments in time. That is, human feelings are assigned a source in *qi*. *Qi* is also inferred from clinical observations. For example, the traditional conception that the *qi* of environmental phenomena can penetrate the body's defensive *qi*, overwhelming its right *qi*, producing illness, is not a description of a single, actual flow. It is, instead, the description of a predictable relationship. In fact, the one *qi* that is actually discussed in terms of flow is *ying qi*, channel *qi*. Thus, this is one research subject where electrical and electromagnetic energies certainly play a role. As this is the *qi* mostly discussed in the West, it has come to stand for *qi* in general and is typically the central focus of basic science research in acupuncture. However, as in the example of modern ideas of the extraordinary vessels, when all forms of *qi* are thought of as channel *qi*, as a material flow, Chinese ideas are obscured.

On the whole, *qi* was, and is, too broad a concept to be covered by the idea of energy in either lay or scientific terms.[7] The word 'energy' is a convenient short-hand that allows us to talk about the responses we observe. It is also a description that attracts positive attention. However, it also tends to overwhelm the thought process essential to proposing an explanation for how acupuncture works. The search for *qi* energy obscures acupuncture, because no *qi* can be absolutely equated with energy in any scientific sense, or even in any colloquial sense. Thus, if the scientific validation of acupuncture is exclusively pursued as a search for a measurable energy, many of traditional acupuncturists' actual skills will be ignored.

Although understanding or knowing *qi* is to most Westerners a matter of abstract knowledge, Asians who practice traditional disciplines often understand *qi* as a matter of personal culture. For example, the Japanese honored as their greatest sword masters those whose *qi* was so powerful that they never needed to draw their swords. In China, the greatest clinicians are those whose individual mastery of *qi* benefits their patients directly. *Qi gong*, China's newly restored traditional medical art,[8] all the martial arts, cooking, flower arranging, calligraphy, and even crafts such as carpentry have all been practiced as matters of *qi* cultivation. Each has been seen as a benefit to the health of at least the practitioner.

We can no more hope to equate *qi* to a single energy than we could equate, as Paul Unschuld notes, *gui*, an illness-causing ghost or demon, to a 'virus.'[9] Some conditions that tradition ascribed to *gui* could be viral in modern terms. Nonetheless, 'virus' can no more replace 'demon' in the traditional context than 'demon' can replace 'virus' in bioscience. But, when we look at Western acupuncture research, what we see is that, as *qi* was translated to 'energy,' people made a further, implicit translation based on their ingrained ideas of how energy behaves. *Qi* became energy, and then, because it is measurable neurological energies that are most intuitively analogous to *qi* in Western thought, acupuncture was investigated as a nervous system function.

If we are to truly explore a rationale for acupuncture, we cannot shortcut the process. The depth and breadth of traditional East Asian medicine must be explored before its full potential for adaptation can be understood. Its statement for Western science cannot be abbreviated. Acupuncture is a tradition, not a modern discipline. It is thus diverse, complex, and not uncommonly inconsistent. It was not newly designed to our Western standards of evidence, but evolved to meet the needs of vast populations. It is not a monolith built to satisfy the criteria of biostatistics. Instead, it is organic; it has been defined through the people and events of its history. We cannot jump to the conclusion,

we must begin with the observations. We cannot answer 'How?' so easily because the question is really a host of interrelated questions that depend on the interests and biases of those who ask them.

THE PROBLEM OF DIVERSITY

The second related and considerable problem is the diversity of acupuncture. In the preceding chapters we saw how a variety of approaches to the practice of acupuncture evolved. In following chapters we will describe approaches that accept traditional models, and approaches that reject them entirely. There are people who accept a direct, empirical approach, and people who insist on a scientific rationale. We will also find a wide variety of diagnostic methods and associated treatments. In therapy, some use strongly stimulating needling, others use techniques where needles barely touch the skin. This variety of techniques, this great diversity, raises the uncomfortable question: 'What is acupuncture?' Is it only needling to produce a strong stimulus? Is it only needling to produce a light stimulus? Is it needling at all? Put another way, if we ever hope to answer how it works, we must first describe what it is without eliminating too much of what we know it to be and to have been. This requires finding experimental models that embrace the variety of approaches and techniques that exist in the field.

Again, we must ask difficult questions. If we can describe a model of acupuncture that embraces the approaches we explore in this book, does any subsequent conclusion apply to only those methods? Does it only apply to those approaches that share techniques included in those models? If only a few approaches share qualities with the model proposed, how can we generalize the entire field? Is it not possible that different mechanisms are activated by different techniques? Why is it not likely that, because different schools of thought learned to evaluate different phenomena, they developed different means and methods of responding to a patient's complaints? If this is true, can the same research method be generalized for every school of thought? Likewise, if we cannot describe a model that embraces all approaches, how can we apply a limited answer to the general question of how acupuncture works? In other words, in a field of such enormous diversity, it is very difficult to formulate the type of precise model that analytic science requires.

Furthermore, within this diversity every model will ignore some aspect of acupuncture, particularly as it becomes more and more precisely stated. Because what researchers test is whether or not their hypothesis successfully predicts what actually happens, the answer each researcher discovers is prejudiced by how they formulate and test their assumptions. Thus, it is logically possible that there is no single model that describes the entire field. Each different research model must explore only a part, a narrow range. To understand any researcher's work these limits must be clearly known. In practice, the question 'How does it work?' is a series of questions, each of which will require acceptable means and methods, as well as an acceptable outcome, before acupuncture is scientifically understood.

THE PROBLEM OF SUFFICIENT PROOF

The problem of sufficient proof is at least in part a problem of communication. A lack of interaction among acupuncturists, academics, and scientists has given each too little opportunity to understand the others' needs and potential contributions. It is natural for those who treat or who are treated by acupuncture to feel that their experience is sufficient and that the ideas behind acupuncture are therefore valid. Traditionally oriented practitioners believe acupuncture works for reasons their colleagues have accepted for millenia — by regulating and rectifying the flow of qi in the channels, regulating the qi associated with the functions of the organs, and by draining the qi of stressors such as cold, wind, and damp. Because these ideas work in practice, it is not surprising that some believe that acupuncture requires no proof.

Thus, for many acupuncturists it is useless to pursue the question of how acupuncture functions. If it is a 'black box' to Western science, what happens inside that black box is irrelevant. The accretion of several hundred years of clinical efficacy is all that matters. For some in science and biomedicine this is an arrogant stance. There are several reasons for this opinion, but three are often cited. First, logically something cannot define itself. You cannot define acupuncture as affecting qi and then claim it works because it affects qi. Instead, the mechanisms of qi must be clearly demonstrated. Second, effects in practice do not constitute proof of a theory. Because the observations are uncontrolled and unscrutinized, so-called 'clinical experience' proves little unless it is gathered precisely and repeated systematically. Finally, the experience of individuals cannot be generalized without evidence of consistency. Thus, from a scientific viewpoint, acupuncturists' claims for clinical evidence are suspect.

For example, imagine that we were able to gather every acupuncturists' written evidence of successfully treating backache. We could not offer that experience as scientific evidence without showing that a statistically significant majority of those practitioners had identified the same condition, and used relatively similar acupoints and scientifically defensible outcome measures. In technical terms, without evidence of inter-rater reliability any improvement in patients' conditions could be the result of other factors. Without first demonstrating that clinical success depended upon the identification and treatment of particular patterns, it would be impossible to demonstrate that pattern recognition, or even acupuncture, was unquestionably linked to treatment success.

When these problems were solved, there would still be a problem of sufficient proof. Because any explanation for acupuncture's function might logically be countered by any other, a mechanism would still need to be demonstrated. Thus, there is no practical shortcut around the basic science. The long continuance of acupuncture's clinical practice does not establish that it works in terms other than its own. Rather, it establishes that acupuncture satisfies enough patients to support a population of practitioners. What the so-called 'test of time' proves is viability. Practically, of course, this is unwise to ignore. Although practical viability cannot replace scientific demonstration of function as part of acupuncture's scientific trial, once there is a base of acceptable science, acupuncture's viability is powerful evidence and incentive.

To some acupuncturists these opinions seem harsh and unfairly biased. However, in medicine no treatment works in many cases. Whether this is called the body's natural healing power, qi, the power of suggestion, or the placebo effect, the possibility that an outcome has been determined by more than any particular treatment is too great to be ignored. This reasoning fuels another extreme — the opinion that acupuncture requires no further attention because it has already failed. This opinion has its roots in the Western tradition of scientific inquiry. In this milieu questions must be formulated in terms that are reliably observable, rigorously quantified, and logically tested. Traditional acupuncture never developed methods of quantification, and it is therefore difficult for some who are trained in the Western tradition to think of it as a valid medicine. These critics demand that acupuncture be tested against Western knowledge of the body, just as the validity of any new idea is usually established in relation to already known or 'established' facts. Some of these skeptics dismiss acupuncture's survival, arguing that it was culturally, not clinically determined, and that religious, social, and political forces allowed it to avoid rigorus examination. Although, as we saw in Chapter 2, this argument has little basis in the 20th century, it often goes unchallenged.

THE PROBLEM OF 'NOT INVENTED HERE'

Although the argument that there is no reason to pay attention to acupuncture because it is nonscientific is too extreme for most scientists today, many people do feel that acupuncture cannot become an acceptable medicine without a scientifically determined rationale. Naturally, they feel that understanding the effects of acupuncture means understanding its action on the nervous system, the cardiovascular system, or the endocrine system. What is important to scientists is how acupuncture fits the models of human function they already trust. In every culture in which biomedicine is dominant, its principles are the obvious truths.

When concepts such as qi and yin-yang were incorporated into the language and the thought processes of East Asian cultures, these ideas seemed intuitively true. However, biomedical ideas are no longer foreign in China.[10] In fact, in all of Asia today traditional ideas are no longer exclusively accepted truths. Biomedicine is world dominant; science is pervasive. As we found in our review of the Asian history of acupuncture, many Chinese look to biomedical science exactly as do people in the West. As regards traditional medicine, important Chinese institutions provide a powerful impetus toward modernization.

Ironically, there is now an opposite process in the West. Disillusionment with biomedicine has increased. Not everything that is scientifically acceptable works or is without discomfort or pain. Biomedical mistakes are dramatic; iatrogenic illness and malpractice are feared; antibiotic-resistant bacteria are a frightening prospect. Millions seek alternative treatments. There are more and more people willing to accept explanatory models that use terms like qi and yin-yang in place of scientific language. Thus, the cultural processes at work are complex, and the science of acupuncture cannot be understood, nor can progress be made, without sensitivity to both Eastern and Western cultural, social, and political trends.

THE PROBLEM OF WHERE TO BEGIN

We have asked an obvious, simple question to show that its answer is neither simple nor obvious. No matter how content anyone may be with the idea of energetics, qi is neither a single energy nor a single entity. It is a class of phenomena inferred from observations with the naked human senses. There is no obvious way to describe an energy that does everything *qi* is said to do. Indeed, thus far, attempts to define *qi* based on the assumption that it is an energy have done acupuncture serious harm by limiting research. So too have simplistic definitions of acupuncture. Although acupuncture's defining characteristic is the insertion of needles at particular points, there is nothing about the tradition of acupoints or channels that irrevocably ties acupuncture to needling. Thus, although needling can be tested and different types and methods of needling can be scientifically compared, needling and acupuncture are not the same thing. In fact, it is not clear that acupuncture is intrinsically related to any one technique.

In both the East and the West, acupuncture cannot be examined outside the culture that asks the questions. Acupuncture is a human invention riding a wave of social and cultural change. It is a shifting target moving ever more rapidly as it blends with the cultures into which it is being absorbed. Science too is in constant change. It is now broadly understood that the dominant Newtonian model of nature gave way to the current relativistic model when the questions asked in the 19th century produced experiments that revealed inexplicable anomalies. These anomalies were not accepted until the older Newtonian model gave way. When the new models provided an acceptable explanation, the results were no longer anomalies. It is possible that the same will be true for the traditional explanations of acupuncture. They may be neither proven nor disproven until our view of nature changes. Thus, we must also be aware that paradigmatic issues could affect our understanding of acupuncture.

For the purposes of this book we have chosen some fairly basic and stable points of departure. First, and most importantly, as the cynical expression goes, things that are said to be 'too good to be true' probably are. Easy answers are often wrong and extreme opinions frequently lead the way to error. Thus we have

addressed neither the positive nor the negative extremes. The odds that acupuncture contains nothing useful are about the same as the odds that it contains nothing useless. The idea that longevity is scientific dispensation, that practitioner reports are all that is required, is no more likely to prove true than the idea that everything about acupuncture must be proven with legalistic precision. Thus our opinion is that acupuncture will need to be set upon some generally acceptable scientific footing. But, as is increasingly common in many areas of medical science, it is unlikely that anyone will wait until every question has been answered in exquisite detail. Once the positive evidence has begun to mount, utility will become the operative criterion. Economic utility may not have the prestige of scientific proof, but it is a powerful motive force for change.

Practically, sufficient proof will be whatever creates a working agreement in the peer-review system. It is thus likely that what will prove most useful to the Westward migration of acupuncture is scientific work that tests its validity while explicitly recognizing the logical complexities entailed in that venture. The Western scientific approach has grown so fast and so broadly that it will probably absorb acupuncture as well. Thus, an acceptable rationale will almost certainly be stated in Western terms. However, because of the problems created by that bias, we have highlighted incidences where scientists have tested acupuncture with models that have little to do with acupuncturists' skills, along with research where the weakness of acupuncture literature has been a negative contributory factor.

In general, we suggest that the scientific study of acupuncture can be discussed as several related areas: First, there are explorations of how well acupuncture works and for what problems. This is often called 'clinical research,' and is discussed in Chapter 5. It is meant to describe how acupuncture can be reliably used, not why it works.

Second, there are attempts to reveal the mechanisms by which acupuncture can be shown to do something. For example, what happens when you needle or heat an acupuncture point? This research concerns the basic science of acupuncture, and provides a foundation for further research. Studies fit several major subcategories:

- the effect of acupuncture on the central, peripheral, and autonomic nervous systems
- related humoral effects, such as changes in the biochemicals that circulate in the blood (e.g. the endorphins)
- the effects of acupuncture on the vascular system
- other physiological effects of acupuncture.

Third, there is research that seeks to discover whether traditional acupuncture theories and concepts can be measured or observed. These resolve into several major investigations:

- research on acupoints
- studies of the channels
- studies of *qi*, *yin-yang*, and the five phases.

Research in this last area is aimed at developing methods and technologies relevant to the investigation or application of acupuncture. Because this variety of research can directly affect the reputation of traditional claims, it is often thought of as proving or disproving acupuncture itself.

MECHANISMS BY WHICH ACUPUNCTURE HAS BEEN SHOWN TO BE FUNCTIONAL

Most Western research into the mechanisms of acupuncture followed Richard Nixon's diplomatic visit to China and reporter James Reston's *New York Times* article concerning his post-appendectomy pain relief by acupuncture. This event inspired Western researchers to attempt explanations of how acupuncture could treat pain and replace anesthetics in surgery, and how major surgery could be performed on patients who were still awake. The films from the 1970s were as astonishing to Western researchers as they were to the general public. This is as true today as it was then. For example, people often talk about a segment in

Bill Moyers' 1994 television documentary, 'Healing and the Mind,' showing in conjunction a woman awake and talking during brain surgery in which acupuncture was used with an analgesic instead of a general anesthestic.

The idea of acupuncture analgesia inspired a generation of medical researchers who wanted to understand the extremely common but elusive phenomenon of pain. The events were not only newsworthy, but also closely fit a field of research that was already generally accepted as worthy of attention and funds. Algologists raced to understand how acupuncture could produce an analgesic effect. However, researchers were not seeking to adopt acupuncture, or to change anesthesia as a clinical protocol, but to discover new avenues of pain research. One of China's experts, Ji Sheng Han, was explicit in stating that he realized that acupuncture 'could be the perfect tool for understanding more about how the brain kills pain.'[11] Other researchers in the West, if asked, would probably admit to the same opinion. So it is not surprising that slowly and inexorably acupuncture research became an effort to map and measure pain, pain-related phenomena, and mechanisms that could explain acupuncture analgesia.

Researchers asked: What was it that acupuncture was doing? Could it be measured? Would it reveal the answers to unexplained areas of pain research? For many researchers, the question 'How does acupuncture work?' became 'How can acupuncture be used as a research tool for exploring pain control?'

This was also true in clinical research. The first US university clinical trial using acupuncture featured renowned Chinese practitioner Tin Yau So in a pain control study.[12] There was, and is, plenty of stimulus in this direction. The statistics on pain are dramatic; 80% of all visits to US physicians every year are for pain-related problems.[13] Over 11% of all visits to a physician in the USA are for the problem of low-back pain alone.[14] Nearly 10% of all Americans have problems of pain that persist for more than 100 days per year.[15] The cost of pain treatment is probably over $100 billion annually, with low-back pain accounting for $16 billion alone.[16] Every insurance-paying employer knows they are paying these bills. The USA is not unique. Pain is such an enormous burden on the world's health-care systems that acupuncture quickly found a place in a broad research spectrum encompassing modalities from medication to meditation.

The question 'How does acupuncture work?' transformed into 'What can studies of stimulating the body with needles (acupuncture?) tell us about pain and how we can best treat it?' This was neither a deliberate subterfuge nor an attempt to ignore acupuncture. Indeed, many of these studies are extremely useful, interesting, and important, and have given credibility to acupuncture in the eyes of the biomedical community. But the practical reality of doing research in hospitals and research institutions inevitably influences the design of the research performed. Thus what determined the outcome was not that researchers were insincere, but that grants were their bread and butter. What gets funded gets investigated, and what gets investigated must fit the current professional consensus and have known social and economic consequences. Merely explaining some exotic therapy was never likely to be a priority in the 1970s and 1980s.

A secondary and strongly related influence on these investigations was the nature of the information available about acupuncture. It is an often-stated tenet of scientific culture that research that disproves a possibility is as important as that which produces a broadly heralded discovery. However, it is a fact of a career in science that recognition by one's peers contributes to tenure and advancement. Therefore, the risk that a researcher's assumptions about acupuncture would be found in error, or even just less than precise, greatly dissuaded scientists from studying acupuncture itself. Again, there was nothing unseemly in these decisions. Who would want to invest their time or limited funding on studies that could be critically flawed by a single bad assumption? Investigating an idea for which there is no acceptable Western foundation is not a conservative career investment. As we have just discussed, acupuncture is not only very diverse, but also presents many difficult choices.

In the 1970s and early 1980s there was very little reliable information on acupuncture available in English.[17] The literature on acupuncture was largely the product of Chinese government presses or the reports of enthusiasts. Because China was only a few years from the Cultural Revolution, anything Chinese was still suspect. For many in the West, China was still a 'red peril.' Beyond prejudice, many books in Western languages were not based on Chinese or Japanese sources. When scientists consulted sinologists they learned that most of what was written about acupuncture in English had never been subject to peer review or even standard methodologies.

Although information about acupuncture has since both improved and increased, scholars still list only a dozen or so books as having met academic translation and documentation standards. As a result, during the 1970s, when a sizeable body of significant research was done and the groundwork laid for what is accepted today, efforts to study how acupuncture worked were profoundly limited by inconsistent and inadequate information.[18] Efforts to investigate acupuncture as thoroughly as possible were impractical, and the research that was undertaken was often more limited than researchers knew. Although this in no way invalidates the research that has been done, it has sometimes limited the value or generality of its conclusions.

Neurologic and humoral effects of acupuncture analgesia

Given these influences and limitations, the obvious and safest research target for algologists (pain specialists) was the nervous system. They could draw upon a body of basic science and foundation research that was easily available and highly trusted. Furthermore, the information required from East Asian sources (e.g. acupoint locations) seemed simple, and hardly controversial. Thus, the need for acupuncture literature would be minimal and studies could be relieved of the dangers inherent in using informally transmitted information. However, even if the technical literature had been perfect, nervous system investigation would have been the most likely choice. After all, from the biomedical perspective, any analgesic effect had to be mediated through the nervous system. So, what was undertaken were studies that focused on either the underlying features of the nervous system or the chemicals released by, or active in, its functions.

The assumption that acupuncture produces analgesia via stimulation of the nervous system leads to some immediate questions: Which nerves are stimulated and at what locations? What stimuli give the best responses? There have been a variety of studies and a variety of answers. Felix Mann and others have suggested that acupunctural affects are brought about by stimulation within a neural dermatome that affects other areas within the same dermatome.[19] A dermatome is a region of the body surface defined by the innervation pattern of spinal nerve branches (Fig. 4.1). George Ulett, C. Chan Gunn, and others have suggested that these effects are brought about by stimulating 'motor points.'[20] These are the sites where where nerves insert into muscle bundles. Ronald Melzack, Peter Baldry, and others have suggested that the effects are caused by stimulating underlying 'trigger points.'[21] These are points under the skin where chronic pain results due to degenerative changes in muscular tissues, often as the result of another bodily event. Others have added various peripheral nerves to the list of candidates.[22]

Some researchers have suggested that acupuncture is a 'counterirritant.' This closely parallels the suggestions of Rougemont in 1798. One of the leading proponents of this idea is Daniel LeBars, who has written most about the phenomenon of 'diffuse noxious inhibitory control' (DNIC).[23] In this model, any noxious stimulus is believed to cause the relief of pain elsewhere in the body. LeBars and others have mapped the neurologic bases of these claims (see Box 5.2 in Ch. 5).

What is clear is that there is no area of skin where some underlying nerve cannot be found. The tissues under the skin are richly innervated by tiny nerve branches. Thus a needle placed anywhere in the body will affect some nerve.

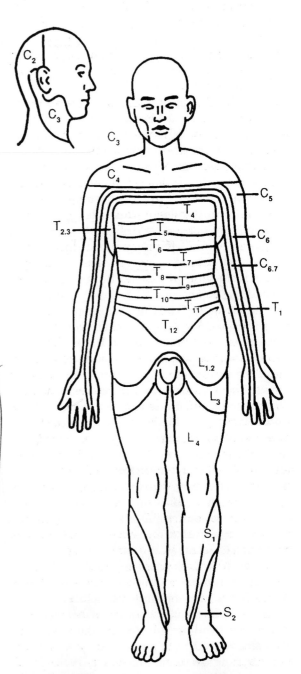

Figure 4.1 Dermatomes.

The vital question vis-à-vis acupuncture thus becomes, 'How point specific is the neurological response?' Except for counter-irritation theorists, everyone agrees that the needles cannot be randomly placed. Thus research looks beyond the omnipresent superficial nerve endings, to larger, more specific neurological structures. Acupuncture is presumed to work because neural structures and acupoints are related. In effect, research of this class attempts to explain acupuncture by locating the nerve structures that are the acupoints. Acupoints are assumed to be functions of the nervous system that the ancient Chinese discovered but failed to understand because their naked-sense view of the human body never accomplished a nervous system concept. It is not only researchers in the West who have made these assumptions, but also many in Asia. For example, in a study supposedly examining the relationship between acupuncture point locations, needling sensations, and afferent nerve fibers, Chinese researcher Wang Ke-mo and his colleagues defined the location and depth of the acupuncture points as the needling locations that elicit the strongest afferent nerve discharges.[24]

At many places on the skin there will be larger nerve structures lying beneath, for example, larger peripheral nerves, trigger points, and motor points. The key issue is whether there is an organized correlation between these nerve structures and acupoints, or whether the correspondence is only that of chance. If some aspect of the nervous system had very nearly always been found beneath the classical acupoints, scientists could have safely assumed that acupoints were nervous system features or, at least, were functionally tied to the nervous system. This was a clear, simple answer that would have opened many avenues of research, generated more research, more grants, more clinical technologies, and patentable measurement and treatment machinery. It was the perfect solution, except that it failed.

As we will see in the example below, these studies were seriously biased and this bias was their undoing. They set out to look for known neurological structures beneath each acupuncture point. This is a bias because it prejudices the scope of the information gathered. But, equally importantly, the idea of an acupoint was neither clearly defined nor well located. Thus, the correlation criteria were flawed, and the ensuing attempt to define acupuncture points by reference to neural structures failed. In other words, correlations were accepted when the distances between the acupoints and the supposedly related neural structures were far greater than working acupuncturists would accept. Had these scientists been taking their acupuncture examination in the 12th century, they would have needled the bronze man and seen no drops of water.

In fact, even using easily satisfied location criteria, the correlations were not all that exciting. Some researchers solved this dilemma by simply denying the existence of any acupuncture point that did not correlate with their chosen structure. If a classically described acupoint failed to correlate with a known neurological structure, it was dismissed as invalid or not useful.[25] On the other hand, some researchers used these studies to develop new therapies, for example, 'trigger point needling' or 'motor point needling.' In these systems acupuncture needles can be applied without learning any of the traditional methods for choosing acupoints.[26]

Perhaps the best example of this research approach is the 1977 study by Ronald Melzack and his coworkers.[27] This study is usually called a 'landmark study,' because the researchers' announcements had such a defining effect. What they announced was a 71% correspondence between acupuncture points and trigger points. Based on these findings, many researchers directed their attention to the neurological effects of acupuncture. Extensive neurological models were developed. In addition, reports of such a high correlation affected the design of clinical trials. This, as we will see later in this chapter, created considerable confusion, because this study was flawed. In fact, the correlation between the two classes of points is neither so dramatic nor significant.

Careful re-examination of these claims shows that, not only was there a problem with the structures to which correlations were claimed, but also that the correlation was maximally in the range 20–40% and was more realisticaly less than 10% (Box 4.2). This study is an excellent example of one of the primary difficulties in acupuncture research — the irregularity and inaccuracy of information transmitted between cultures.

The second major search for a neurological explanation of acupuncture has been the cataloging of the biochemicals released by the nervous system in response to needling acupuncture points. Notice that this research

also implicitly assumes that acupuncture and the nervous system are related. However, unlike research meant to explain acupoints as neural structures, this assumption does not rely on a one-and-only physical relationship. In other words, the working hypothesis is still that the effects of acupuncture are nervous system products, but the mechanism is openly explored. The possibility that the relationship is complex is not discarded by the study design.

Some very elegant work has been done in this area. Researchers such as Ji Sheng Han of

---

Box 4.2   Problems with the acupuncture point–trigger point correlations

There are several problems of inaccuracy with the study conducted by Melzack and his colleagues.[28] These problems show how difficult it can be to transmit medical information between cultures. Although the study is important because it maps potential correlations between a class of acupoints and certain features of the nervous system, it has nonetheless misdirected the scientific understanding of acupuncture. When you speak to scientists they remember the claim that there is a 71% correlation between acupuncture points and trigger points. Some even remember the study's conclusion that 'trigger points and acupuncture points for pain, though discovered independently and labeled differently, represent the same phenomenon.'[29] Simply stated, the study is the source of a belief that acupuncture points are trigger points, nothing more or less, and that acupuncture has been experimentally reduced to a set of anatomical locations. The problems with this conclusion are best revealed by examining Melzack's assumptions.

The first assumption is that all acupuncture points, and specifically the channel points, are defined by the presence of pressure pain. This was a very useful assumption for Melzack and his colleagues, because pressure pain is the defining characteristic of trigger points. However, there is only one set of acupuncture points that is entirely defined by the presence of pressure pain. These are the a-shi ('it's there') points, and these have never been considered part of the channel system. That is, these are not the acupoints to which acupuncture theory and practice apply.

The study's second major assumption compounds this problem. By assuming that pain conditions are treated predominantly or exclusively by needling the acupuncture points found close to the source of pain, just as trigger points or a-shi points are used, a large set of acupoint indications were arbitrarily excluded from the study. For example, a review of six English-language acupuncture texts[30] discovered that 30–50% (mean 42.5%) of the acupoints

recommended for the treatment of pain are located nowhere near the painful region. Had these points, known as 'distal' or 'distant points,' been included in the study's calculations, it would have been anything but memorable. In more modern translations, particularly those that do not translate traditional acupoint indications as biomedical conditions, the number of potentially relevant points is even larger. In other words, compared to the treatment options available in traditional treatment texts, Melzack's assumptions vastly understate the practice of acupuncture. Before the study began, the odds of arriving at its conclusion were more than doubled by ignoring traditionally indicated acupoints that were neither painful nor close to the area of pain. Accounting for this bias alone would have rendered the study less than convincing.

There are also other arbitrary assumptions in the study procedures. For example, an anatomical proximity of 3 cm was used as the criterion of sufficient proximity. If an acupuncture point and a trigger point were within 3 cm of each other, the points were considered identical. This is an extreme allowance. In contrast, for example, a recent World Health Organization proposal for standardizing data in acupuncture suggests a 2 cm radius.[31] Even this allowance is immense when compared to the location criteria demanded by actual systems of practice. In addition, this single absolute measure is itself arbitrary. The closeness of acupoints varies from body area to body area and patient to patient. In practice, acupuncturists actually use a variable measure for point location, the cun. It is individual to each person and each area of the body. Again, the probability of reaching the study's conclusion was at least doubled (the area of a 3 cm radius circle is more than twice that of a 2 cm radius circle) by the study design. Compared to the location criteria acupuncturists use, the study's correlation assumptions are measurably biased.

This was not all. There are three major classes of acupuncture points on the body: the channel points,

Box 4.2 Problems with the acupuncture point–trigger point correlations *(cont'd)*

the 'extra' points, and the *a-shi* points. Thus, even if a 3 cm proximity criteron was acceptable, the study's assumption would still be wrong. Acupuncture books have listed approximately 361 channel points and hundreds of extra points, and described the existence of *a-shi* points for the last several hundred years. Yet, Melzack and his colleagues only considered correlations with locally painful channel points. This is not only arbitrary, but almost perfectly misrepresents what acupuncturists actually do.

When an acupuncturist needles painful points near the location of a pain condition, which is by no means always or even usually the case, they needle tender *a-shi* points, not channel points. This class of points is associated with the *jing jin,* or 'channel sinews.' These are associated with the body's muscular structures and are almost exclusively used to treat pain, in particular the bodily aches and pains associated with physical activity, and minor traumas such as bumps and bruises. In some systems the *a-shi* points are thought to come and go as the body's condition changes. Again, the study design reduces the probability of reaching any other conclusion by ignoring basic facts about acupuncture. This bias is further compounded because it is the traditional description of the *a-shi* points, not the channel points, that most clearly matches trigger points.

Furthermore, when we examine the acupuncture points that are used to justify the study's concluding correlation of 35 acupoints with 50 trigger points, we find that few of these acupoints are significant, and some have absolutely no reputation or traditional indication for the treatment of pain. Again, a review of the same six acupuncture texts shows that of the 35 acupoints the study scores as correlated, a minimum of six and a maximum of 29 (mean 20.2, 57.7%) are not mentioned at all for the treatment of pain conditions. From none to 20 (mean 6.7, 19.1%) are mentioned for the treatment of pain, but are not among the 50 acupoints most commonly used for pain treatment. In fact, only 4–12 (mean 8.2, 23.4%) are mentioned as being among the 50 points most commonly indicated for pain conditions.

From acupuncturists' viewpoint, only 4–9 of the 35 points (11–26%) on which Melzack bases his conclusion are even among those that they would consider for the treatment of pain. Put bluntly, the 35 points for which Melzack and his colleagues claimed a correspondence are not much used for the treatment of pain. Again, the study design increases the odds of arriving at its conclusion by another 300–500% by prejudicial definition. The actual correlation level is only 23.4% with typically used points and 42.5% with the addition of points that are sometimes used. Had these figures been announced rather than the correlation of 71%, it is doubtful that

the study would have had much influence at all. Even if the study's correlations had been accurate, the figure of 71% depends on yet another, almost unbelievable, error. To say that 71% of acupuncturists are under 40 years of age, you must show that 71 of every 100 acupuncturists are 39 years old or younger. To say that channel acupoints and trigger points are 71% the same, you must find 256 trigger points in correlation with the 361 channel points. Even allowing the greatly exaggerated matches scored in this study, there were only 35. The study's 35 of 361 is really less than 10%, and is closer to 2% if realistic point associations are used. The more dramatic number was accomplished by reversing the expected comparison, thus producing an impression that virtually the entire body of acupuncture points had been correlated to trigger points.

What the study really shows is that of 50 trigger points studied, 35 were found to be locally painful acupoints. The study concluded otherwise because its inherent bias is that trigger points are real and acupoints are an ancient fantasy. In this study, to be real an acupoint had to be local and painful; in other words, it had to be a trigger point. All considered, the correlation between the main body of acupuncture points and trigger points is, at best, a chance correlation. However, what goes unmentioned is an equally impressive evidence of bias, because the study never mentions the possibility that *a-shi* points are a traditional observation of what modern anatomists call trigger points. That 35 of 50 trigger points correlate with locally painful acupoints would be more fairly interpreted to indicate that trigger points are at least a very significant subset of *a-shi* points. Assuming that the 35 points continue to correlate when more accurate correlation criteria are applied, this study is a justification of the traditional observation. Thus a study that has been widely quoted as discrediting traditional acupuncture can be more fairly interpreted as evidence that Chinese observers had already identified what we now call trigger points and defined their function rather well.

This may be little consolation for researchers who have taken this study at its announced value, assuming that a neurological basis for acupuncture has been definitively proven. Although the practices based on the observations made in this research are logically as valid as any other system of practice (in fact, traditional experience supports an assumption of validity), the conclusions of this study are unacceptable. This aspect of the neurological model is questionable, and it is by no means convincing evidence that trigger points explain away the traditional forms of acupuncture.

China, Bruce Pomeranz and Richard Cheng of Canada, C. Richard Chapman of the USA, Kazuo Toda and Chifuyu Takeshige of Japan, and others have contributed to this knowledge.[32] This work follows from the discovery in the 1970s that acupuncture initiates the secretion of naturally occurring human biochemicals with molecular characteristics like those of the pain-killing drugs called opiates. These compositional cousins of morphine are called endorphins. Like morphine, they kill pain. Since that discovery, there have been studies that reveal a complex of different secretions that increase in bloodstream or cerebrospinal fluid concentration following acupuncture. These secretions are known as neuropeptides and monoamines. Among these are the endorphins, enkephalins, dynorphins, serotonin, and norepinephrine. Researchers such as Bruce Pomeranz, who is the best known Western researcher in this area, have used this information to construct complex models of how acupuncture could affect the nervous system.[33] These models are now broadly accepted by the biomedical community. In his presentations and publications, Pomeranz documents 17 convergent lines of evidence supporting the claim that acupuncture releases endorphins, producing acupuncture analgesia.[34] No other hypothesis is supported by so many convergent lines of research, making the general conclusion that acupuncture causes the release of endorphins virtually impossible to repudiate. Among these convergent lines of evidence are the following:[35]

• Four different opiate antagonists are able to block acupuncture analgesia. Microinjection of endorphin antibodies blocks acupuncture analgesia.
• Mice genetically deficient in opiate receptors show poor acupuncture analgesia.
• Rats deficient in endorphin production show poor acupuncture analgesia.
• Reduction of pituitary endorphin suppresses acupuncture analgesia.
• Acupuncture analgesia can be transmitted to a second animal by transfer of cerebrospinal fluid or by cross-circulation, and this effect is blocked by administration of naloxone to the second animal.
• Acupuncture analgesia is enhanced by protecting endorphins from enzyme degradation, prolonging their action.

Box 4.3 summarizes further aspects of the model that Pomeranz describes.

The general neurochemical model proposes that acupuncture stimulates sensory nerves in the skin and muscles. These nerves send signals to the spinal cord, which signals the midbrain.

Box 4.3   Primary neurological pathways for acupuncture analgesia

Low-frequency, high-intensity acupuncture analgesia by electro acupuncture

The needle receives a slowly pulsing but intense current that activates sensory receptors in the surrounding muscle tissues. These receptors initiate impulses that travel to the spinal cord and ultimately act at one or more of three neural sites:
1. Within the spinal cord, where receptors control the release of enkephalin or dynorphin, neurochemicals that inhibit the transmission of pain signals.
2. In the midbrain, where exciting cells in the periaqueductal grey matter release enkephalin. This enkephalin then causes descending signals to be sent from the raphe nucleus to the spinal cord, where serotonin and norepinephrine are released. These substances block pain signals.
3. In the pituitary–hypothalamic complex, where reception of signals results in the release of beta-endorphin, which blocks pain, and

adrenocorticotrophic hormone, which in turn releases steroids from the adrenal cortex that help to reduce inflammation.

High-frequency, low-intensity acupuncture analgesia by electro acupuncture

The needle receives a rapidly pulsing but relatively small current that activates sensory receptors in the muscle, sending impulses to the spinal cord. These impulses ultimately act at two neural sites:
1. Within the spinal cord, where they activate nonendorphinergic transmitters such as γ-aminobutyric acid. These block pain signals.
2. In the midbrain, where they cause the raphe nucleus to release serotonin and norepinephrine that block pain signals.
For further reading, see note 36.

There, some messages are relayed to the hypothalamus and pituitary, while others are routed to the thalamus and cerebral cortex. In each of these areas brain tissues release neuropeptides in response to those signals. In other cases the nerves are thought to send a signal that blocks reception of further pain. This is a simplification of the model, but it describes the essential elements for which the evidence is good. Pomeranz has the best referenced description of this model.[37]

This model is still not the whole story, because there are questions that it does not answer. For example, to activate these mechanisms the stimulation must be very strong. In fact, virtually all research into these mechanisms employs electro acupuncture, because these levels of stimulation can be produced manually only by laborious, continuous, needle manipulation. (Electrical stimulation of the needles gives an easier, better quantified, and reproducible stimulation.) These needling techniques produce a strong sensation that is usually related to the Chinese idea of de qi. However, these sensations are reported as a 'noxious stimuli' by many researchers, and have recently been characterized as 'sharp, pulling, electric, tingling, heavy, pulsing, spreading, pricking, aching, or hot.'[38] Many researchers have concluded that if these heavy techniques are not applied to activate the biochemical mechanisms, then acupuncture will not work.[39]

This assertion prompts the question, 'What is the minimum necessary de qi?' This is important, because if only a strong stimulus (heavy needling) activates this chain of actions, the neurologic model can only explain certain modes of practice. If electro acupuncture is the only practical way to generate these levels of stimulus, what have practitioners been doing for the last several hundred years? In other words, either the model is partial, or all other forms of acupuncture could never have worked. The problem is that in the patient or practitioner's view, this discards the great majority of treatments.

In part because modern Chinese acupuncturists have been influenced by neurological ideas, and in part because acupuncture in China generally features stronger stimulation, this model will most likely apply to modern Traditional Chinese Medicine (TCM) acupuncture. Even this generalization is overly broad, because the needles used, the depth of insertion, and the stimulation sought are varied relative to the problem treated. Historically, it appears that strong stimulation is related to China's need to rapidly train many practitioners during the modern era.[40] Different stimulation levels have been more or less common at different times.[41] Also, European or American patients do not tolerate as strong a needle stimulus as do Chinese patients.[42] Western practitioners who try to obtain de qi with every insertion do not use nearly so strong a stimulation. In fact, the Japanese needles and insertion tubes that are very widely used in the USA make insertion nearly painless and patients describe de qi as a 'dull ache,' and only rarely mention the more dramatic responses that neurochemical researchers describe. Even practitioners who preferentially use electrical devices try to avoid administering 'tingling, heavy pulsing' sensations, because these are often accompanied by muscle spasms, which disconcert patients. Indeed, muscle spasms are actually included in the list of adverse side effects attributed to acupuncture.[43]

We cannot help but wonder whether acupuncture researchers have experienced much acupuncture. Personally, having experienced most forms of acupuncture many times, we have found this degree of stimulus only in procedures mislabeled 'acupuncture anesthesia.' For example, when we have each used electroacupuncture during dental procedures, the stimulus has needed to be strong, constant, and heavy. In fact, the stimulus required is so strong that even healthy teenagers who are inured to acupuncture do not tolerate it well. Otherwise, acupuncture analgesia is generally the only clinical technique that produces sensations like those pain researchers describe. The experience of such treatments is also very different from that usually produced by acupuncture. Instead of feeling relaxed and energized, you feel something like the lump of insensitivity that novocaine produces. There is also a lingering after-effect like a hangover. Compared to these sensations, even acupuncture from Chinese practitioners like Tin Yau So, who is world-renowned for his powerful *de qi*, is quick and light.

Other questions also arise because the research on which this model is based has been almost exclusively conducted using electro-acupuncture. The electric current virtually guarantees that the nervous system will be affected. In fact, researchers have found that one range of frequencies causes the release of one neuropeptide, and another range of frequencies causes the release of another neuropeptide.[44] Thus the relationship to other modes of practice is even less convincing. For example, it is a common clinical experience that a Japanese *hinaishin*, or 'intradermal needle,' inserted to an appropriate point relieves pain instantly, and can increase a patient's range of motion almost as quickly. A *hinaishin* is very thin and is inserted painlessly to a depth of only 1 mm. There is nothing like heavy needling, and the speed at which the pain disappears is so great that it is difficult to believe that it is a result of neuropeptides circulating in the blood.

Logically, however, the neurological models are very important and useful. Although they probably explain some of the effects of acupuncture, they are probably more limited than their proponents at present believe. These models help explain the heavier stimulation modes of acupuncture, but it is unclear how applicable they are to the acupuncture routinely practiced throughout the world. Some researchers recognize these limitations. Bruce Pomeranz came to the same conclusion. As he stated a few years ago: '... there is more to acupuncture than endorphins and chronic pain.'[45] Recently, he has been researching the actions of acupuncture in morphine withdrawal, in accelerating nerve regeneration, and in speeding wound healing.[46]

Autonomic nervous system effects

In Japan and Europe, where heavy needling is rare and more people had experience with acupuncture in the 1970s, Melzack's claims were less believable. In addition, a different neurological model had already evolved to explain how acupuncture and auricular acupuncture worked. As early as Soulie de Morant's writings in the 1930s, Europeans focused on parallels with another aspect of the nervous system — the autonomic nervous system.[47] The model proposes that symptoms and diseases are so often a result of an imbalance between the sympathetic and parasympathetic nervous systems that acupuncture must work by correcting that imbalance.

Together, the sympathetic and parasympathetic nervous systems comprise the autonomic nervous system, and each regulates much of the body's physiology. The effects of one are counterbalanced by the effects of the other. What one increases, the other decreases. For example, chronic stress will cause a relative activation of the sympathetic system. This in turn tends to cause relative inaction in the parasympathetic system. Thus, in this model, needling is seen as affecting different aspects of this two-sided system. Acupuncture therapy is thought to help orchestrate a desired response. Research by Lee and others has clearly demonstrated the effects of acupuncture.[48]

In Japan the concept of autonomic nervous imbalance is currently accepted as the basis of several East Asian medical systems. Each of these has proponents. For example, the *Ryodoraku* system uses the electro diagnosis method developed by Yoshio Nakatani. Today it is proposed and researched by practitioner-researchers such as Hirohisa Oda[49] and the late Masayoshi Hyodo.[50] They support their claims for the autonomic nervous system imbalance theory with diagnostic and therapeutic methods that measure the status of the autonomic nervous system. These will be discussed along with other electrical measurements later in this chapter.

Vascular effects

There is reasonably strong evidence that acupuncture affects the circulatory system. Using methods such as color thermography[51] and microphotoplethysmography,[52] various studies have demonstrated the effects of acupuncture on peripheral circulation. In one experiment that Felt observed, thermography revealed an immediate increase in the temperature of the back muscles, due to an increased blood flow. In this case it was nothing more than the pressure of tennis balls on acupoints that produced the necessary stimulation.[53] This suggests a pressure-initiated signaling mechanism, for example, a piezoelectric (pressure electric) response. Although this line of research has not yet been systematically explored, the sequence of events that follows the insertion of a needle is predictable. Some of these events have already been demonstrated. Evidence is mounting that what Birch calls the 'splinter effect' is very real.

When a splinter pierces the skin, a series of biological responses occur (Box 4.4). First, the body recognizes that the integrity of the skin has been compromised. The mechanism by which this occurs is probably the 'current of injury,'[54] the electrical effect of cell damage, in addition to signals from local nerves. In response, the brain initiates a general peripheral vasoconstriction, a narrowing of the body's blood vessels. This serves several func-

tions. It reduces the blood loss that frequently accompanies breaking of the skin and aids clotting at the site of the injury. This reduction in the flow of blood to the wound also helps slow the spread of microbes that accompany penetration of the protective skin barrier, by an unsterilized object.

Somewhat later, an increase in the diameter of the vessels, vasodilation, begins.[55] This too serves several functions. It aids the migration of the white blood cells (immune and defensive system cells), which were activated by the current of injury, to the injury site. White blood cells help scavenge microbes (bacteria). Vasodilation also allows more nutrients to reach the tissues, thus aiding, for example, the reparative functions of fibroblasts and increasing the speed with which waste products are carried away.

In addition to vasoconstriction and vasodilation, a third effect has been observed in experimental acupuncture studies. This phenomenon is called 'vasomotion.'[56] This is a pumping of the microscopic blood vessels. It can be seen to flush the damaged cells and blood that collect around an injury. Vasomotion thus further aids healing.

In general, the first stage, vasoconstriction, lasts for aproximately 20 minutes. The second stage, vasodilation, has been observed for several hours, and the third stage, vasomotion, for an hour or more.[57] This is a predictable sequence of biological responses to the insertion of a splinter or any other object that pierces the skin, including an acupuncture needle. In fact, this sequence of events has been clearly observed with the insertion of an acupuncture needle. This is entirely to be expected, because there is no reason why the body should differentiate a needle from a splinter. Of course, acupuncturists use presterilized needles so that needle wounding is negligible. The insertion of an acupuncture needle also has been shown to produce biological changes that none previously suspected. The late Yoshio Manaka and his coworker Kazuko Itaya found that the insertion of a needle in the back of a rabbit produced profound effects on the circulation observed in the ears.[58] In fact, they actually filmed these changes. These experiments demonstrated that

---

Box 4.4   The 'splinter' effect

1. The 'splinter' (needle) is inserted.
2. Vasoconstriction occurs to prevent blood loss, assist clot formation, and prevent the spread of invading microbes. This continues for as long as 20 minutes.
3. Vasodilation begins, helping white blood cells migrate to the area where they will neutralize invading microbes. This also helps other cells arrive to help heal the wound, bring nutrients to the injury site, and eliminate waste products. This continues for as long as 2 or 3 hours.
4. Vasomotion begins, helping to bring nutrients to the tissues and to eliminate waste products. This begins after approximately an hour and has been observed for an hour or more.

   These vascular changes participate in basic defensive, repair, and metabolic processes that comprise the body's response to a wound. They have been observed to occur distant from the site of insertion, and are thus theorized to occur throughout the body. However, these effects probably occur most strongly in the insertion region.

the insertion of a needle brings about the splinter effect, not only at the insertion site, but also at distant sites. In addition, the results of other studies suggest that the effects can be site specific. In other words, choosing where to insert the needle influences where the vascular changes occur. Although these effects have been observed to occur far from the insertion site, it is possible that they may also be predictably targeted to specific tissues or locations. More research is needed in this area.

This leads to a broader understanding of the possible physiological effects of acupuncture. The vascular changes observed have their most profound effect at the microvascular level, the levels at which the microscopic vessels (the capillaries) exchange nutrients and waste with the cells and lymph. This is also the level at which physiologic activity takes place. Thus, acupuncture potentially can have general effects on the most basic biochemical processes of the body.

In the preceding discussions we noted that certain white blood cells are activated by needling. This implies that the immune system is also affected. This too would be a natural part of the splinter-effect scenario. A nonspecific immunologic response should be observed when any object punctures the skin. However, acupuncture not only alters the activities of white blood cells, it also seems to alter immunological responses more generally.[59] In the developing field of psycho-neuroimmunology (the study of the interrelated effects of the endocrine, immune, and nervous systems) there is research that shows certain nervous-system chemicals bind to, and alter the behavior of, white blood cells.[60] Since acupuncture can affect the nervous system and the biochemical messengers that communicate between the nerve cells and the white blood cells, there exist means by which it could affect the immune system. Research into general immunological effects might explain some of the positive observations made when immune-compromised patients receive acupuncture treatment, as well as some of the immunologic effects of acupuncture observed in basic research.

Other effects

There are further studies that suggest acupuncture produces predictable physiologic responses. It is well documented, for example, that needling a specific point on the leg below the knee increases gastric acid secretion.[61] This correlates with the historic reputation of this acupoint as a 'stomach point.' A variety of gastrointestinal effects has been observed in response to acupuncture, including effects on gastric motility[62] and intestinal motility.[63] The association of acupuncture points on the limbs with internal systems was also shown, dramatically but accidentally, in a completely unrelated field of study.

Mstislav Volkov and Oganes Oganesyan are specialists in trauma, orthopedics, and orthopedic surgery. They have developed original external devices for fixing in place broken bones, and bone and joint deformities. In this external fixing procedure mechanical devices are implanted partially in and partially out of the body. This is how they accidentally discovered that these reposition–fixation devices sometimes caused internal disturbances. These disturbances included acute-onset diabetes insipidus, angina-like pain, and gastrointestinal disorders. On further investigation, Volkov and Oganesyan discovered that these problems only occurred when the external fixing mechanisms were placed at acupuncture points. When they avoided the acupuncture points, these complications did not occur. They concluded from their clinical experimentation that:

we should like traumatologists pay attention to the necessity of avoiding the acupuncture points when inserting the pins. ... When this technique was included in the application procedure, there was not a single case of general complications.[64]

This study is intriguing for scientists because accidents are unbiased. Because noone began with any assumption relative to acupuncture, attentions and intentions were turned elsewhere and bias played a minimum role. Thus, this evidence has a particularly strong impact. If the acupoints, stimulated by the pressure or electrical potential of a medical device, can produce an illness in someone who was formerly free of that illness, it is hard to deny that acupoints could predictably influence bodily processes. These events lend credence not only to acupuncture, but also to old stories of the discovery of acupuncture (for example, when arrow wounds led to cures).

Other acupuncture studies have shown that needling certain points on mice decreases liver toxicity from mercury.[65] Other experiments have demonstrated that acupuncture can stimulate the expulsion of gallstones[66] and the improvement of bladder tonus in incontinent patients.[67] Several theories have been used to explain these findings. For example, the 'viscero-cutaneous reflex theory' posits a reciprocal relationship between an organ and an anatomical region at the body surface.[68] Although this observation has been made in non-Asian cultures and is also seen in modern Western ideas such as reflexology, these theories seem inadequate to account for all the findings.

The neurologic, vascular, and physiologic effects just described can be used to explain many acupuncture techniques; however, as we have seen, the field is tremendously diverse. It is difficult to imagine, for example, how the splinter effect would be initiated by techniques that do not require penetration of the skin, or by electrical stimuli that have the potential to overwhelm such subtle and local biologic responses. What, for example, are the effects of pressure, moxa, lasers, colors, the slight current produced between two different metals, or microwave radiation? All these forms of stimulation are used somewhere in acupuncture (see Ch. 7). Is it not likely that different mechanisms are involved? What might all these techniques have in common? Clearly, if a comprehensive model is to be developed, more research is required.

For us, Yoshio Manaka's idea offers a fascinating possibility for future research, because it is a comprehensive model. Manaka was a Japanese medical doctor who had ample opportunity to apply his pre-Second World War interest in traditional medicine while an army surgeon, a prisoner of war, and civilian doctor in post-War Japan. During the War, especially when Manaka was on Okinawa during the American landings, he found himself treating war-injured patients, particularly those who had been badly burned, without the facilities and supplies that his physician's training required.

Manaka was extremely inventive. Later in life he was known for leaving colleagues while he unexpectedly disappeared into hardware stores. He would often emerge with some gizmo that had caught his eye as a potential part for a new invention. Typically, his response to the frustration of his medical skills was creative. He developed various techniques, finally settling on a diode in a wire which passed current in only one direction. This he used to 'pump' the concentration of ions (partial molecules with an electrical polarity) which Western research had suggested might concentrate at the site of burns.[69] By experimenting with traditional acupuncture concepts, he was able to discover methods that greatly relieved his patients' pain and enhanced their recovery. Thus began the now famous and broadly used 'ion-pumping cords,' and a career that would produce one of Japan's *Dai Sensei* (great teachers) of acupuncture (Box 4.5).

In his book with Birch and Itaya, *Chasing the Dragon's Tail*, Manaka describes his exploration of different acupuncture techniques and how it led to one of the most ambitious explorations of the validity and utility of traditional medical ideas.[73] Although it is important to note that these experiments have not yet been rigorously reproduced by others, his results are supportive of the traditional models of acupuncture, and his experiments are often so simple that anyone can perform them. He investigated channel, acupoint, yin-yang, and five-phase ideas. Based on his findings, he developed a broad model of the function of acupuncture.

Manaka's theory is that the clinical principles of acupuncture describe a set of software rules. By using these algorithms one can access a deep-lying signal system, which Manaka called the 'X' or 'unknown' signal system, that operates within the body.[74] This idea is rooted

Box 4.5 Manaka's X-signal system

After over 40 years of studying, practicing, and researching acumoxa therapy, Yoshio Manaka formulated a theory that bridges traditional explanations and scientific methods. The subject of his theory is what he called the 'X-signal system.' Manaka was unusual because he was fluent in many languages, read classical and modern acupuncture works from several nations, and continuously studied with his colleagues, among whom were many of the most famous acupuncture practitioners in Japan, China, Korea, and Europe. He was highly educated and knowledgable, bringing to bear not only his experience as a physician and physiologist, but also treatment skills that became near legendary, even when he was a relatively young man.

Essentially, Manaka formulated a neutral description of traditional acupuncture theories. His goal was to protect those theories from reduction by allowing them to be tested on their own terms. He did not doubt that the dominant neurologic models of acupuncture were useful for understanding analgesic techniques when strong stimulation was applied, but he was keenly aware that these research studies involved stimuli that were rarely employed by expert traditional practitioners. To Manaka, it was obvious that none of the then currently proposed models could explain the variety of methods found in real-world clinical practice. Thus he concentrated on understanding what all methods had in common and what was unique to each.

Looking for what each system has in common is like looking for the lowest common denominator in a sequence of numbers. Among 2, 26, 56, 98, 158, and 1004, the lowest number that can divide evenly into all the other numbers is 2. Similarly, what every acupuncture technique has in common with every other acupuncture technique, ranging from the very strong to the unbelievably delicate, is the subtle influences produced by the finest methods. Just as in our example of a numeric sequence, where each larger number is a multiple of 2, the effects of each method of acupuncture build from those of the finest techniques. In other words, if the traditional acupuncture model is correct, then it is the most subtle influences common to each approach that are most probably related to those traditional concepts.

When there is a stronger stimulus, other physiologic influences are activated, each according to the technique employed. For example, when electro acupuncture with strong *de qi* is used, neurologic pathways and neurochemical exchanges are activated. With the non-inserted needles of the Toyohari method it is not possible to invoke these neurologic explanations, thus other mechanisms must be activated. Manaka named these undefined pathways the 'X-signal system,' after 'X,' the generic variable to be solved for. He looked for examples not only in acupuncture but also in biomedicine and the natural sciences.

He eventually concluded that there was a subtle, low-energy signal system operating in humans which, according to his research, seemed to reflect the foundation principles of traditional models of acupuncture. Specifically, the X-signal system was activated and functioned according to 'biases' or 'influences.' These he saw as being essentially polar (i.e. either positive or negative). For example, a particular positive bias would establish a trend leading to an opposite bias. Each bias is a particular trend in a complex system that increases the probability of one outcome rather than another. He argued that these biases were information that the body employed. Thus, when the stronger stimulation seen in electro acupuncture or the acupuncture analgesia that had recently emerged in China were applied, the effects of the signaling system were overwhelmed. The higher-level signals associated with the nervous system and physiologic processes would dominate. Even though the more subtle effects were still occurring, they would be masked. Just as we do not see the red components of visible light when viewing a white light source, we do not notice the finer, difficult-to-measure effects when the nervous and endocrine systems are at work. Manaka stated this thus:

> There is a primitive signal system in the body that has embryological roots but it is masked by the more advanced and complex control (regulation) systems. Thus the original signal system is hard to find or see. This primitive system is able to detect and discriminate internal and external changes and plays a role in regulating the body by transmitting this information. This system serves as the *modus operandi* of acupuncture.[70]

Manaka suggests that the systems operating in acupuncture are those characterized by the ancient Chinese as *qi, jing-luo, yin-yang*, and the five phases. It is implicit in Manaka's writings that these are 'software systems' that express the functions of the X-signal system. In Manaka's view they are not the signaling system itself (the as yet undescribed hardware), but are the operating procedures that describe how the hardware will respond. Manaka argued that this system necessarily would have evolved before the nervous system because primitive organisms without a nervous or endocrine system cannot survive without self-regulation and adaptation. As early-stage embryos are in fact primitive organisms, where, if the primitive system were operating it would be most obvious, Manaka used events and anomalies in embryological development to support his theory. He further proposed that, as the more evolved and efficient nervous and endocrine systems developed, the primitive signaling system retained a background role. It never ceased to function, and continues to operate unseen.

In essence, Manaka suggests that the X-signal system helps regulate the body's physiology. It is not, for example, the metabolism but a regulator, a metabolic control. It is not the 'flap' that turns the airplane, the gears that raise the flap, or the energy that runs the motor that turns the gears. It is the signal that sets the motor to turning. He thought that *qi* was how ancient naked-sense observers explained the X-signal system's operation. In effect, the signal system explains *qi* in the clinical sense. He thought that channels were part of this system, and that *yin-yang* and the five phases were the observed rules by which this system was seen to regulate itself and the physiologic processes that Manaka thought tended to mask it.

Manaka's idea is not unique; in fact, it is highly congruent with research in other fields that have examined acupuncture. Robert Becker suggested a similar system in his studies of primitive DC current systems that operate in the body. These are involved in growth, healing and regeneration:

...living organisms have self contained, automatic, feedback regulated, growth control systems utilizing direct electrical currents as the data transmission and cellular control signals.

From an evolutionary point of view this system may be viewed as the original, primitive analog data transmission and control system, which later developed specialized elements (neurones) operating in a digital fashion.[71]

When each of the many disciplines that compose the field of sinology have examined *qi*, *yin-yang*, and the five phases, ideas of information, influences, and governance often arise. Thus, the X-signal system also fits nicely with what scholars find in their research. The theory of the X-signal system helps put acupuncture into a broader perspective so that more relevant methods of study can be brought to bear on the traditional explanatory models. However, the resources necessary for this are not small, and progress will take time.

For further reading see note 72.

not only in traditional concepts but also in modern biology. Before the nervous system develops in a human embryo, considerable communication occurs as the fertilized egg divides, producing embryonic layers, then fetal features, and finally all the structures and organs of the body.[75] Manaka proposes that the communication pathways that operate in these very early stages remain functional even after the central nervous system has assumed overall control. This system may utilize the electrically active large molecules of the body as its communications network. In other words, certain body structures such as the fascia may also be communications lines. Manaka proposed that the human body carries with it all the capacities that it developed during the course of its growth from a single cell to maturity. Manaka's work coordinates well with the research of molecular biologists, such as James Oschman, who see in the body's connective tissues and fascia the ground substance of a powerful system of cellular communication.[76]

Stated simply, this theory proposes that the acupoints and channels are expressions of potential. In other words, they are not wires through which some current is constantly flowing, but circuits that become active when

stimulated. When the signal is strong enough, the nervous system responds and its actions predominate. However, signals not strong enough to activate the central nervous system are received by the X-signal system. Manaka proposed that the body's communications systems have become specialized, just as other systems in the body have. The X-signal system automatically handles the low-level responses typical of, for example, changes in the immediate environment, just as the autonomic nervous system controls respiration and digestion. In this regard, Manaka's idea is an extension of how we already see bodily functions.

The idea is not hard to understand. Think of a landscape with which you are very familiar. In dry weather, there are obvious waterways, perhaps trenches or valleys. By analogy, the landscape is the human body and the waterways are its nervous system. Now imagine a light rain, such as a morning mist or fog. The waterways do not change, but there are inumerable small features where water vapor condenses, many small depressions into which droplets flow, and many tiny rivulets collecting the larger trickles. The water is not distributed evenly, the terrain is not glass-like and flat, but neither is the water condensing or flowing randomly. Gravity and the shape, slope, and material of the terrain control the distribution of the water droplets. However, once a strong rain begins, the volume is too great for the smaller features to absorb; these are washed over as the rain flows into the established waterways. These collect and carry the greater volume of rain into the larger features of the terrain.

In this model all Western medical knowledge applies. Everything we believe we know in biomedicine is operative. In our analogy these medical principles are like the laws of gravity, and the physical laws of movement that predict the flow of water. Everything functions as expected. Thus, this theory of acupuncture conflicts with none of what we know about the nervous system. In fact, it simply adds to that description an idea of how the body responds to slight stimuli (e.g. environmental stimuli that do not appear to affect the nervous system, the subtle internal changes that accompany our emotional lives, or the lighter stimulus techniques of acupuncture).

Light stimuli influence the X-signal system through differences in potential, in particular through their polarity.[77] Just as two metals with different electrical potentials can create a current in a conductive medium, any area of the body that internally or externally acquires what Manaka called a 'bias' (using the term after the fashion of electrical engineers) will be recognized through the X-signal system. However, like the rivulets in our imaginary landscape, these flows will not be random. Rather, the topography of the body, its native electrical potentials, and the nature of the stimuli will determine the flow of the signal.

In this conception acupoints and channels are seen as the predictable outcome of potentials created within the bioelectrical nature of the body. In this schema, *yin-yang* and the five phases are not in conflict with scientific knowledge. Instead, they are traditional methods of predicting what happens when certain signals occur. Put another way, these traditional ideas are software 'rules of thumb.' As we will discuss later, this model takes on the features of a mathematical model; that is, particular responses can be predicted from a set of initial conditions.

This model has potentially far-reaching implications for research in acupuncture. It requires no biologically unlikely energies or events; it rationalizes known responses that current nervous system theories cannot explain. It requires neither the reduction nor elimination of either modern or traditional observations. Although it challenges the idea that *qi* is an energy constantly flowing in the channels, it neither ignores nor reduces the utility of the traditional concept which, as we saw in Chapter 3, serves acupoint selection. It also provides a reasonable foundation for selecting those aspects of the *qi* concept that might best fit the channel model without supposing a 'one and only' acupuncture. Manaka's proposal that there are multiple layers of effects that occur in the practice of acupuncture encourages refinement of research methodology so that the more subtle aspects begin to be investigated. The layers activated depend on the technique applied, an observation that is consistent with generations of clinical experience. There are relatively heavy stimulation effects, such as heavy *de qi* needling and electrical stimulation of the needles; these can be researched and modeled in neurological terms. There are relatively light effects, such as those found with the use of intradermal needles or very thin shallowly inserted needles, that can be researched using tiny polar stimuli.

Although it will require considerable research to test and validate this model fully, thus far clinical experiments with slight stimuli tend to support traditional concepts. What Manaka and those who have repeated his clinical tests have demonstrated is that traditional observations, such as acupoint pressure pain, can be reliably altered by applying slight magnetic or electrical influences to acupoints related by traditional *yin-yang*, five-phase and channel theory. The X-signal concept is thus very powerful and can be very broadly applied because traditional acupoint indications can be understood as the naked-sense observation of the influence of a low-energy signal system on physiology. This is particularly practical because most traditional indications for acupoints are not precise biomedical conditions, but are instead lists of reactions such as changes in color, temperature, and function. These are precisely what careful observation with the human senses reveals.

This theory is important if only because it allows for the development of a testable biological model of acupuncture that embraces traditional concepts and the most subtle techniques of their practice. Although it can be said to have been found to be consistent (i.e. it makes sense within itself and predicts nothing that we already know to be untrue), many observations and rigorous studies will be required before it can be considered proven. However, it poses an even greater research challenge than do studies based on heavier stimulation, because of the problems involved in obtaining convincing measurements.

MEASUREMENT AND OBSERVATION OF TRADITIONAL CONCEPTS

There have already been efforts to demonstrate and measure the phenomena described by the traditional medical model. These have included the use of measurement technologies to find correspondences between traditionally described ideas such as *xue* ('holes' or acupuncture points) or *jing luo* (channels) and, for example, lowered electrical resistance. Investigators have also tried to develop instruments that quantify traditional naked-sense observations such as radial pulse palpation and tongue inspection.[78] The assumption driving such studies is that quantified and experimentally demonstrated correspondences will provide for legitimacy and acceptance of traditional diagnostic techniques.

As we have already discussed, many traditional concepts are very difficult to demonstrate objectively because they are the outcome of an approach to natural science that focuses on quality not quantity. This, combined with overly enthusiastic pronouncements about the 'energetic' nature or trigger point correlations of acupuncture, makes it difficult to attract

funding for the relatively sophisticated research required. Manaka's work points to the need for foundation studies, effective instrumentation, and interdisciplinary cooperation. Fortunately, there are scientists willing to face the problems of rigorous research. Nevertheless, there are complex theoretical and social problems to be resolved. For example, if the qi paradigm describes a subtle global operating system, if it describes human software not human hardware, how do we know what technology is right for its measurement?

In many respects, the problems confronting the scientific measurement of acupuncture are similar to those that destroyed electromagnetic medicine at the turn of the century. In the early 20th century the measurement devices needed properly to measure and test weak electric and magnetic fields did not exist. At the same time pharmacological medicine was popular and gaining power. Broadly acceptable means of testing drugs put pharmacotherapy on a firm scientific footing. There were institutions that had the money, technology, and intent to fund research. There were many young scientists interested in a pharmacological career. In all, it was easy to forget research into the electromagnetic medicines of the day. Put simply, the lack of an appropriate technology led to the idea being dismissed without rigorous research. This left the entire field typecast and hobbled by the derogatory label of 'vitalism.' Was this good science? No, it was prejudiced science. What was lost by dismissing a whole field of inquiry as unscientific? None know. Yet, until recently, electromagnetic medicine was nonetheless dead.

This parallel is particularly poignant because it is electromagnetic theory and technology that are often called upon to test, measure, and explain acupuncture. Despite the mountain of evidence that electromagnetic phenomena are very significant in biological systems, they are still dismissed by 'anti-vitalists.' The careers of respected scientists such as Robert Becker bear witness to these problems. Any association with electromagnetic theories and measurement technologies can still draw ridicule.[79] However, it seems that, while there are legitimate questions about what electromagnetic technology has revealed, those questions render these measures no more unscientific than the closed-mindedness that dismisses them out of hand.

Measurement of acupoints

Researchers around the world have attempted to demonstrate objectively the existence of the acupuncture points. By far the most effort expended on measuring these has been the attempt to make electrical measurements of the skin. The basic hypothesis is simple: if the channels and acupuncture points are real, and if they circulate or conduct a *qi* that is an energy, it will be possible to measure that energy electrically. Of the traditionally defined *qi* it is *ying qi*, the *qi* traditionally said to flow in the channels, that is labeled by Chinese names rooted in an analogy to waterways and currents. Thus, it is here where it is legitimate to look for an actual energy flow. If *ying qi* is an electrical energy that flows in the channels, then acupoints and channels should manifest as sites of lowered electrical resistance and increased electrical conductance. This they do.

Although electrical measurement technologies have been applied to the body surface throughout this century, it was not until the 1950s that significant efforts were made to explore explicitly the electrical characteristics of acupuncture points. Nakatani of Japan and Niboyet of France were the first to use electrodermal measurement devices to study acupuncture points.[80] Their findings prompted many in Germany, France, China, and elsewhere to repeat the measurements. Today, not only is there a substantial body of literature showing that the acupuncture points have lower electrical resistance than the surrounding skin, but whole systems of diagnosis and treatment have been based on those observations.[81] Many other researchers have looked at the various microsystems of acupuncture, such as those of the ears and hands, and have found that the points described by those systems also have lower electrical resistance than the surrounding skin.

The significance of these observations is that these points of lowered electrical resistance may serve to conduct electrical signals, energy, or information around the body. Robert Becker has suggested that there is a primitive DC electrical signaling system in the body and that this system serves a number of biological functions, especially in healing.[82] He also notes that the acupuncture points appear to be part of this signaling system. In fact, this, or something like Becker's and Manaka's descriptions, is becoming a more commonly encountered hypothesis.

This idea implies that the acupuncture points are anatomically real, but are not necessarily features of the nervous system. Rather, they may be part of a non-neurological communications system. It further implies that what was traditionally described as *ying qi* is in fact an energetic event, although probably not the 'current in a wire' that has been popularly assumed. *Ying qi* may refer to an electrical flow, or a transmission that is electrical in nature or which has electrical characteristics. However, it behaves less like a flowing current that feeds a human motor and more like a signaling network that carries information throughout the body. The analogy appropriate to acupoints and channels may not be the distribution grid of a power company, but a computer network where messages that start, stop, and modify biological events are sent, routed, and received.

The results of electrical measurement studies are accepted by many acupuncturists and researchers. However, there are questions about what has been measured.[83] The readings of electrodermal diagnostic instruments vary with the strength of the measurement current applied, the frequency of the current, whether the current or voltage is constant or varied, and with pressure variations in the measurement probes and their chemical composition.[84] Because of these measurement variables, different instruments produce different readings. For example, in the 1970s, Manaka and Itaya mapped the location of low-resistance points in the ears.[85] When they varied the strength and frequency of the current, differences emerged. In fact, with each different measurement setting the low-resistance points changed.[86] William Tiller of Stanford University has precisely described how different measurement devices actually measure different things, in particular the resistance of different layers of skin.[87] Thus, when two different measurement devices, for example, Voll's 'Dermatron' and Motoyama's 'AMI' machines, are used to measure the same point, they produce different findings (e.g. different point locations).[88] How then can we tell which measurement, if any, is the actual point, the traditionally described point? At present, this is a very difficult and unresolved technical problem.

The problems associated with the electrical measurement of acupuncture points are compounded further by the fact that measurements made with different instruments are made at different speeds. When a current is applied to the body, the local tissues polarize. This occurs in milliseconds (thousandths of a second). Thus instruments that start measuring resistance after approximately 2 ms are not measuring the original state of the tissues. Rather, they are measuring the body's response to the measurement current. Put another way, by the time the device reads the result of its own test, the state it intended to measure no longer exists. Instruments that measure in microseconds (millionths of a second) avoid this problem.[89] Thus, claims that microsecond-speed instruments tell us something about the state of the body before the test began are on firmer ground. Some researchers believe that measurements made on the millisecond scale are actually measuring the status of the autonomic nervous system,[90] making interpretation relative to the channels more difficult. In other words, they suggest that by measuring the response to an electrical current we are learning about the system that controls that response. Researchers such as Nakatani, Oda, and Hyodo, who use the *Ryodoraku* system, explicitly recognize this phenomena and assert that *Ryodoraku* measurements assess the response of the autonomic nervous system.[91]

Although the claims from this research are not completely unequivocal, all in all, the evidence from electrical measurement research does support the claim that the acupuncture points have electrical characteristics; in particular, they have an electrical resistance that is lower than that of the surrounding skin. However, there is as yet no consensus for how this fact should be interpreted, and more research with improved technologies is required. At the Yale University School of Medicine, Birch, Chun Falk, Arthur Margolin, and Kelly Avants attempted to determine the best and most objective method of locating acupuncture points in the auricles.[92] The study explored visual, palpatory, and electrical differences at the site of each acupuncture point. To conduct the study properly it was first necessary to test various electrodermal-measurement instruments and to build an appropriate measurement device. Working closely with Chun Falk, a reliable measurement methodology was developed.[93] It is hoped that this methodology will be useful for investigating the electrodermal properties of skin, and thus of acupuncture points and channels.

Measurement of channels

Many people feel that objective measurement of the acupuncture channels is crucial to proving the validity of acupuncture. In China, Japan, and elsewhere, there are fierce debates about whether the channels are real, whether they conduct *qi*, or whether they are just imaginary lines used to remember acupoints. The central question is whether or not the channels are something in and of themselves. Many feel that, if the channels are real, they must be objectively measurable.[94] Some researchers feel that clinical utility supports the idea that the channels are a real phenomenon, but that this will be very difficult to measure. A few are convinced that particular measurements have resolved the matter.

At conferences in China, Yoshio Manaka of Japan and Li Ding Zhong of China cooperatively proposed that a reasonable first step toward resolving this debate would be to demonstrate *jing luo* phenomena,[95] that is phenomena that at least appear to be related to either *jing luo* pathways or theories. They proposed cataloging these events and phenomena (e.g. channel-following rashes). They then suggested that the next step should be a rigorous exploration of those observations to determine whether there is a conclusive commonality or relation to the channel system.

To date, most investigations of the channels have accomplished the first suggestion put forward by Li Ding Zhong and Yoshio Manaka. Although some researchers would agree with this statement — noting that the findings are, as yet, imperfect — others would suggest that the investigation has already progressed further. Various methods have been used to measure and observe the channels. Electrical measurements like those described above have been used to investigate whether the channels correspond to lines of lowered electrical resistance. Several studies suggest that this is the case,[96] but the research is open to the same questions as the electrical measurement of acupoints.

In general, it would be better to use more sensitive equipment to measure the electrical characteristics of channels and acupoints without imposing currents sufficiently strong to change their initial state. Were extremely sensitive magnetometers, such as the superconducting quantum interference device (SQUID), to be employed, it would be possible to find out whether there are magnetic fields associated with the channels. If the channels have electrical characteristics, they will produce magnetic fields; however, these fields will be extremely small. Although the ability of low-power magnets to alter acupoint palpatory sensitivity (as shown in Manaka's clinical experiments) suggests a polar, magnetic component to channels and acupoints,[97] to date sensitive equipment has only rarely been employed. Because such devices are very expensive, they are unavailable on the budgets allotted for acupuncture research at present.

Channels have been imaged by other methods. Li Ding Zhong of China documented many dermatological problems that manifest along channel pathways.[98] Although interesting and provocative, creating the statistical correlations necessary to eliminate observational variability from this type of evidence is very difficult. Thus it will probably be difficult to interpret this evidence and develop further research.

In Japan and China it is known that a small percentage of the population is sensitive to needling channel points.[99] When needles are placed in an acupuncture point, these subjects describe propagating sensations, and their descriptions often match the traditional channel pathways. Some of the most extensive research of this variety was done in China,[100] and much of that by Li Ding Zhong and his colleagues.[101] Their studies found that sensitive individuals who know nothing of the channels describe needle sensation pathways that coincide with traditional channel descriptions.[102] Although intriguing, information on this phenomenon, like that on dermatological manifestations on channel pathways, is difficult to gather in a manner that will convince skeptics. However, it is part of a growing body of evidence, and is particularly interesting because it is exactly this variety of naked-sense observation that might have contributed to the historical development of the channel concept.

A related and equally interesting area of research has emerged in China — investigations of sound conduction along channel pathways. If sound (e.g. light percussion) is applied to the body at an acupuncture point, that sound can be measured at a distance from the site of percussion. If the measurement is made on the pathway of the percussed channel, optimal sound spectra can be measured. If the measurement is not on that channel, minimal sound spectra are measured.[103] Like the phenomenon of propagated sensation, this research is intruiging and raises interesting questions about the physical nature of the channels, but it is not yet sufficiently documented or understood to convince sceptics.

Interesting research on the channels has also been performed using radioactive tracers and X-ray imaging. In the late 1970s, Jean Claude Darras and his coworkers started a series of studies in which they injected radioactive tracers into a subject and used specialized imaging techniques to map the migration trails.[104] When the radioactive tracer was injected into an acupuncture point or a channel, it migrated along the channel pathway. If it was injected into tissues that were not near a channel, it migrated only into the surrounding tissues. If the tracer was injected close to a channel, it initially diffused only into the surrounding tissues, but as soon as it contacted the channel it migrated along the channel pathway. The rate and degree of migration were enhanced by needling an acupoint on the channel studied.

Various researchers in Romania, France, and China have reliably repeated these studies. However, there are still several ways to interpret the results. Some believe that the radioactive tracers merely follow the blood and lymph vessels, and thus that the movement which Darras recorded has nothing to do with channels. However, there is some evidence that this is not the case. Darras and his coworkers hypothesize that the migration follows vascular nerve packs in the connective tissues.[105] Again, this evidence is not yet unequivocal, but the results are visually very striking and strongly suggest that the channel system has a basis that can be understood in biomedical terms.

Taking the evidence from these diverse investigations, following Manaka and Li Ding Zhong's suggestion we can say that the number of *jing luo* phenomena are building and have yet to be explained away by skeptics. There is evidence of scientific correlation to the traditional channel system that seems to be valid — electrical measures, responses to a magnetic stimulus, dermatologic phenomena, propagating sensations, X-ray images, and sounds. However, our understanding of what channels might be and how they may best be measured is not yet adequate. Understanding the channel system from a scientific perspective is difficult and technically challenging. Channels are a subtle phenomenon, and thus are difficult to measure. It will take more appropriate technologies and carefully structured studies to bring clarity to the issue.

From a practical point of view, the channel system remains a good explanatory model. It is used in daily clinical practice by thousands upon thousands of acupuncturists. Specific points are routinely chosen for treatment, for the reason that they are on a channel or channels associated with a patient's complaint. It is a routine clinical strategy to needle a point on the hand to affect the teeth, because that point is on a channel traditionally described as passing through the mouth. Yet this is hard to explain through neurological knowledge. Needling a point on the leg to affect the stomach is easy to explain based on a knowledge of the channels, but nearly inexplicable by any other means. Thus, it is important to keep in mind that the ultimate justification of the channel concept and its scientific validation are two distinct issues. If acupuncture based on channel logic performs well in clinical research, the channel concept is useful software, whether or not its hardware can be found.

Measurement of *qi, yin-yang,* and the five phases

Most attempts to measure *qi* have focused on studying the claimed emissions of *qi gong* therapists. In the realm of acupuncture not much has been done to measure what people propose *qi* to be. Hiroshi Motoyama claims to have measured *qi* in his experiments but, as with most of the electrical measurement research, it is not clear exactly what has been measured.[106] The possibility that he measured what he terms 'propagating *qi*' cannot be completely denied, but neither can it be affirmed. Again, technological uncertainty is the defining factor.

The idea of measuring *qi* lends itself to misunderstanding, because *qi* is not a unitary entity. All things are *qi*, and thus to discuss measuring *qi* we need to specify exactly which traditionally described *qi* we are studying. Again, what Westerners are usually discussing when they use the term *qi* is *ying qi*, that which is traditionally said to circulate in the channels. However, *ying qi* and the *qi* that propagates as a result of needling are not the same entity simply because they share the name '*qi*.' Either could be a discrete energy in combination with an orchestrated chain of biological responses, one or more electrical events, or a set of responses keyed to a signal. For now, there is no clear answer. The same is true of the *qi* for which *qi gong* is named. There are two types of *qi gong* studied in *qi* research: 'internal *qi gong*' and 'external *qi gong*.' Most research is focused on external *qi gong*, because what is claimed is that *qi gong* masters emit a *qi* that affects things at a distance. Remember David Eisenberg's story of experience with a *qi gong* master:

> Then it happened. Though he was three feet away, the tassels moved – all six of them. Slowly, the lantern began to move back and forth. I was speechless. Either I had been tricked or this was my first exposure to forces that Western science had not yet defined.[107]

The idea that something emitted under the willed control of a human can effect the physical universe is so alien to Western science that it quickly grasps attention, often by skeptics, for whom these claims are a favored target. In addition, compared to the *qi* of a mountain, a melon, or an honored guest, this emanating *qi* easily fits Western ideas of how energy should behave. It is linear (point to point), temporal, and measurable because it affects matter.

The techniques employed to find what is emitted by *qi gong* masters concentrate on electromagnetic phenomena. The Human Body Field Research Group at Shanghai Jiao Tong University measured near-infrared radiation emitted from the hands of the *qi gong* master.[108] Akira Seto and coworkers of Showa University, Japan, have measured magnetic fields emitted from the hands of *qi gong* therapists.[109] These fields are of the order of hundreds to thousands of times stronger than the strongest fields normally measured at the body surface.

This research is fascinating because it recalls the Western religious tradition of 'palm healing' or 'laying-on of hands.' Bernard Grad from McGill University researched this technique in the 1960s and John Zimmerman from the University of Colorado undertook its study in the 1980s and 1990s. Grad studied the effects of palm healers on cell cultures in sealed containers. He found that cell growth could be affected by whatever it was that a palm healer emitted.[110] He also found that near-infrared radiation seemed to be involved, a finding similar to that of the Shanghai group.

John Zimmerman is an expert in the use of the SQUID and biomagnetic field measurements. He studied gifted palm healers, and found that they emitted magnetic fields that were hundreds of times stronger than the strongest fields normally found in humans.[111] These findings are similar to those of Seto and coworkers in Japan. Similar findings have been reported in China in response to the efforts of *qi gong* practitioners.

Thus it appears that researchers in the West, Japan, and China have independently found similar phenomena when studying *qi gong* practitioners and palm healers. This suggests a link, particularly as both are so strongly rooted in a healing tradition. This research will need to be repeated many times before it becomes widely accepted. Because it is associated with human religious experience rather than the conceptions of medical science, it is by definition an expression of 'faith,' a phenomenon that skeptics often use to dismiss unexpected results. Regardless, this is another area of research that may be important to understanding the *qi* that is reported to circulate in the channels and those *qi* affected or elicted by acupuncture. Perhaps work in the area of 'therapeutic touch,' a method used by increasing numbers of nurses, can lend support to this research.[112]

William Tiller of Stanford has proposed that the *qi*-related effects of acupuncture and *qi gong* are related to a 'magnetic vector potential.'[113] He has developed a theory of how these phenomena work, and we are looking forward to the book he is writing in which he will explain his theories. Another area with research potential is the measurement of the effects of *qi* and *qi*-related phenomena, rather than attempts to measure the *qi* directly. By working backwards from the observed effect, models and tests might be devised that will allow elucidation of the nature of '*qi*' itself. Again, very little work has been done so far in this area. It seems that magnetic measurements would be another area for future research. This is virtually unexplored territory that demands work and resources, especially money.

The investigation or observation of *yin-yang* and five-phase related phenomena is an even more complex issue. *Yin-yang* and the five phases describe relationships between things, processes, and qualities that are common to theoretically every class of phenomena. Thus, they do not refer to things that can be measured. In fact, because they are qualitative assessments traditionally perceived by human senses, they not only share measurement problems with *qi*, but also introduce complex problems of observational reliability. To study these concepts scientifically we will need to focus on correlations between what is described by these theories and what is observed in rigorously controlled experiments.

Studies that seek to find a correlation between, for example, a particular clinical observation or diagnostic pattern and biomedical data are useful because they help establish greater acceptance for traditional concepts. Just as English is the arrival language of translations in English-speaking countries, biomedicine is the arrival language of medical ideas in Western cultures. Thus, if it were possible to relate a traditionally described condition such as 'kidney *yin* vacuity' to a particular set of biomedical measures, acceptance for that concept would be greatly enhanced. The trust placed in biomedical quantifications would then be grafted onto the traditional pattern. In the biomedical community such studies will play an important role; however, to date few studies have been conducted, so there are far too few data to suggest any conclusion.

In China, researchers such as Xie Zhu-fan of the Beijing College of Traditional Chinese Medicine have investigated the correlation between observed diagnostic findings, such as a red tongue or a rapid floating pulse, symptom profiles, and biomedical conditions.[114] These studies help establish links between traditional diagnostic findings, the underlying theories, and corresponding biomedical observations. That is, they help bring the validity of the traditional observations to the attention of the biomedical community. Logically, these studies do not test traditional theories. They are undertaken in contexts where the goal is attachment of traditional techniques to biomedical practice, what is known as 'integrated medicine' in the Peoples' Republic of China.

A different, but related, study type looks at the diagnostic agreement between practitioners who use traditional concepts. These studies measure the reliability of traditional methods. This follows the Western diagnosticians' standard that conditions that are not diagnosed by absolutely objective criteria (e.g. psychiatric syndromes) must be proven reliable before they can be used professionally. Bluntly stated, if practitioners who are trained in the same system of practice cannot examine the same group of patients without statistically significant agreement on diagnosis and treatment, those diagnoses will not be considered valid. Without this 'inter-rater reliability' it is essentially impossible to design an acceptable controlled clinical trial using traditional patterns. Traditional acupunctural diagnoses will need to be proven reliable before they can be used in clinical trials. Because such reliability cannot be tested without written instruments that can be anonymously scored, acupuncturists' clinical experience will continue to constitute unacceptable evidence so long as acupuncturists' terminology is inconsistent.

In traditional East Asian medicine, Chinese provides the terminological standard, and thus reliability research is more easily accomplished. This goal has been furthered by considerable efforts in lexography during the 20th century.[115] In Japan, researchers such as Akio Debata and Yukio Kurosu performed preliminary reliability studies of pulse diagnosis as early as the late 1960s and early 1970s.[116] But the small size and infrequency of these studies make it hard to justify any conclusion. Birch has been conducting studies in this area for several years in order to generate enough data to make convincing statements.[117] In one study he found what may be the first case of statistically significant agreement among acupuncturists using traditionally based diagnoses, in this case *Toyohari* practitioners.[118]

Inter-rater reliability studies do not test or prove the traditional theories as such; rather, they help test the utility of theories and build a firm foundation for clinical research. Unless acupuncturists can complete successful reliability trials, they will have failed to demonstrate that they have mastered traditional diagnostic skills. This is critical, because without terminological consistency and observational reliability to a degree practically sufficient for use in controlled clinical trials, acupuncture will remain totally dependent upon biomedical diagnostic authority. The legal and economic consequences of such dependency could be profound.

To actually test the theories of *yin-yang* and the five phases, an entirely different approach is required. That approach is neither immediately obvious nor intuitive. Again, because many people believe that the long history of continuous practice of acupuncture is proof of validity, they suppose it to also be sufficient proof of the theories applied. This is understandable. It is also wrong. The fact that good clinical results can be obtained is not precisely or absolutely linked to the veracity of the theory used. Obtaining good results makes patients come for treatment and causes people to pay attention to acupuncture, but it does not show that traditional ideas are valid. Indeed, to our knowledge, other than Yoshio Manaka's experiments,[119] there has yet to be a single study designed to test traditional theories. The issues involved are complex, but are probably surmountable.

Birch and Mark Friedman of the University of Alabama have developed a strategy for addressing this issue. If the traditional theories are to be tested, what is first required is a clear statement of those theories. As we have seen throughout this examination of research in acupuncture, the concepts of *qi*, yin-yang, the five phases, channels, and *zang fu* are difficult to state precisely. Models framed purely in the traditional terms cannot be quantified directly by instruments capable of measuring any body process, because these models describe qualities and relationships, not quantities. Even a basic traditional clinical observation such as 'hot' is not based on a thermometer reading but on a subjective assessment of an individual patient's current state. 'Hot' is identified by a complex of subjective and objective signs that are related by qualitative similarity. For example, all the following qualities can indicate a 'hot' state for the traditional diagnostician:

- reddish coloration
- increased activity
- increased speed of activity
- irritability
- presence or preponderance of upbearing bodily events
- presence or preponderance of *yang* bodily events or products.

As each of these qualities — redness, activity, irritability, and upbearing — are perceptions, a basis of perceptual reliability must first be established. Because each is in fact a Chinese-language label that has been subject to historical and cultural variation, there must be a firm definition for each of these qualities among English-speaking clinicians. To complicate further the assessment of these qualitative measures, the correspondences to quantitative measures is relative to the individual. The thermometer reading, color, and physiological and psychological temperament that is 'hot' for you may be normal for someone else. As you can see, it is not easy to reliably measure phenomena that clearly correlate to *yin-yang* theory.

The method that Birch and Friedman have chosen to ameliorate this problem is mathematics (Box 4.6). If precise models of traditional concepts can be stated in the language of mathematics, these models can be linked to instruments. Just as mathematics is used in neurobiology, Birch and Friedman have been developing 'phenomenological mathematical models' of traditional theories. 'Phenomenological' indicates that these models are based only on what is described. The ideas are taken

Box 4.6 The potential utility of mathematical modeling in the understanding and testing of acupuncture

Although there are numerous theories and concepts in acupuncture, some of which are contradictory, a basic model and several key concepts can be isolated. It is these ideas that most essentially characterize the traditional qi paradigm. The problem of investigating this model is two-fold. First, it is very difficult to formulate clear statements from which hypotheses and predictions can be made. Because these concepts have a 'fuzzy nature' and come from a language that is highly evocative and symbolic, these ideas are easily reinterpreted. Secondly, it is very difficult to make reliable measurements, to select appropriate and relevant physiological events to measure, or to select measurable related events from which accurate inferences might be made. In other words, these studies are difficult because the correlations needed to follow a scientifically rigorous approach are as yet unclear.

Although we can formulate verbal descriptions of the traditional model and its key concepts, these are hardly precise. Because verbal descriptions are often expressed in terms that are familiar to Western readers, but are only vaguely defined, these descriptions are further removed from the original concepts by the preconceptions of Western thought. The logic system of acupuncture is alien enough that if we understand a Chinese idea as something with which we are familiar, we have probably missed the point. Because the qi paradigm describes things that are related by qualities (something that is rare in modern Western thinking), the first step in testing and validating the traditional qi paradigm must be the creation of a set of clearly stated relationships. This is where mathematical modeling is helpful. Mathematics provides a language and discipline for expressing the relationships of traditional ideas. Traditional thinkers defined things by their results, by what happened that they could see, feel, or touch. Because mathematical statements represent relationships in an exact way, mathematical language is an ideal intermediate language for the expression of traditional ideas.

This approach to modeling the basic concepts of acupuncture has the additional, but not inconsequential, value of being a standard research tool. Thus Steve Birch and mathematician Mark Friedman from the University of Alabama have begun to formulate mathematical descriptions of traditional ideas. The basic principle is to find the simplest and most concise mathematical description of each seminal concept. This is accomplished by stating in mathematical terms which phenomena that traditional concepts predict will occur in what specific circumstances. Thus far they have accomplished working models of five-phase interactions, the flow of qi in a channel, the moderations produced by needling five-phase acupoints, how flow stagnates, the various interactions between the 12 channels (yin-yang, five phases, etc.), and a general model of how health is restored by acupunctural manipulation.

These models have been linked to electrical circuit diagrams of a channel. These diagrams are based on electrodermal channel measurements. There is also a formulation of how the whole channel system interacts and regulates itself according to yin-yang, five-phase, and other traditional ideas. Because each aspect of this complex model can be tested against real clinical events, it is not only possible to ensure that it accounts for clinical practice, but also to ensure that the concepts are not being forced into a Western mold. Because this approach thoroughly recognizes that the traditional model is a dynamic system, which is without question an essential characteristic of the qi paradigm, it is possible to avoid the reduction of these dynamic traditional ideas to familiar concepts with definitions that are too fixed in Western use to fairly represent the traditional system.

The following differential equation represents the five-phase model:

$$\frac{dw_i}{dt} = aw_{i-1} - bw_{i-2} - cw_i - dw_{i+1} - ew_{i+2} \qquad (1)$$

where w_i is the energy of phase i ($i = 1$ to 5), t is time, and a to e are constants. Here the rate of change of energy in the phase w_i is dependent on the relative level of energy in each phase according to the phase cycles (engendering, restraining, etc.). The interaction of the spleen channel (Q_4) with the other channels can be represented as follows:

$$\frac{dQ_4}{dt} = a_{5,4}Q_5 + a_{9,4}Q_9 - a_{12,4}Q_{12} - a_{1,4}Q_1$$
$$- a_{8,4}Q_8 + a_{1,4}\frac{dQ_1}{dt} - a_{2,4}\frac{dQ_2}{dt} - a_{3,4}\frac{dQ_3}{dt}$$
$$- a_{10,4}\frac{dQ_{10}}{dt} - a_{4,4}Q_4 + C_{9,4}(Q_9 - Q_4)$$
$$+ C_{1,4}(Q_1 - Q_4) + C_{5,4}(Q_5 - Q_4)$$
$$+ C_{12,4}(Q_{12} - Q_4) + C_{8,4}(Q_8 - Q_4)$$

Here the rate of change of energy in the spleen channel (Q_4) is affected by the spleen channel five phase relationship to the other five yin channels (first five items) yin-yang relationships to the other channels (next four items) a homeostatic effect, and the effect of the extraordinary vessels (last five items). Predictions are made from the completed models. Once appropriate measurements have been selected they are then made to see if they match the predictions. If they do, this helps validate the mathematical model. By this method the underlying qi paradigm may start to become more believable, and parts of it may be shown to be valid. This is one of the best ways of testing the traditional models on their own terms.

For further reading see note 120.

at face value without prejudgement. In practice, the qualitative relationships on which traditional theories are based are translated into mathematical statements of relationship. Just as expert translators of Chinese medicine look for words that express all the qualities associated with every use of a Chinese character, these mathematical expressions attempt to model all the events that traditional theories describe. Just as translators must avoid words that overly concretize the logic of Chinese medicine, these models try to avoid reducing the fluid events that traditional theories predict to arbitrarily permanent states.

The advantage of this approach is that it becomes possible to use experimental data without distorting Chinese ideas. The first model so far prepared is one for five-phase interactions.[121] The second model proposed describes a channel based on the electrical findings of Motoyama and Tiller. These mathematical models take into account traditional theories of the channels, treatment methods, Manaka's experimental findings, and modern treatments that utilize the channels.[122] By incorporating this information, traditional explanations of how *qi* flow is increased or decreased by five-phase acupuncture treatments can be logically tested. The third equation models *yin-yang* and five-phase interactions so that these ideas may be tested against the results of actual cases[123] (see Box 4.6). The fourth model examines how different styles of treatment can be accounted for within previous models or by expanding previous models, and how the general physiological state of the body can be altered to produce health.[124]

The goal of these models is to mirror traditional explanations of the channel, *yin-yang*, and five-phase theories, and how *qi* flow is altered and controlled. Once accomplished, experiments to test the mathematical models can be designed. If the traditional theory is correct, a precise mathematical expression of that theory will predict the experimental measures. With the appropriate measurement tools, measurements of the body can be made to confirm or contradict what the models

predict. If the results match the theoretical predictions, the traditional theories will have begun the lengthy road to validation.

Although it will take a long time to produce significant results, this approach not only has the advantage of testing traditional concepts on their own terms, but also the practical advantage of eliminating controversy. In other words, this approach does not simply validate a treatment; it also validates an approach to the design of treatments through traditional logic. Its major disadvantage is that research funds are hard to find because there is no commercial or academic demand for the validation of traditional theories.

CONCLUSION

We have seen that there are conventional biomedical approaches to testing and understanding how acupuncture works. Much of this research is important, but is likely to be found more limited in effect than its proponents have hoped because of limited knowledge and inadequate experimental models. Other findings, for example the vascular effects of acupuncture, appear to be verifiable; what is observed is what we expect. In other areas, outcomes are sensitive not only to the initial conditions of the experiment but also to the measurement approach. Thus experimental models need to be more carefully constructed. Electrodermal measurements of acupuncture points and channels need to be improved and validated through a different approach (e.g. biomagnetic measurements with a device such as the SQUID). The preliminary models and data regarding other traditional concepts such as *yin-yang* and the five phases are too new to justify conclusions. Everyone researching traditional explanatory models of acupuncture needs money, more money, more often.

Our discussions here, although at times critical of earlier conclusions, should not be taken as a blanket critique of the researchers who have devoted their time to these problems. Often enough, it is the acupuncture community that has failed to formulate adequate models and explanations. Ironically, the assumption that *qi* is a single, undefined energy has contributed as much to the reductionism of current scientific research as has the economic emphasis on pain. Without reasonable models, researchers cannot ask appropriate questions. What is clear is that the understanding of how acupuncture works is in the very earliest stages of development and requires more resources and talent if it is to be explored properly.

Regardless of the current state, negative conclusions are unjustified. Put in the vernacular, there is too much smoke to discount fire. Indeed, given how few resources have been dedicated to acupuncture research, there is so much smoke that most researchers refuse to discount the likelihood of fire. However, until more of the flames' light is revealed, skepticism will control scientific and biomedical opinion and the flow of human and financial resources. The current situation thus needs to be seen in terms of its process. Observing the failures to integrate Traditional Chinese Medicine within the Chinese biomedical establishment, Paul Unschuld has proposed that integration should begin with the simple sharing of facilities and resources. Only later, through a series of intervening stages, can genuine conceptual integration be achieved.[125]

Such sharing has begun now in the West because science professionals and acupuncturists have backed away from earlier, more combative characterizations of each other. Within the nascent acupuncture profession, some have begun to support the idea of providing the scientific community with what it needs. Rigorously translated texts, both primary and secondary, and publicly available standardizations of term sets and nomenclature, now provide reliable access to information from which truly well-founded research may be designed. Without such, the translation at scale which is required for sinological, scientific, and clinical research will never be financially feasible. The Society for Acupuncture Research's annual symposia have provided a prototype for the exchange of information between different disciplines. Again, without academic and scientific participation it will be very difficult to develop the trust required for effective cooperation. All these projects and more must succeed if coexistence is to grow toward cooperation.

We hope that the Office of Alternative Medicine at the National Institutes of Health, Bethesda, MD, USA, the Centre for Complementary Health Studies, University of Exeter, UK, and other centers like these around the world will be the beginning of a new stage of communication, one that will see appropriate resources brought to the investigation of these issues. We hope that the levels of funding for these centers will greatly surpass what Joe Jacobs, former Director of the Office of Alternative Medicine, has called 'homeopathic levels of funding.'[126] For, as thick as the smoke may be, it is still not certain that acupuncture will continue to contribute warmth to the hearth of humankind.

NOTES

1   Kleijnen J, Knipschild P, ter Riet G 1992 Clinical trials of homeopathy. British Medical Journal 302:316–323

2   Reported by CS Cheng in a P-AL posting 1/16/1998. The JAMA report is available at http://www.ama-assn.org/sci-pubs/journals/archive/jama/vol_278/no_21/jmn71154.htm

3   Unschuld PU 1998 Chinese medicine. Paradigm Publications, Brookline, MA, p 113

4   Wiseman N 1990 Introduction. In: Wiseman N, Boss K (eds) Glossary of Chinese medical terms and acupuncture points. Paradigm Publications, Brookline, MA

5   Sivin N 1987 Traditional medicine in contemporary China. Center for Chinese Studies, University of Michigan, Ann Arbor, MI, p 47

6   See 'spleen' in: Wiseman N, Feng Y 1998 A practical dictionary of Chinese medicine. Paradigm Publications, Brookline, MA, pp 552–554.

7   See 'qi' in note 6, p 475

8   Miura K 1989 The revival of *qi*; *qi gong* in contemporary China. In: (eds) Taoist meditation and longevity techniques. Center for Chinese Studies, University of Michigan, Ann Arbor, MI, p 335

9   Unschuld PU 1989 Approaches to traditional Chinese medical literature. Dordrecht, Kluwer Academic, p 105

10 Chen Keji, President of the Chinese Association of the Integration of Traditional Chinese and Western Medicine, stated that 'We believe fundamentally that the outside world will only take us seriously if we modernize.' The

Wall Street Journal Interactive Edition, December 3, 1997

11 Interview with Ji Sheng Han. Omni February 1988: 81 ff

12 Felt R. Interview with Tin Yao So

13 Turk DC, Melzack R 1992 The measurement of pain and the assessment of people experiencing pain. In: Turk DC, Melzack R (eds) Handbook of pain assessment. Guildford Press, New York

14 Hanson RW, Gerber KE 1990 Coping with chronic pain. Guildford Press, New York

15 See note 14

16 See note 14

17 Birch S, Tsutani K 1996 A bibliometrical study of English-language materials on acupuncture. Complementary Therapies in Medicine 4:172–177

18 See note 17

19 Mann F 1972 Acupuncture; the ancient Chinese art of healing and how it works scientifically. Vintage, New York

20 (a) Gunn CC 1988 Reprints on pain, acupuncture and related subjects. Vancouver
(b) Ulett G 1992 Beyond *yin* and *yang*. WH Green, St Louis, MI

21 (a) Baldry PE 1989 Acupuncture, trigger points and musculoskeletal pain. Churchill Livingstone, Edinburgh
(b) Melzack R, Stillwell DM, Fox EJ 1977 Trigger points and acupoints for pain: correlations and implications. Pain 3:3–23

22 Dung HC 1984 Anatomical features contributing to the formation of acupuncture points. American Journal of Acupuncture 12(2):139–142

23 Le Bars D, Willer JC, de Broucker T, Villanueva L 1989 Neurophysiological mechanisms involved in the pain-relieving effects of counterirritation and related techniques including acupuncture. In: Pomeranz B, Stux G (eds) Scientific bases of acupuncture. Springer-Verlag, Berlin

24 Wang KM, Yao S, Xian Y, Hou Z, 1985 A study on the receptive field of acupoint and the relationship between characteristics of needling sensation and groups of afferent fibres. Scientica Sinica (Series B) 28(9):963–971

25 See, for example, note 20(b)

26 See, for example, notes 20(b) and 21(a)

27 Melzack R, Stillwell DM, Fox EJ 1977 Trigger points and acupoints for pain: correlations and implications. Pain 3:3–23

28 Birch S Trigger point–acupoint correlations revisited. Unpublished

29 Melzack R, Stillwell DM, Fox EJ 1977 Trigger points and acupoints for pain: correlations and implications. Pain 3:3–23

30 The following sources were reviewed:
(a) Anon 1980 Essentials of Chinese acupuncture. Foreign Language Press, Beijing
(b) Mann F 1974 The treatment of disease by acupuncture. Heinemann, London
(c) O'Connor J, Bensky D 1981 Acupuncture: a comprehensive text. Eastland Press, Seattle, WA
(d) Shiroda B 1986 *Shinkyu Chiryo Kisogaku* 6th edn. Ido No Nippon Sha, Yokokusa
(e) So JTY 1987 Treatment of disease with acupuncture
(f) Yang J-Z 1982 Zhen Jiu Da Cheng 1601 Da Zhang Guo Tu Shu, Taipei in Matsumoto K, Birch S 1986. Extraordinary Vessels. Paradigm Publications, Brookline, MA, pp 77–12

31 World Health Organization 1991 A proposed standard international acupuncture nomenclature; report of a WHO scientific group. WHO, Geneva

32 See: (a) Chapman CR, Chen AC, Bonica JJ 1997 Effects of intrasegmental electrical acupuncture on dental pain; evaluation by threshold estimation and sensory decision theory. Pain 3:213–227
(b) Cheng RSS 1989 Neurophysiology of electroacupuncture analgesia. In: Pomeranz B, Stux G (eds) Scientific bases of acupuncture. Springer-Verlag, Berlin, pp 119–136
(c) Han JS 1987 The neurochemical basis of pain relief by acupuncture. Beijing Medical University
(d) Han JS 1989 Central neurotransmitters and acupuncture analgesia. In: Pomeranz B, Stux G (eds) Scientific bases of acupuncture. Springer-Verlag, Berlin, pp 7–33
(e) Han JS 1997 Physiology of acupuncture: a review of thirty years research. Journal of Alternative and Complementary Medicine 3(suppl 1):S101–S108
(f) Pomeranz B 1991 Scientific basis of acupuncture. In: Stux G, Pomeranz B (eds) *Basics of acupuncture*. Springer-Verlag, Berlin, pp 4–55
(g) Pomeranz B 1996 Scientific research into acupuncture for the relief of pain. Journal of Alternative and Complementary Medicine 2(1):53–60
(h) Takeshige C 1989 Mechanism of acupuncture analgesia based on animal experiments. In: Pomeranz B, Stux G (eds) Scientific bases of acupuncture. Springer-Verlag, Berlin, pp 53–78
(i) Toda K, Suda H, Ichioka M, Iriki A 1980 Local electrical stimulation: effective needling points for suppressing jaw opening reflex in rat. Pain 9:199–207

33 See, for example: note 32(f)

34 (a) Pomeranz B 1996 Scientific research into acupuncture for the relief of pain. Journal of Alternative and Complementary Medicine 2(1):53–60
(b) Presentation at the Consensus Development Conference on Acupuncture, National Institutes of Health, November 3–5, 1997

35 See note 34a

36 (a) See Pomeranz & Stux, note 32(b)
(b) See Stux & Pomeranz, note 32(f)

37 See note 32(f), pp 4–55

38 Vincent CA, Richardson PH, Black JJ, Pither CE 1989 The significance of needle placement site in acupuncture. Journal of Psychosomatic Research 33(4):489–496

39 See, for example, note 20(b)

40 See the discussions in Chapter 2. Acupuncture with a needle stimulus requires less experience. The patient can report the needle sensation, its direction, and quality, thus confirming point location and stimulation. Techniques that require the practitioner to note a subtle needling sensation, which the patient cannot so easily sense, or to verify location and stimulation by pulse-taking or palpation, requires more training.

41 See the discussions in Chapter 7

42 This is based on our discussions with acupuncturists in the USA, Europe, and Australia, information on needle use gathered via a practitioner questionaire, and the themes evident in practitioner brochures and advertisements. However, to our knowledge, there is presently no statistically reliable source for this information.

43 Lytle CD 1997 Safety and regulation of acupuncture needles and other devices. Presented at the Consensus Development Conference on Acupuncture

44 Ji Sheng Han 1997 Physiology of acupuncture. Review of thirty years research. Journal of Alternative and

Complementary Medicine 3(suppl 1):S101–S108

45   Pomeranz B 1993 Change in the medical science of acupuncture. In: Abstracts of the Third World Conference on Acupuncture. World Federation of Acupuncture and Moxibustion Societies, Kyoto

46   Pomeranz B 1989 Research into acupuncture and homeopathy. In: Energy fields and medicine; a study of device technology based on acupuncture meridians and chi energy. Proceedings of a symposium sponsored by the John E Fetzer Foundation, pp 66–77. Quite recent evidence from preliminary studies have shown actions of acupuncture in specific regions of the brain. A small study by Alavi, LaRiccia, Lee and colleagues at the University of Pennsylvania in Philadelphia used a SPECT (single photon emission computed tomography) scan to visualize the brain of volunteer patients. They selected patients that had already shown a positive response to acupuncture treatment for their pain. SPECT scan images were taken of their brains before and after an acupuncture session. The researchers could clearly show changes in the brainstem and thalamus as a result of treatment (Alavi A, LaRiccia PJ, Sadek AH, Newberg AB, Lee L, Reich H, Lattanand C, Mozley PD 1997 Neuroimaging of acupuncture in patients with chronic pain. Journal of Alternative and Complementary Medicine. 3(suppl 1):S47–S53). A more recent small study by Zang-Hee Cho and colleagues of the University of California, Irvine, found even more specific results. Using a functional MRI (magnetic resonance imaging) machine to visualize the brain, they found that needling points on the leg that are reputed to be good for eye problems, produced specific changes in the visual cortex (Dold C 1998 Needles and Nerves. Discover. September pp 59–62). While these preliminary results are based on small studies, future work will be able to build on this and possibly produce confirmation and other interesting results. A team of researchers from the National Institute on Alcohol Abuse and Alcoholism has set up research laboratories that will use PET (positron emission tomography) scans to visualize the effects of acupuncture on the brain (Joseph Hibbeln, personal communication). This may prove to be a very fertile area for research into the neurophysiological effects of acupuncture.

47   Soulie de Morant G 1994 Chinese acupuncture. Paradigm Publications, Brookline, MA, pp 46, 273–275

48   Lee MHM, Ernst M Clinical research observations on acupuncture analgesia and thermography, in Pomeranz & Stux, note 32(b), pp 157–175

49   Oda H 1989 Ryodoraku textbook. Naniwasha, Osaka

50   Hyodo M 1975 Ryodoraku treatment. Autonomic Nerve System Society, Osaka

51   Liao SJ, Liao MK 1985 Acupuncture and tele-electronic infra-red thermography. Acupuncture and Electro-Therapeutics Research International Journal 10:41–66

52   Itaya K, Manaka Y, Ohkubo C, Asano M 1987 Effects of acupuncture needle application upon cutaneous microcirculation of rabbit ear lobe. Acupuncture and Electro-therapeutics Research International Journal 12:45–51

53   This was an informal trial conducted by Marc Coseo as part of the research for his text. See: Coseo M 1992 The acupressure warmup. Paradigm Publications, Brookline, MA

54   Becker RO, Marino AA 1982 Electromagnetism and life.

State University of New York Press, Albany, NY, pp 40ff

55   See notes 48 and 52

56   See note 52

57   Based on Itaya et al, note 52

58   Based on Itaya et al, note 52

59   Impression work has been done in China. See, for example: Cao XD 1997 Protective effect of acupuncture on immunosuppression. NIH consensus development conference on acupuncture. Program & abstracts. National Institutes of Health, Bethesda, MD, pp 129–133

60   See, for example: Carr DJ, Blalock JE 1991 Neuropeptide hormones and receptors common to the immune and neuroendocrine systems: bidirectional pathway intersystem communication. Psychoneuroimmunology 573–588

61   Sodipo JA 1979 Acupuncture and gastric acid studies. American Journal of Chinese Medicine 7(4):356–361

62   See, for example: Guelrud M, Rossiter A, Souney PF, Sulbaran M 1991 Transcutaneous electrical nerve stimulation decreases lower esophageal sphincter pressure in patients with achalasia. Digestive Diseases and Sciences 36(8):1029–1033

63   See, for example: Li Y, Tougas G, Chiverton SG, Hunt RH 1992 The effect of acupuncture on gastrointestinal function and disorders. American Journal of Gastroenterology 87(10):1372–1381

64   Volkov MV, Oganesyan OV 1987 External fixation: joint deformities and bone fractures. International Universities Press, Madison CT. This reference was kindly provided by Dr Sharon Rubrake

65   Yoshio Manaka Y. Personal communication

66   Guo QT, Wu SQ, Chen TR 1991 Clinical and experimental observation on treating cholelithiasis by earpoint pressing. International Journal of Clinical Acupuncture 2:1

67   Chang PL 1988 Urodynamic studies in acupuncture for women with frequency, urgency and dysuria. Journal of Urology 140:563–566

68   See, for example: Ulett GA 1982 Principles and practice of physiologic acupuncture. WH Green, St Louis, MI, pp 118–121

69   Manaka Y. Personal communication

70   Manaka Y, Itaya K 1986 Acupuncture as intervention in the biological information system (meridian treatment and the X-signal system). Address given at the annual assembly of the Japan Meridian Treatment Association, Tokyo, March 29–30. Published in English in the Journal of the Acupuncture Society of New York 1994, 1(4) 9–18 and 1995, 2(1) 15–22

71   Becker RO 1984 Electromagnetic controls over biological growth processes. Journal of Bioelectronics 3(1/2):105–118

72(a) Manaka Y, Itaya K, Birch S 1995 Chasing the dragon's tail. Paradigm Publications, Brookline, MA
(b) Becker RO, Selden G 1985 The body electric. William Morrow, New York
(c) Matsumoto K, Birch S 1988 Hara diagnosis, reflections on the sea. Paradigm Publications, Brookline, MA
(d) Oschman JL 1994 A biophysical basis for acupuncture. Proceedings of the first symposium of the Society for Acupuncture Research. Society for Acupuncture Research, Newton, MA

73   See note 72(a), chs 3–6

74   See note 72(a), ch 2

75 This development has been one of the most puzzling areas in biology for a long time, with many models put forward to explain these complex processes. See, for example, discussion in:
(a) Campbell NA 1987 Biology. Benjamin Cummings, Menlo Park, CA, pp 935–943
(b) Sheldrake R 1981 A new science of life: the hypothesis of causative formation. JP Tarcher, Los Angeles

76 See note 72(d)

77 Manaka's publications detail the use of polar stimuli. See note 72(a), chs 2–6

78 See, for example:
(a) Chen ZL 1988 Development of research on tongue diagnosis. Chinese Journal of Integrated Medicine 8(special issue 2):104–108
(b) Broffman M, McCulloch M 1986 Instrument assisted pulse evaluation in the acupuncture practice. American Journal of Acupuncture 14(3):255–259

79 See note 72(b)

80 See discussions in: Zhu ZX 1981 Research advances in the electrical specificity of meridians and acupuncture points. American Journal of Acupuncture 9(3): 203–216

81 For references to many of the publications in this area, see:
(a) Tiller WA 1989 On the evolution and future development of electrodermal diagnostic instruments. Energy fields in medicine; a study of device technology based on acupuncture meridians and chi energy. Proceedings of a symposium sponsored by the John E Fetzer Foundation, pp 257–328
(b) Falk CX, Birch S, Margolin A, Avants SK (submitted) Measurement of electrical resistance of the skin: mapping resistance at auricular acupuncture points

82 See note 81

83 Tiller WA 1987 What do electrodermal diagnostic acupuncture instruments really measure? American Journal of Acupuncture 15(1):15–23

84 See note 81(b)

85 See note 72(a), pp 344–348

86 See note 72(a), pp 344–348

87 See note 81(a)

88 See note 81(a)

89 See note 81(a)

90 See note 50

91(a) See notes 49 and 50
(b) Nakatani Y, Yamashita K 1977 *Ryodoraku* acupuncture. Ryodoraku Research Institute, Tokyo

92 This study was conducted as part of Birch's work to standardize point location for a multicenter trial of acupuncture run by Herbert Kleber of Columbia University: Margolin A, Avants SK, Birch S, Falk CX, Kleber HD 1997 Methodological investigations for a multisite trial of auricular acupuncture for cocaine addiction. A study of active and control auricular zones. Journal of Substance Abuse Treatment 13(6):471–481

93 See note 81(b)

94 See, for example, note 20(b)

95 Manaka Y. Personal communication

96 See note 72(c), p 206, especially footnote 4

97 See, for example, note 72(a), pp 31 ff, 43 ff, 52 ff, 62 ff

98 Li Ding Zhong 1984 *Jing luo* phenomena, vol 1. Yukonsha, Tokyo

99 See discussions in note 72(a), pp 52–53

100 This phenomenon has been frequently reported on by researchers in China. In the National Symposia of Acupuncture and Moxibustion and Acupuncture Anesthesia, Beijing, June 1–5, 1979, there were over 30 papers reporting on studies of this phenomenon (over 6% of the papers). In the Selections from Article Abstracts on Acupuncture and Moxibustion, Beijing, November 22–26, 1987, from the first World Federation of Acupuncture and Moxibustion Societies Conference, there were over 30 papers reporting on studies of this phenomenon (over 5% of the papers)

101 Li Ding Zhong 1985 *Jing luo* phenomena, vol 2. Yukonsha, Tokyo

102 See note 101

103 See, for example:
(a) Sun PS, Zhao YZ, Li YL, Yan QL, Liu H 1987 The study of acoustic information along channels. Selections from article abstracts on acupuncture and moxibustion, Beijing, Nov 22–26, 334–336
(b) Sun PS, Li YL, Yan QL 1987 Analysis on the forming factors and the changing regulations of the background sound in measuring the sound information along the meridian. See note 103(a), pp 336–337
(c) Sun PS, Zhao YZ, Li YL, Yan, QL, Liu H 1987 The spectrum analysis on the propagation of sound information along meridians. See note 103(a), pp 337–338
(d) Zhao YZ, Sun PS, Li YL, Yan QL, Liu H 1987 Study on the relations between the production of the sound information along meridian and the exciting pressures. See note 103(a), pp 339–340
(e) Sun PS Zhao YZ, Tian QN, Zhu FS, Wang DS 1987 Contrast observation between sound information along meridians and muscular electricity. See note 103(a), pp 340–341
(f) Sun KF, Li YL, Liu H, Yan QL, Sun PS 1987 The experimental study on conduction of quantitative acoustic frequency signals along the large intestine channel of hand *yangming*. See note 103(a), pp 341–343
(g) Zhu FS, Peng JS, Wang PS, Wan YG 1987 Transfer of sound signals along acupuncture meridians an experimental study. See note 103(a), p 343
(h) Wang PS, Ma YR, Zhao Y 1987 The experimental observation on sound information of propagated sensations along channels (PSC). See note 103(a), pp 344–345

104 Darras JC 1989 Isotopic and cytologic assays in acupuncture. In: Energy fields in medicine; a study of device technology based on acupuncture meridians and chi energy. Proceedings of a symposium sponsored by the John E Fetzer Foundation, Kalamazoo, Michigan, pp 44–65

105 de Vernejoul P, Albaïède P, Darras JC 1992 Nuclear medicine and acupuncture message transmission. Journal of Nuclear Medicine 33(3):409–412

106 Motoyama H 1986 Biophysical elucidation of the meridian and ki energy. What is ki energy and how does it flow? Research for Religion and Parapsychology 7:1–78

107 Eisenberg D, Wright TL 1987 Encounters with qi. Penguin, New York, p 139

108 Qian CZ et al 1981 Simulated human body information in bio-medical therapy: experimental investigation in 'human body field' (II). Shanghai Jiao Tong University

109 Seto A, Kusaka C, Nakazato S, Huang WR, Sato T,

Hisamitsu T, Takeshige C 1992 Detection of extraordinary large bio-magnetic field strength from human body during external qi emission. Acupuncture and Electro-Therapeutics Research International Journal 17:75–94

110 Reported in: Zimmerman J 1990 Laying-on-of-hands and therapeutic touch: a testable theory. Newsletter of the Bio-Electro-Magnetics Institute 2(1): 8–17

111 See note 110

112(a) See, for example: Krieger D 1979 Therapeutic touch: how to use your hands to help or heal. Prentice Hall, Englewood, Cliffs, NJ
(b) For a brief review. See: Fugh-Berman A 1996 *Alternative medicine: what works*. Odonian, Tucson, pp 155–157

113 See note 81(a)

114 See, for example: Xie Zhu-fan 1988 Researches on 'cold' and 'heat' in traditional Chinese medicine. Chinese Journal of Integrated Medicine 8(special issue 2): 93–96

115 Wiseman N 1998 Eighty years of Chinese lexicography: response to modern challenges. Internet research paper at http://www.paradigm-pubs.com/refs/eiyech-1.pdf

116(a) Debata A 1968 Experimental study on pulse diagnosis of *rokujuboi*. Japanese Acupuncture and Moxibustion Journal 17(3): 9–12
(b) Kurosu Y 1969 Experimental study on the pulse diagnosis of *rokujuboi* II. Japanese Acupuncture and Moxibustion Journal 18(3): 26–30

117(a) Birch S, Jamison RN 1993 The importance of assessing the reliability of diagnosis in traditional acupuncture. Abstracts of the third world conference on acupuncture. World Federation of Acupuncture and Moxibustion Societies, Kyoto
(b) Birch S Preliminary investigations of the inter-rater reliability of traditionally based acupuncture diagnostic assessments (submitted)

118 See note 117(b)

119 See note 72(a), chs 3–6

120(a) Birch S, Friedman M 1989 On the development of a mathematical model for the 'laws of the five phases. American Journal of Acupuncture 17(4): 361–366
(b) Friedman M, Birch S, Tiller WA 1989 Towards the development of a mathematical model for acupuncture meridians. Acupuncture and Electrotherapeutics Research International Journal 14:217–226
(c) For more general discussions, see: Friedman MJ, Birch S, Tiller WA 1997 Mathematical modelling as a tool for basic research in acupuncture. Journal of Alternative and Complementary Medicine 3(suppl 1):S89–S99

121 Birch S, Friedman M 1989 On the development of a mathematical model for the 'laws' of the five phases. American Journal of Acupuncture 17(4): 361–366

122 Friedman M, Birch S, Tiller WA 1989 Towards the development of a mathematical model for acupuncture meridians. Acupuncture and Electrotherapeutic Research International Journal 14: 217–226

123 Birch S, Friedman M 1990 Towards the development of a mathematical model describing the interactions of the twelve channels (*jingluo*). Unpublished

124 Friedman MJ, Birch S, Tiller WA 1997 Mathematical modelling as a tool in basic research in acupuncture. Journal of Alternative and Complementary Medicine 3(suppl 1):S89–S99

125 Unschuld PU 1985 Medicine in China: a history of ideas. University of California, Berkeley, CA, pp 260–262

126 Jacobs J 1994 Presentation at the Wellness Conference, Washington DC

How acupuncture is practiced

5

What does acupuncture treat?

In the 20th century this is really three questions: Is acupuncture safe? What has acupuncture been proven to cure or ameliorate? For what conditions is acupuncture an economically practical alternative? The first of these questions can be answered with a definite 'yes.' Without question or controversy acupuncture is safe. The second and third questions can be answered, often positively, but with less certainty. A Western consensus has only recently begun to form because the answers to these questions involve dealing with the variability of acupuncture, the vagaries of its current transmission, the lack of funds for researching nonbiomedical modalities, the difficulty of adapting acupuncture to biomedical trial designs, and the natural Western bias against something so often presented as 'exotic.'

IS ACUPUNCTURE SAFE?

If acupuncture provided effective relief but had severe side-effects, it would never be widely adopted. The evidence indicates that this is far from the case. At the Consensus Development Conference on Acupuncture at the US National Institutes of Health, the documented side-effects of acupuncture were acknowledged to be 'extremely low.'[1] In the presentation by David Lytle, a researcher at the US Food and Drugs Administration, four major areas of adverse effects were identified through case reports and surveys:[2]

- infections (transmission from patient to patient or local infections)

- damaged tissue (nerve damage, punctured organs)
- broken needle remnants that migrate
- less serious transient events.

In the documented literature from more than 25 years of worldwide use, the total number of incidents reported was 3778. These included seven deaths, 97 punctured lungs, and 170 cases of hepatitis transmission. The vast majority of events were less serious transient effects, such as fainting during treatment, nausea and/or vomiting, skin irritation, muscle spasm, and local skin infections.[3] An Australian survey estimated that there were 4.2 adverse events per 1000 consultations.[4] In a Norwegian survey, 0.21 adverse events were reported for each practitioner-year of full-time practice.[5] Lytle concluded that 'acupuncture is a relatively safe therapeutic procedure.' The total of 3778 reported events occurred over a 25-year period during which hundreds of millions of treatments were performed. This gives an adverse-effect rate of less than 1%. The real percentage is probably lower because of the reporting bias created by the legal status of acupuncture during this period. For example, during the years when US laws required acupuncturists to be supervised by physicians, the legal and financial pressures on supervising physicians increased the probability that any adverse effect would be fully reported. However, since there was no mechanism for recording the cases treated by acupuncturists, the records available to researchers are probably understated.

Compared to the adverse-effect rate of modern pharmacotherapy, acupuncture is very safe. For example, MedWatch routinely reports information about adverse events in standard biomedical practice. It is reported that 3–11% of hospital admissions were attributed to adverse drug events and that hospitalized patients have a 1–44% chance of an adverse drug reaction.[6] It is thus obvious that acupuncture is relatively safe, provided it is administered by a properly trained practitioner.[7] The deficits that either physician or specialist acupuncture training may have had during this formative period have clearly not resulted in an epidemic of side-effects. Acupuncture is a medical option that may be tried or recommended with no appreciable risk. In addition, the specific training of acupuncturists in proper needle handling, the extensive use of single-use presterilized needles since the mid-1980s, and the current almost exclusive use of these needles, has significantly lowered the rate at which the more serious adverse events are likely to occur.

WHAT CONDITIONS HAS ACUPUNCTURE BEEN PROVEN TO CURE?

Although limited in scope, for the first time in the history of the westward migration of acupuncture, there are some unequivocal answers to this question. After reviewing the literature on the performance of acupuncture in controlled clinical trials, the Consensus Development Conference panel concluded that there was substantial evidence for the efficacy of acupuncture in the following four conditions:[8]

- postoperative nausea and vomiting
- chemotherapy-associated nausea and vomiting
- pregnancy-associated nausea and vomiting
- postoperative dental pain.

In addition, the panel noted other conditions for which the evidence of effectiveness is good but requires further substantiation. These conditions are:

- headache
- low-back pain
- fibromyalgia
- myofascial pain
- tennis elbow
- osteoarthritis
- carpal tunnel syndrome
- postoperative pain
- addictions
- stroke rehabilitation
- menstrual cramps
- asthma.

Why only this short list and not the earlier and larger list reported by the World Health Organization (WHO)? Why not the hundreds or thousands of conditions noted in traditional and modern acupuncture texts? Why not simply accept the claims of Chinese clinical experience? Why not the results of studies that were not controlled clinical trials? There are many reasons, but most evolve from the adaptability and clinical logic of acupuncture.

In both historic and modern literature, acupuncture is described as useful for an extremely wide range of symptoms and disorders. Gao Wu's famous *Zhen Jiu Ju Ying* (1529) lists 208 indications for just eight pairs of treatment points.[9] George Soulie de Morant's *Chinese Acupuncture* is based on 4 decades of research into major Chinese and Japanese clinical manuals. It compiles treatments for more than 5500 conditions in more than 700 categories.[10] Tin Yau So's text *Treatment of Disease with Acupuncture* specifies treatment protocols for over 125 symptoms or disorders based solely on his own and his teacher's experience.[11] Modern Chinese texts list anywhere from just over 50 disorders to more than 100.[12] In a four-page appendix to Bunshi Shiroda's Japanese text, *Shinkyu Chiryo Kisogaku (The Fundamentals of Acupuncture and Moxibustion Therapy)* there is a list of 110 diseases said to be treated by moxibustion alone.[13] In Wu Yan & Fischer's *Practical Therapeutics of Traditional Chinese Medicine* over 100 current Chinese hospital protocols are detailed; each of these conditions suggests one or more correspondences to biomedically defined symptoms or diseases.[14] Why not accept these? Could everyone in so large a health-care system as that of the People's Republic of China be completely deluded as to the efficacy of acupuncture? Could millions and millions of patients all have been placebo responders?

People who are aware of the extent of the current and historical application of acupuncture do not doubt that it is effective for a considerable variety of conditions. What is lacking is not a record of successful treatment by acupuncture, but a generally acceptable means of relating two substantively different systems of knowledge — the East Asian and Western logical systems. Practically, this creates three related difficulties. First, there are problems with the cross-cultural identification of what has been treated and how success in treatment

has been determined. Second, clinical experience in acupuncture is difficult to transmit, because it is experienced and recorded in the language of human observation. Finally, there are significant cross-cultural differences in how treatments are verified.

Identifying what has been treated

In modern books, the indications for the use of acupuncture sometimes go well beyond the suggestion of Western medical correspondences by actually translating Chinese or Japanese terms as symptoms or diseases defined by biomedicine. This relieves translators of considerable linguistic research, because Chinese monolingual medical dictionaries can be used. Furthermore, except in cases where the terms are archaic, this is potentially more acceptable in biomedically dominated circles. This also follows Chinese trends. We have already noted the dominance of biomedical diagnoses in the PRC.[15] However, this also adds an additional complexity to the question 'What does acupuncture treat?' because there is little scientific evidence to support the relationship between traditional diagnoses to biomedically defined diseases.

Some experts feel that direct, one-to-one equivalence is rare, perhaps non-existent.[16] However, the biomedicalization of Chinese medicine has been continuous since biomedicine arrived in China, and various degrees of correspondence have been noted by many writers.[17] Indeed, one of the first attempts to establish correspondences was a Chinese medical encyclopedia that Soulie de Morant researched in the first decade of the 20th century. In this encyclopedia, Chinese traditional and biomedical concepts were already mixed.[18]

There also are many practical barriers to formulating accurate equivalences between the two systems. No bilingual dictionary has been consistently used in the westward migration of acupuncture. Thus, English-language clinical records are discursive and practically useless as a source of biomedical equivalence.[19] References to Chinese monolingual dictionaries also create complex practical problems. For example, when some Chinese biomedical dictionaries were compiled, Chinese intellectuals considered traditional Chinese medicine unworthy of preservation. Therefore, they appropriated the characters used in traditional medicine for biomedical concepts. Because it is difficult to create new Chinese characters, traditional characters were simply assigned new, biomedical meanings. For example, the character that had traditionally labeled an entire class of illnesses (*lin*) became a single biomedical disease (gonorrhea). Characters that once meant 'a spot suddenly arising in the flesh, as big as a beam, or as small as a red seed, and in serious cases as big as a plum,' were recycled as 'felon' or 'melanotic fingernail tumor.' It is easy to see how these dictionaries can be misleading.[20]

The problem is also deeper than one of recycled characters. In the example just given, even had the characters not been recycled, association with the biomedical condition could have been just as inaccurate. The descriptions used in acupuncture predominantly depend on observation with the naked senses — something is so big, so located, colored in a certain way, and accompanied by certain other observations in a pattern of relationship. Phenomena are described not by their cause, as in Western science, but by relation to events that share qualities. Western diagnoses predominantly depend on precise measurements of microscopic biological events; patterns depend upon systematic recognition by human observers. For example, 'melanotic' means an excess of cells containing darkly pigmented melanin. As a biochemical measure, this is useful when it references physiological research that sets quantitative standards for what is normal. However, melanin pigments skin and hair in the West as well as in the East. Thus, naked-sense evaluations are not only possible but are also probably an integral part of some physicians' clinical experience. The problem is not that biomedicine makes exclusively quantitative assessments and acupuncture makes exclusively naked-sense observations. There are indeed observations that both systems share. The

problem is that the differences in the assessment methods make it difficult to establish a standard by which to equate the two. Thus any equivalence is difficult to justify, particularly to the degree necessary for controlled clinical trials.

Another common result of these differences is that diagnoses based on traditional principles often relate to several different biomedical symptoms or diseases. It is also difficult to equate even just a symptom (remember Paul Unschuld's reasoning for the term 'pathocondition,' see Ch. 3, p. 131) not only because East and West see symptoms differently, but also because Eastern and Western patients respond differently to similar states. Thus, from the viewpoint of biomedically trained physicians who approach acupuncture unaware of its cognitive character, acupuncturists are often claiming to treat a multiplicity of symptoms, or even several diseases with a single treatment.[21] This is one of the reasons why Western physicians are so tempted to think of acupuncture as a placebo – its effects do not correspond to their experience.

This characteristic is not exclusive to one system or another, but is general to the field. In Denmei Shudo's *Introduction to Meridian Therapy, Japanese Classical Acupuncture*, the five-phase channel diagnosis of lung vacuity is associated with as many as eight primary symptoms and 16 secondary symptoms.[22] In the modern Chinese *yin-yang ba gang bian zheng* system of acupuncture, the pattern of ascendant hyperactivity of liver yang can have as many as 13 related symptoms.[23] In Manaka's system of *yin-yang* balancing and channel therapy, a *yin qiao-ren mai* pattern can have up to 13 different symptom correspondences.[24] In each of these cases, the listed symptoms are really only those most commonly associated with the pattern. In principle, many symptoms can develop when lung vacuity, ascendant hyperactivity of liver yang, or *yin qiao-ren mai* problems occur.

Transmitting clinical experience

Making this multiplicity of claims even more difficult to understand, traditional East Asian acupuncture has undergone radical change in the modern period. The history of practitioners who lived and worked up to the middle of this century describes a role for acupuncture that is greatly different from that of post-Liberation China. A biographical example illustrates the issues.[25]

Tin Yau So, a Christian minister, began to practice acupuncture full-time in 1939 in China when his church was forcibly closed after the Japanese invaded China. Although Dr So is not a medical doctor, he is called 'doctor' because so many people respect and are grateful for his skills. He was often the primary health-care provider for a considerable community. In fact, some accounts of his treatments are so dramatic that skeptics will probably never accept them.

In the early 20th century, diseases such as cholera still swept through China. Dr So's Chinese students tell of an epidemic, when he administered acupuncture to as many as 200 patients every day. In one such report, Dr So triaged the sick from the dying in a Hong Kong epidemic by administering acupuncture or moxa to points indicated by the specific symptoms he observed. If the patient responded appropriately, Dr So would complete the treatment. If not, he knew the victim was too weak to survive. Dr So cured so many people of cholera using acupuncture that he describes it as a disease requiring only one or two treatments.[26] Although skeptics discount such stories, this is exactly what Soulie de Morant reported from Bejing in 1901: 'I saw a Chinese doctor quickly stop the dangerous cramps, vomiting, and diarrhea — whose grave significance I immediately recognized — without using European medicines.'[27]

Dr So is among the last of generations of practitioners who studied through apprenticeships with a teacher who transmitted clinical knowledge as a style of practice that they knew to be effective for a range of conditions which, however broad or narrow, was determined by individual experience. Dr So's teacher, Tsang Tien Chi, was a high-school teacher. Because neither Western medicine nor Chinese herbal medicine rescued his family from the diseases

he describes as 'asthma, dysentery and dropsy,' he undertook the study of acupuncture. In 1930, Tsang sold his property, quit teaching, and went to Shanghai to study with Cheng Tan An, one of the most famous acupuncturists of the early 20th century.[28] In 1934, 2 years after returning from Shanghai, Tsang opened a school in Canton, the school Tin Yau So would attend. There, training was by doing; Dr So treated more than 200 patients, including his own father, before graduation. Graduating in 1941, he opened his own school in Hong Kong, graduating 500 students by 1972, when he went to the USA.

What we learn from this brief biography is that the question, 'What can acupuncture treat? has very often been answered as 'Whatever my teachers and I know how to do, in whatever terms we choose to use.' As we see in this example, conditions were recorded as Western disease names. However, they were recognized without biomedical technology or training. 'Dropsy,' an older biomedical term for edema, is used in this story to describe a cold evil condition of the kidney and lung.[29] Were an unsuspecting translator to translate 'dropsy' as 'edema,' its Western dictionary definition,[30] the relation to the symptom set by which So and his teachers described dropsy would be lost. Because there are several traditional patterns that evidence edema, the biomedical term cannot transmit the necessary information. The condition that So refers to is actually 'water swelling' in Chinese. It is treated though the lung, triple burner, and kidney. However, application of those acupoints to an edema traditionally treated through the spleen and kidney would be inappropriate.[31]

Traditional schools were more like large clinics than formal educational institutes. Teaching was not standardized by a formal curriculum, and written materials were the notebooks of apprentices, not the didactic texts of Western-style classrooms. Dr So's books existed only as handwritten notes until formalized to meet the demands of his Western students in the early 1980s. The notes of one of Felt's Japanese teachers were hand copied from his teacher's notes, and so backward in a one-on-one process; it was claimed that they had lasted for 300 years.

As you can see from these examples, traditional clinical knowledge often developed from relatively short periods of hands-on training. Learning was confirmed as the master and apprentice worked together. It was preserved by long periods of communication, and occasionally augmented by notes and more broadly distributed literature such as books of rhymes. Practically, what counted for helping patients and earning a living was understanding the local definition of terms, how to recognize patterns, and how to apply techniques that were learned one-on-one. Clinical definition was not guaranteed by formal systems, but assured by the need to repeat accurately a teacher's hands-on skills. Although this can be a highly effective method, and it is doubtful that some skills can be transmitted in any other way, it is not an approach that is easily translated into biomedical terms, or transmitted without reference to the naked-sense details.

Dr So's treating of 200 patients as a student intern represents a larger base of experience than was previously common in Western acupuncture schools. It is a level of experience (approximately 4 new cases per week, perhaps 40 treatments per week) that demanded continuing development through on-going teacher–student and student–student interchange. For example, today, at 86 years old, Dr So still spends much of his time consulting with his students about their cases — asking the questions they did not ask, and seeking the clues he would have sought himself. As you can imagine, when these personal-experience chains are broken, it is very difficult, if not impossible, to salvage all the knowledge contained within them, much less relate it to modern medical language.

Modern acupuncture practice is different and there is a genuine potential for practical biomedical correspondence and efficacy research. Because most patients have biomedical records, modern clinical experience is theoretically easier to conform to formal acupuncture systems. However, individual experience is still very difficult to assess, because today's practitioners use acupuncture for an extremely wide range of disorders that is delimited, and sometimes defined by, the socio-economic milieu in which they practice, personal interest, and their reputation for success. A review of Birch's clinical records reveals the extent of the biomedically diagnosed conditions with which his patients have presented.

In American, British, and European settings, Birch has successfully treated patients who have been diagnosed with a broad range of musculoskeletal conditions (back, neck, head, shoulder, hip, leg, arm, and multiple joint pains), as well as arthritis (especially osteoarthritis), Morton's neuroma, and plantar fascitis. There were also successful treatments for a number of internal conditions such as gastritis, hepatitis, asthma, diarrhea, constipation, irritable bowel syndrome, dysmenorrhea, irregular menstruation, prostatitis, complications from diabetes (e.g. peripheral neuropathy), Parkinson's, infectious and immunological problems (e.g. allergies, rhinitis, sinusitis, pneumonia, bronchitis, chronic and acute otitis media, pharyngitis, tooth abscess, iritis, and cystitis). He has also helped many patients whose main complaints were fatigue, insomnia, anxiety, and stress. Similar practice scopes are common. Thus, even today, the lists of what acupuncture treats can be long and include many conditions that a naive observer might not expect.

Although clinical experience within biomedically dominated health-care systems is a potential source of information, the lack of central records systems for acupuncture makes accessing that information nearly impossible. Furthermore, without inter-rater studies to set reporting standards and a formal terminology for traditional symptoms and patterns, the development of the questionnaires, recording forms, and information systems on which such assessments would depend is seriously impeded. The same is true for 'data mining' in East Asian health-care systems. Because a methodologically consistent and sufficiently extensive Chinese–English terminology is now available, this is one area where ideas of what acupuncture can treat may be informed by statistical research.[32]

In sum then, answering the question, 'What does acupuncture treat?' requires a sensitivity to precision on several levels. First, we need to be aware that English translations can err and that no broadly agreed and demonstrably reliable associations with biomedical diseases have been accomplished. When these appear in Western languages we must not only be sure that we are not chasing a translational chimera, but we must also carefully assess the assumptions underlying the writer's sources. So too we must approach long oral histories with care, particularly if there are no living practitioners with whom to discuss cases. We need to be guided by historians, anthropologists, and sinologists, who can help us understand whether the reports we use are valid representations of acupuncture at a particular time or place. In blunt terms, we must make sure we are not making formal assumptions about idiosyncratic ideas plucked from the immense pool of Chinese literature to fit fixed assumptions. Finally, we must be aware how the varying terminology and skill sets of individual practitioners and schools of thought impact on reports of clinical success.

Verifying treatment success

The first recognized Western attempt to verify historic Asian claims of clinical efficacy was made by Soulie de Morant and his French colleagues who set out to verify acupuncture treatment using the knowledge and procedures of early 20th century biomedicine.[33] Although this had a considerable effect in France, it was a list of indications for acupuncture attributed to the WHO that brought the question of verifing acupuncture treatments to the attention of Western medico-legal authorities worldwide. The story of the WHO list introduces what is perhaps the most critical problem in determining what acupuncture can be said to treat successfully.

The WHO, a division of the United Nations, is often credited with a list of disorders and conditions for which acupuncture is supposed to be effective.[34] The list, as first published in 1979, is shown in Table 5.1. Many around the world still point to this list when asked what acupuncture can treat. Even today there are repeated internet requests for the 'List of diseases, published by the WHO, of conditions successfully treated by acupuncture,' and in November 1997 presenters and panelists at the NIH Consensus Development Conference on Acupuncture cited and discussed the list. However, the WHO has been actively distancing itself from this list, almost from the day it was published. In the recent words of one WHO official:

Table 5.1 WHO list (1979) of disorders and conditions for which acupuncture is effective

System	Disorders
Upper respiratory	Acute sinusitis, acute rhinitis, common cold, acute tonsillitis
Respiratory	Acute bronchitis, bronchial asthma (most effective in children and patients without complicating diseases)
Eye	Acute conjunctivitis, central retinitis, myopia (in children), cataract (without complications)
Mouth	Toothache, post-extraction pain, gingivitis, acute and chronic pharyngitis
Gastrointestinal	Spasms of esophagus and cardia, hiccough, gastroptosis, acute and chronic gastritis, gastric hyperacidity, chronic duodenal ulcer (pain relief), acute duodenal ulcer (without complications), acute and chronic colitis, acute bacillary dysentery, constipation, diarrhea, paralytic ileus
Neurological and musculoskeletal	Headache, migraine, trigeminal neuralgia, facial palsy (early stage, within 3–6 months), paresis following a stroke, peripheral neuropathies, sequelae of poliomyelitis (early stage, within 6 months), Ménière's disease, neurogenic bladder dysfunction, nocturnal enuresis, intercostal neuralgia, cervicobrachial syndrome, 'frozen shoulder,' 'tennis elbow,' sciatica, low-back pain, osteoarthritis

Some years ago — December 1979 — the Journal *World Health* published an article [now out of print] listing a wide variety of conditions which participants at a seminar considered might be treated by acupuncture. However, this list was not based on controlled clinical research and *cannot* be considered authoritative nor does it reflect WHO's views in any way.[35]

Why would an official of WHO want so bluntly to distance that organization from a list so often and persistently attributed to it?

In 1977, the 30th WHO Assembly put forward the celebrated 'Health for All by the Year 2000' program. By 1978, the organization had recognized that, if this goal were to be achieved, traditional medicines such as acupuncture must become an integral part of the world's health-care systems. Since then, the WHO has been a consistent advocate for traditional medicines, including traditional East Asian medicines. So, why did the WHO back away from their list? Was this an implicit admission of error? Did they succumb to some political pressure? Surely, if practitioners feel that the list is accurate and East Asian medical historians back their claims, it would be better for the 'Health for All' program if this list were widely promoted. The reasons for this tactical retreat are, of course, complex and might go beyond science alone. Elements of international politics might have been involved, although we have no evidence that this was the case. Regardless, the essence of the problem is clear, and it is the essence of the deciding scientific issue — what can establish sufficient scientific proof of the efficacy of acupuncture? This becomes clearer in a 1980 reiteration of the 1979 list, where WHO officials explicitly state:

The inclusion of specific diseases in the list is not meant to indicate the effectiveness of acupuncture therapy, but rather the extent to which it is currently being applied. Furthermore, the derivation of this list of indications is based on clinical experience and not necessarily on controlled clinical research.[36]

At first, a distinction between 'effectively treats' and 'commonly applied' may seem mere semantics. However, it is the dividing line between what is and is not to be scientifically acceptable. Put bluntly, the problem of diversity in acupuncture, and the scholarly challenges of its translation and transmission, are to be resolved by 'starting from scratch.' Although modern clinicians understandably feel that their clinical experience is broadly applicable and clearly indicative of the value of acupuncture, as we discussed above, claims of successful treatments by individual practitioners are subject to so many variables that they cannot be the source of proof. For the West the emphasis is on the method of research known as the 'controlled clinical trial.'

This standard becomes more explicit in later, even more cautious statements about clinical research into acupuncture. A 1985 WHO document states that one of the objectives of the traditional medicine program was to:

...assess traditional practices in the culture concerned in order to identify those that are safe and effective ... criteria for evaluating the efficacy and safety of therapies should include both the biomedical and socio-medical aspects. The basic concepts of traditional practices must be taken into account. Since opinions differ about what constitutes a demonstration of therapeutic efficacy, extensive discussions are needed to establish guidelines on the matter.[37]

In 1991, the WHO stated that:

...an authoritative list of what conditions can effectively be treated by acupuncture can only be drawn up after each claim has been examined and either verified or rejected. There is, so far, no such agreed list, although research aimed at establishing clinical indications for acupuncture is being pursued in institutions around the world ... putting acupuncture on a firm scientific basis requires rigorous investigation of the claims made for its efficacy.[38]

These more recent WHO proposals on how such an authoritative list could be achieved are only now beginning to be addressed.

In 1993 a revision of the 1979 list was used as a point of departure for claims that were to be more systematically and rigorously validated. Birch participated in further discussions with other participants of the Workshop on Acupuncture.[39] In this meeting, as well as in the scientific community in general, the crux of the issue was and is this: Many books, practitioners, and organizations claim long lists of conditions that have responded or routinely respond to acupuncture therapy, but where is their proof? This question is now critical to the future of acupuncture in the West. In effect, when the WHO inadvertently gave the list of indications for acupuncture a patina of truth through publication, the scientific community made their opinion known – no matter how old, no matter how generally applied, acupuncture would have to meet modern criteria for safety and effectiveness.

Today, science is not simply society's investigative branch, it is the dominant clearing house for how social resources (governmental and institutional funds) are allocated. With thousands of pharmaceutical drugs, natural drugs, natural and synthetic supplements, medical devices, and medical procedures available, almost all Western patients ask their doctors to decide which therapy to use. How do doctors know which therapy is best? How do insurance companies determine who should be paid and at what rate? How would the WHO know which of the many traditional practices to promote? What could a hospital administrator permit an acupuncturist to do within the limits of malpractice liability? None of these are simple questions. But all are thought to be best answered by the complex protocols of modern medical science.

It is these protocols to which Western institutions turn to verify what is and what is not a legitimate claim of efficacy, and thus what can be labeled as scientifically accepted. Because Western culture considers these means unimpeachable, they are used to decide what is a legitimate claim of efficacy. Failing these methods results not merely in a loss of access to funds, but also in a loss of legitimacy, which confines a practice to the realm of quackery. It is these methods that establish what can and cannot be incorporated into modern Western health care.

Before discussing these protocols in detail, we remind you that the conclusions of the studies that we will discuss say relatively little about clinical practice. In other words, where therapy proves effective, it is effective. An individual cure is a cure, whether or not the therapy has been validated by these methods, but no individual cure is suffcient evidence that other cures are likely in the future.

Statistics are the key to establishing clinical efficacy in scientific testing. What this means is that a very narrow claim of effectiveness is tested in a carefully controlled study. The results are positive if patients who have received the treatment tested improve at a rate sufficiently greater than those who have not. Carefully controlled studies are rarely a mirror image of any clinical practice, and the guarantee of statistical significance neither denies nor affirms that any particular patient will benefit from any procedure. Rather, these studies describe the probability that patients in a general population will benefit. In other words, these studies examine a therapy from the viewpoint of administering and paying for drug treatments. They answer the question, 'What proportion of patients will benefit?' not 'Will this particular patient benefit?'

This produces a related problem; that is, assessing treatments that have not been tested. In other words, when the statistical probabilities that a treatment will be successful have not been determined, how does someone decide what to do? There is, for example, not a shred of scientific evidence that Birch should be successful in treating acute iritis with acupuncture. However, in one patient, the results of treatment were both remarkable and immediate. But, does that success mean that another practitioner, using perhaps a different technique, will obtain a similar result? Will anyone diagnosed as suffering from acute iritis benefit from the same treatment? From any acupuncture treatment? Does it mean that Birch's next patient with an iritis diagnosis will be quickly cured? Hopefully, yes; possibly, no! Uncontrolled individual clinical experience has very little value in science because it is so difficult to establish the extent to which it is generalizable. Finding a therapy effective for the treatment of a particular condition in a carefully controlled clinical trial describes the probability that it will be effective in the future. This gives physicians the confidence to recommend it, and insurance companies the motivation to examine treatment benefits in terms of cost.

In science, repeatability is the critically important criterion. Results become acceptable to the scientific community when they are generalizable. In medicine, the assumption of future benefit is examined by tests known as 'clinical trials.' This explains the WHO's present position. The fact that their original list had not been based on controlled clinical trials is what made the WHO retreat. It is now the explicit intent of the WHO to 'assess traditional practices in the culture concerned in order to identify those that are safe and effective,'[40] and they intend that this be done according to strict scientific guidelines.

Assessing the efficacy of acupuncture following strict scientific guidelines has been difficult. In addition, many of the symptoms and diseases on the WHO list have never been tested following any guidelines, much less those that determine what is a properly controlled clinical trial. Hence, the WHO has difficulty endorsing the list, as do many national health agencies and organizations. Why is this the case? When people have attempted to scientifically prove the efficacy of acupuncture, why have so very few succeeded? Why is it so difficult to make a scientific conclusion one way or the other?

In part, this difficulty is because the long lists of symptoms and conditions reported are results from clinical practice. In some part, it is because it has been too difficult to reconcile the impression of acupuncture conveyed by the popular literature with the scientific communities' sense of truth. In part it is because enthusiasts' emphasis on the ancient and philosophical has tended to mask the significant practical and economic role of acupuncture in modern East Asian societies.[41] It is not solely that the effects of acupuncture are scientifically unproven, it is also that too much of what has been claimed seems too fantastic, too far beyond the expectations of Western scientists.

After all, a number of mainstream therapies have never been tested. Many surgical procedures, for example, have not been studied outside of practice. Many practices in psychiatry and psychology have not been subjected to controlled clinical trials. Furthermore, many therapies are still in use even after cumulative evidence from clinical trials has proven negative. For example, when a negative study is shown to have design inadequacies, the practice continues, despite the negative results.

Neither is biomedical science perfectly applied. Reviews of medical literature frequently discuss the problem of study design, and there is a growing number of reports in the biomedical literature of drugs or other medical interventions that have been found to be ineffective or much less effective than previously thought. Greenberg and his colleagues found that the literature on some antidepressant medications fits this category.[42] The revised treatment effects were only barely beyond those of the placebo. Lipman found similar problems in the pharmacological treatment of anxiety disorders.[43] Yet antidepressant and antianxiety medications are among the prescription drugs most widely prescribed. A study of a pharmacological treatment of alcohol withdrawal by Moskowitz and colleagues showed similar problems,[44] as did the study by Chalmers et al of some anticancer drugs.[45] The clinical trial evidence for the appropriateness of short hospital stays following varicose vein or hernia surgeries was found to be inadequate by Blackburn and colleagues.[46] Recently, questions have surfaced about the efficacy of cognitive–behavioral techniques in the treatment of hypertension, following a literature review by Eisenberg and his colleagues.[47] Yet, all these therapies are still used in biomedicine.

In summary, the standards of research in Western biomedicine are said by a growing number of researchers to be poor.[48] Clinical research presents problems that are not always easy to solve in one try. Thus, drawing solid conclusions from the biomedical literature can, in some cases, be just as difficult as drawing conclusions from the acupuncture literature. The difference is that biomedical treatments are used by a dominant medical establishment that controls its own funding sources and with whom the general population is relatively content. In other words, the anecdotal basis is larger, and thus easier to trust, and research funds are more plentiful. Therefore, if acupuncture, or any part of acupuncture, is to be brought into mainstream health-care systems, it must solve the problems presented by the demand of the scientific community for evidence produced in controlled clinical trials, and do this efficiently with the funds available.

In the USA this process is the explicit domain of the recently established Office of Alternative Medicine at the National Institutes of Health, Bethesda, MD. The creation of this office brings acupuncture to a critical juncture in the West. It has been practiced with varying degrees of prominence for at least 20 years in the USA, and has established a foothold in most Western countries. Now, however, it must prove itself. Like it or not, fair or unfair, for better or not, the controlled clinical trial is a trial by combat

in which acupuncture must succeed if it is to be acculturated fully in the West. Although increasing popular support can help keep the contest funded, and an educated acupuncture community can carefully monitor the scientific referees, these influences are unlikely to change the basic rules of the game.

WESTERN CLINICAL SCIENCE

The standard by which pharmaceutical medicines are tested is the so-called 'randomized double-blind controlled clinical trial.' This is a research process where patients are randomly assigned to one of two or more treatment groups. Patients are not to know to which group they belong, and the treatment providers are not to know which treatment they administer. One treatment group receives an inactive, or placebo, treatment; this is the 'control', the other treatment group receives the 'active' or real treatment (Box 5.1).

Box 5.1 The placebo problem

'Placebo' literally means 'I shall please.' It is the future tense of the Latin verb *placeo* (to please), and is defined both as a 'scientific anomaly' and as a 'nuisance variable' in medicine and medical research. The term was first used in medicine *c* 1780. Then it meant 'to sooth the patient.' By 1811 it was defined as 'an epithet given to any medicine adapted more to please than to benefit the patient.'[49] By the 1950s, the term 'placebo' had acquired a technical meaning related to research methodology. This is the sense in which it is usually used today. However, the term 'placebo' has several definitions, not all of which are identical:

> ...an inactive substance or preparation given to satisfy the patient's symbolic need for drug therapy and used in controlled studies to determine the efficacy of medicinal substances. Also a procedure with no intrinsic therapeutic value, performed for such purposes.[50]

> ...any treatment or aspect of a treatment that does not have a specific action on the patient's symptoms or disease consisting of both subjective and objective changes.[51]

> ...a subjective improvement in the patient's condition that is not directly attributable to the pharmacological or physiological effect of treatment.[52]

The *placebo effect* is thought to involve physiological mechanisms. Among these, the endorphins are thought to be involved because the effects can be reversed by administration of naloxone, an 'endorphin antagonist,' a chemical that blocks the effect of endorphins.[53] Because acupuncture is said to be endorphin-mediated, this link to the endorphins has propelled the idea that acupuncture is primarily a placebo. But there are many unresolved and conflicting ideas about the placebo effect, and many researchers, including acupuncture researchers, evidence some confusion. The placebo effect is generally said to be a therapeutic effect that is due to the enthusiasm or authority of the practitioner, the belief of the patient, patient–practitioner dynamics, or the nature of the procedure tested. It is also related to the severity of the disease.[54] A 1984 review of the research literature found over 30 possible sources of the placebo effect.[55]

The *placebo effect* is regarded as a nuisance variable in research because researchers want to know the effectiveness of a particular treatment. As a therapeutic effect that is not related to the drug or procedure tested, it must be eliminated. This sometimes requires extremely complex clinical trials. The basic relationship is expressed by the equation $T = R + P$, where T is the overall treatment effect, R is the real treatment effect, and P is the placebo treatment effect. Based on the other variables, this

---

Box 5.1 The placebo problem *(cont'd)*

equation will affect the organization of any clinical trial.

Insofar as subjects are concerned, there are said to be 'placebo responders' and 'placebo nonresponders.'[56] Some have even characterized these two groups by psychological type. The placebo effect is commonly said to be found consistently in 30–35% of all people tested.[57] Other researchers are even more precise, giving the placebo effect as 35.2 ± 2.2%.[58] This is often interpreted as meaning that 30–35% of responses are attributable to placebo. However, others note that, with all the possible determinants of the placebo effect, it can affect anywhere from zero to 95% of a trial's participants.[59] Others state the placebo effect in relation to the tested treatment. They say that the placebo effect is consistently 55% as effective as the treatment itself.[60] These levels of effectiveness have prompted some to argue that we should not try to eliminate this effect in clinical practice, but should actively try to promote it and thus help the patient more. This is regarded as an ethical necessity, especially in difficult cases.

The placebo effect is most easily controlled when testing a drug. It is relatively easy to prepare two visually identical pills, one with active ingredients and one without. If the study is properly constructed, the effectiveness of treatment is determined by the difference in effect between the group that receives the active pill and the one that does not.

Some scientists argue that the placebo effect can be measured for a physical intervention such as

surgery or acupuncture. The most famous examples are two surgical trials conducted at Harvard University during the 1950s.[61] In these trials some patients underwent mammary artery ligation in one trial and gastroenterostomy in the other. Other patients were surgically opened and closed while under general anesthesia but no surgical procedure was performed. The so-called 'sham surgery' was found to be significantly effective.

Surprisingly, almost every author commenting on these surgeries argues that the sham surgical procedures were effective solely due to the placebo effect. This is surprising because, as we discussed in Chapter 4, any interference with the integrity of the body elicits many responses. To assume that such physiological responses are equivalent to the placebo effect seems naive, particularly as the patients were anesthetized. An equally valid theory would be that local bloodletting by surgical incision has a specific therapeutic action on the conditions treated. This seems particularly reasonable because the patients' conditions had circulatory components. Bloodletting has been used as a therapeutic tool for centuries in many societies, and is still used in both East Asian and Western medicines. Although prejudice against bloodletting because of its role in Western medicial history might explain why bloodletting was not considered, that is not a valid reason for assuming that the therapeutic effects from sham surgery were solely the result of placebo.

For further information on placebo see note 62.

This methodology attempts to control for the full range of placebo effects, including the influence of practitioners on patients, and the effects of patients' beliefs and expectations. This approach evolved to test pharmaceutical drugs because it is very easy to give an active pill (one containing the medicine to be tested) to one group of patients and an identical-looking but inactive pill (one containing no medicine) to another group of patients. If properly arranged, the effects of the active ingredient can be reliably assessed. Because there is no known active pharmaceutical constituent to the inactive pill, a patient in the control group who improves is said to have improved because of the placebo effect. The difference between the treatment and control groups is what these studies are designed to measure. These results are termed 'statistically significant' if the difference in treatment effect between the

active and control groups is large enough to mathematically eliminate chance. However, these formulas dictate that good results cannot be claimed unless enough patients are included in any particular trial.

This research approach is used to test pharmaceutical drugs, but not invasive physical procedures such as surgery, although in the past a few studies have compared surgical procedures with so-called 'sham surgery.' In the sham procedure, the incisions were made, but the remainder of the surgical procedure was not performed (see Box 5.1). As acupuncture involves the insertion and then further manipulation or stimulation of needles at discrete sites on the body surface, 'sham acupuncture' was conceived as the use of needles at different sites or without the manipulation or stimulation usually applied. However, even from the Western viewpoint, acupuncture may not be an ideal candidate for controlled clinical trials. Were sham acupuncture to produce a wound, it would be considered as unethical as sham surgery. However, because researchers perceive acupuncture as an exotic therapy couched in a language of mystical energies, it is thought to have a tremendous placebo potential. At least they must assume that its placebo potential is greater than that of indigenous psychotherapeutic practices, which are rarely assessed in double-blinded trials. Thus, many researchers have attempted to investigate acupuncture by comparison to sham acupuncture following the model developed in the 1950s for surgical procedures.

Although it is not obvious that the placebo powers of acupuncture are so uniquely profound, or that mysticism figures so strongly in its practice, it is probably these beliefs that the WHO encountered — the judgement that acupuncture is so placebo-prone that it must be tested like a pharmaceutical drug. Nonetheless, there are several questions that must be asked. First, is it possible to successfully blind the acupuncturist in a clinical trial? Where do you find acupuncturists who do not know what acupoints they are treating, how to treat those acupoints, or why those acupoints are generally used? These are requirements for blinding. Acupuncturists in a double-blinded trial must not be able to infer which treatment they are providing. The only way to accomplish this is to use an incompetent acupuncturist, even one specifically trained to know only the mechanics. Unfortunately, someone who cannot tell what points they are needling, who does not know the significance of the way in which they needle the points, has no idea why they needle those points, and who reads no acupuncture literature during the trial, is not qualified to administer acupuncture. And, why would we want clinical trials to be based on the efforts of unqualified practitioners?

This is analogous to testing surgical techniques in a double-blinded trial (which for ethical reasons is no longer done). Would we engage someone with no prior knowledge to perform the control techniques? Would we

train first-year medical students, for example, to cut by diagram? In other words, although woundless acupuncture is dramatically less dangerous than surgery, it is logically no more possible to truly double-blind trials of it. Whether a skill is manual, intellectual, or a combination of the two, a qualified individual will know what is happening and an unqualified individual will break the blind through ineptitude. Although there have been a number of research groups who have announced double-blind studies of acupuncture, an analysis of these claims usually reveals a misunderstanding of what constitutes an effective double-blind.[63]

We must also ask: 'What constitutes an active treatment and what constitutes a placebo treatment?' Which of the multiple techniques of acupuncture should any one study focus on? How can the results of that study then be generalized to the whole field? How can we be confident that one school's inactive treatment is not another school's active treatment? If you test a Chinese treatment developed during the last 20 years, can you make any conclusion about a system from modern Japan? How many English-speaking researchers are certain that they have not tested idiosyncratic translations, individual interpretations, recycled character definitions, informal or inadequate relationships to biomedicine, or inappropriate techniques? A careful look at the published clinical trials reveals a lack of safeguards against all these possibilities. As the authors of the 1993 National Institute on Drug Abuse (NIDA) review state: 'There is a great need for standardized terminology and standardized methodology in the provision and study of acupuncture.'[64]

Furthermore, it is a requirement for a randomized controlled clinical trial that the patients should be unable to tell whether they receive the active or inactive treatment. Thus, the treatment experience must appear to be the same or match similar expectations. This is a minimum requirement for any study to be even single-blinded (i.e. a trial where the patients are unaware of which treatment they have received). Because even the most naive patient expects acupuncture to have something to do with a needle, researchers use 'real' needling at 'real acupuncture points' as an active treatment and 'sham' needling at 'sham acupuncture point' as an inactive treatment. This approach seems straightforward only if you are unaware of the many technical possibilities in acupuncture (the variety of techniques used by acupuncturists are described in Ch. 7). Once these possibilities are considered, sham acupuncture can be very problematic, and many research projects have been rendered less than convincing largely because investigators were inadequately informed about these issues.

Through the influences of basic science research discussed in the preceeding chapter, most clinical trials use the heavier stimulation techniques that are generally typical of modern Chinese needling. Thus, these trials use a *de qi* sensation as a standard of active treatment. This approach involves a number of uncertain assumptions. Since much of the modern Chinese literature on acupuncture states that needling without *de qi* is ineffective,[65] researchers have assumed that needling without *de qi* is all that is required of an inactive treatment. Thus, shallow needling without heavy *de qi* has often been used as an inactive treatment in controlled clinical trials. Researchers who accept this reasoning are not only unfamiliar with the history of insertion depth and technique, but also with the acupuncture commonly used throughout Japan, Korea, Europe, and the USA. They also seem unfamiliar with the results of a clinical trial that were published in 1983, which showed that so-called 'superficial needling' was effective in the treatment of low-back pain. The authors of this report were surprised when good clinical results were found.[66]

In fact, there is no real evidence that heavy stimulus needling is standard treatment.[67] Although stronger stimulation is probably fairly thought to be typical of Chinese needling, stimulus variations (lighter or heavier stimulus, deeper or shallower insertion, longer or shorter duration) are often found in more detailed Traditional Chinese Medicine (TCM) treatment texts.[68] Importantly, although *de qi* is translated or

understood as a painful sensation, this understanding is clearly limited to a single class of acupuncture treatments. The *de qi* or 'obtaining qi' need not be heavy, or even particularly evident to an inexperienced patient. In some acupuncture literature it actually refers to what the practitioner, not the patient, feels.[69]

Even Chinese acupuncturists famous for their powerful needling use only a few acupoints where a powerful *de qi* is unquestionably painful. Tin Yau So is famous worldwide for his use of a powerful stimulus. It is a reputation we know he well deserves. However, he also frequently used less powerful stimuli, when treating patients who were very young, very weak, or extremely ill. Regardless, he achieved good results. In other words, *de qi* is a subjective criterion on which to found a supposedly objective clinical trial, particularly with acupuncturists who are supposed to be blind to the skills of treatment, such as the direction in which the needle sensation should travel.[70]

There are also other problems with the use of *de qi* to qualify the active treatment. Researchers from China, Japan, Europe, Canada and the USA all have claimed that this type of *de qi* needling is a neurological phenomenon.[71] Thus *de qi* needling is another reflection of the neurological bias we discussed in Chapter 4, because even in modern Chinese literature *de qi* is defined as having both a subjective and objective component and differing from the stimulation of the subcutaneous nerves.[72] They nonetheless reason that if *de qi* needling activates well-defined neurological pathways, then it is appropriate to neutralize these pathways as a control treatment. The literature reveals at least one study that was based on this assumption. In this study, the acupuncture treatment was compared with a control treatment that involved the injection of a local anesthetic to numb the insertion sites, followed by the shallow insertion of needles into the numbed spots.[73]

The prejudice of this approach is the idea that neurological pathways are the *only* means by which acupuncture could possibly work. Thus, when researchers find that shallow needling works just as well, they conclude that acupuncture is a powerful placebo. It must be a placebo because the only possible active pathways were blocked! The reasoning is circular, because it is just as logical to conclude that shallow needling is effective, or that *de qi* is not a *sine qua non*. What if bioelectrical signals other than those of the nervous system play a role? Does the anesthetic arrest the splinter effect, inactivate bioelectrical and biomagnetic signals, eliminate electrical potentials, or halt all the possible biological messengers? Could the injection itself have an effect before the anesthetic numbed the local nerves? In some Chinese treatments injections are thought to be the active therapy. Some use what is called 'dry needling'; that is the insertion of an empty hypodermic needle to stimulate, for example, trigger points. In other words, the design of these trials all too clearly reflects their designers' bias, while all too poorly testing acupuncture.

In any controlled clinical trial it is essential that the inactive treatment be as credible as the active treatment.[74] The inactive treatment cannot be more aversive; neither can it be silly or obviously inept. This too is easier said than done. Anyone who has been to an apprentice barber, masseur, or hairdresser knows how easy it is to recognize the 'touch' of inexperience. At present there is not much evidence whether patients who are expecting to receive acupuncture in controlled clinical trials are able to recognize if they are controls. Only a handful of studies, for example, those done by Margolin and coworkers,[75] Vincent and coworkers,[76] Birch and Jamison,[77] Zaslawski et al[78] and White et al,[79] have investigated these issues.

Logically, if the credibility of the control is not assessed, if you cannot be confident that each patient believes that they will benefit from the treatment, you cannot argue that you have controlled for the placebo effect. In many studies it is hard to imagine that anyone would be unaware that they were controls. As human investigation committees at research institutions are demanding increasing frankness about the test and its controls as part of the process of informed consent, sham acupuncture will become even more difficult to accomplish. Furthermore, if the aversiveness of a control treatment is not assessed in advance, it is not possible to argue that any result is not wholly or partially the result of diffuse noxious inhibitory control (DNIC) (see Ch. 4 and Box 5.2). Neither can you always argue that a high dropout rate in the control group is due to ineffectiveness of treatment — how long would you tolerate a painful experience that left you feeling only sore or numb?

Box 5.2 Diffuse noxious inhibitory control (DNIC) 'counter-irritation' models and implications

The diffuse noxious inhibitory control (DNIC) model developed by Le Bars and coworkers theorizes that any noxious stimulus will have a pain-relieving effect.[80] This is a very common idea. We have all 'kicked one leg to take pain from the other' or pinched and squeezed somewhere for the momentary relief it can provide. This model of pain control developed from the European model of counter-irritation first proposed by Rougemont in 1798 as the mechanism by which acupuncture functioned. The DNIC model is potentially devastating to traditional models of acupuncture, because it implies that the sites of stimulation (the acupuncture points and channels) are irrelevant to the effects. In this model, any location is as good as any other, and there is therefore virtually nothing of specific value in acupuncture.

Since *de qi* (*hibiki* in Japanese) needling and electro acupuncture are thought to be relatively noxious stimuli,[81] any treatment that utilizes them will be dismissed as working via DNIC. In other words, where a clinical trial uses these needling methods, it is necessary to control for the DNIC effect. Without this control, there is no way to know whether the specific treatment or the general DNIC effect is responsible for the results. In politico-economic reality, without this control it is nearly inevitable the DNIC theory will dominate acupuncture. The culturally dominant idea will almost certainly replace culturally new concepts such as *yin-yang*.[82]

The presumption that the mechanisms of acupuncture and DNIC are the same is a significant and difficult research bias. In a controlled clinical trial where the control treatment was the shallow non-noxious needling that is typical of clinical practice, it is likely that there would be little to no noxious stimulation. If this were the case, it would be difficult to argue that DNIC was responsible for the treatment effect, although it does not eliminate the

---

Box 5.2 Diffuse noxious inhibitory control (DNIC) 'counter-irritation' models and implications *(cont'd)*

possibility of other diffuse effects (e.g. those resulting from stimulating cutaneous afferents). If the active treatment studied involved *de qi* needling, and was more effective than the control treatment, this would be taken as proof that the effects of acupuncture are mediated by DNIC. In the scientific literature this assumption has already led to suggestions that neither the needles nor the acupuncture theories are relevant. This line of reasoning unintentionally biases both clinical trials and basic science studies.[83] On the other hand, if both the control treatment and the treatment tested utilize methods that elicit noxious stimulation, this further complicates the study design:

1. Reducing the treatment differences between the real and control treatments requires very large patient populations, greatly increasing the funds required and limiting the prospects for research.[84]
2. Because the treatment-effect differences between the two types of acupuncture are less, the probability that there will be a significant difference between the real and control treatments is greatly decreased.

As DNIC effects are active in both the test and control treatments, it is very difficult for studies of this type to test the difference between one set of stimulation locations and another. If one set of locations is shown to be marginally better than another, this does nothing to show that acupuncture

works. Instead it only suggests that there may be some places that are better than others for evoking DNIC. Because counter-irritation can be administered by noxious stimuli such as heat, and electrical and mechanical stimulation, even the needling will be of little consequence.

To forestall this prejudice, and to test acupuncture on its own terms by allowing an exploration of traditional ideas, it is advantageous to use non-noxious stimulation techniques for both the real and control groups.[85] Simultaneously, the level of discomfort associated with both treatments must be measured. This has the following advantages:

1. If the real acupuncture treatment provides statistically better results than the control treatment and there is no significant difference in the pain associated with the two treatments, then we can argue both that acupuncture is effective and that the results are not DNIC mediated.
2. If there are improvements in both groups, and little or no discomfort associated with either treatment, we can still argue that the effects are not DNIC mediated.
3. As the dominant neurological models have been avoided by using shallow needling, then traditional explanatory models may be considered. In other words, by eliminating the culturally dominant bias, researchers can be encouraged to study other, perhaps even traditional, explanations.

Even if these practical problems could be discounted, there is still a very significant problem with the sham acupuncture research model. Typically, the comparison of an active acupuncture treatment with an inactive acupuncture treatment assumes that the inactive treatment has no effect beyond placebo. But, as we saw in Chapter 4, needling anywhere produces measurable physiological effects. These will be in addition to any placebo effect. In other words, sham needling is not the same as a pill placebo. Essentially, there are three coexistent effects that many researchers mistake for two, as described below.

The extent of treatment effect

The three coexisting treatment effects are (Fig. 5.1):

1. the true placebo effect
2. the placebo effect plus a nonspecific physiological response to needling

3. the placebo effect plus nonspecific and specific physiological responses to needling.

Many researchers assume that effects 1 and 2 are identical. This makes it difficult to find statistically significant differences. Furthermore, since the researchers who design these studies assume that effects 1 and 2 are the same, they calculate the number of patients required based on that premise. Thus their studies rarely enroll enough patients to produce a clear conclusion. The smaller the treatment-effect differential, the larger the number of patients required. Lewith and Machin demonstrated this as early as 1983,[86] but many researchers still ignore this critical point. Thus, whether positive or negative treatment effects are obtained, the results are inconclusive.

The crucial issue is the selection of active and inactive treatments. A scientifically conservative assumption is that the 'inactive' treatment is really a 'less-active treatment.' Otherwise, the placebo effect and the less-active-treatment effect

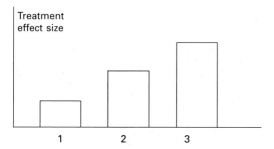

Figure 5.1 The three coexisting treatment effects. 1: true placebo effect. 2: placebo effect plus nonspecific physiological response 3: placebo effect plus nonspecific physiological response plus specific physiological response.

will be confused and an insufficient number of patients will be enrolled. In addition, great care is required to select the most appropriate treatment possible. In other words, there must be more than just incidental evidence for the selection of an active treatment. Likewise, the most irrelevant, and therefore least-active treatment, must be given to the control group. Again, there must be more than just incidental evidence for the selection of the treatment used as the control. It must not be obviously silly, inappropriately painful, aversive, or otherwise unbelievable. Furthermore, the less-active treatment must first be tested in a pilot study to assess its relative efficacy, and must be carefully researched to avoid the scholarly errors we discussed earlier and thus the inadvertent selection of a highly effective treatment as control.[87]

In summary, the larger the treatment-effect difference, the smaller the number of patients required for statistical significance. This is important, because smaller studies will be less expensive and funding is the *sine qua non* of research. Unfortunately, very few published studies have attended to these issues. Although there have been a few good clinical trials, for example, Bullock et al's landmark alcohol recidivism study,[88] most studies have enrolled an insufficient number of patients, often because there were insufficient funds. Thus few clinical trial outcomes have been found statistically significant, despite positive clinical results. This is the paradox of the relationship between acupuncture and science — is science ready to pay for what science demands?

In a deeper sense, the primary problem is inadequate knowledge of what constitutes acupuncture among medical researchers and inadequate knowledge of what constitutes research among acupuncturists. The price of this failure to communicate is that the National Institutes of Health panel was unable to endorse more than a few studies. There are studies where completely inadequate and even ridiculous treatments have been tested.[89] In some, the more powerful treatment has been selected as a sham treatment because researchers misunderstood the literature. An otherwise elegant study of acupuncture for menopausal hotflashes,[90] compared a real acupuncture treatment with a sham acupuncture treatment. However, a review of the acupuncture literature shows that the supposed sham treatment was more frequently recommended for menopausal hotflashes than was the treatment tested.[91] Just as importantly, real treatment groups rarely receive adequate numbers of treatments, much less the treatment and follow-up they would receive from an experienced acupuncturist (see the examples in Box 5.3). Often, sham treatments are selected because they fit the neurological model rather than because they are known to be ineffective. A study that collects pilot data for the sham treatment is exceedingly rare. In fact, the inactive treatments frequently give the same or only slightly less-positive results than the real treatments.

The outcome of these and other problems of design is that, with the exception of those studies that the National Institutes of Health panel cited, current studies do not conclusively demonstrate that acupuncture can or cannot treat anything. As recently as 1993, a US Food and Drug Administration report concluded: 'the present level of human clinical trial evidence favors efficacy for pain control and the treatment of alcohol recidivism, but it is not compelling.'[104] The 1991 NIDA technical review of acupuncture for substance abuse similarly concludes:

There is no compelling evidence for the efficacy of acupuncture in the treatment of either opiate or cocaine dependence. The work of Bullock in the field of alcohol dependence represents the only methodologically sound suggestion of efficacy for the use of acupuncture for any dependence disorder.[105]

Box 5.3 Examples of poor clinical research

Ralph Coan first raised some of these points in 1981. There have been many studies that claim to test the efficacy of acupuncture in single- or double-blind placebo-controlled clinical trials where the real treatment was completely inadequate.[92] In other words, however it was derived, it was not a valid treatment for the condition studied. For example, chronic conditions such as pain demand the use of several acupoints in each session and several sessions in a course of treatment, the length of which is typically proportional to the age of the patient, their general health, and the severity and longevity of the pain. Although it is true that many currently popular English-language clinical manuals are often vague about how many acupoints are used in a single treatment, or how many treatments constitute a reasonable course of treatment, a relatively brief review of the available texts does provide some indication of what might be required. For example, the average number of points and the average number of treatments recommended for chronic pain in five English-language textbooks are as follows:

Text	Average No. of needles	Average No. of treatments
Anon[93]	>10	
O'Connor & Bensky[94]	>8	≥10
Nanjing Seminar[95]	>8	
So[96]	>9.5	9.3
Chen & Wang[97]	>14.5	20.8–23.5

The text by Chen & Wang is a book of Chinese case histories from the PRC, (i.e. authentic treatments). It is included, and is significant because English-language texts seem to state generally smaller numbers of points and treatments.

In contrast, the following table summarizes the point and treatment regimens of five research studies. This clearly shows that researchers administered both inadequate treatments and foreshortened courses of treatment. Thus, their conclusions concerning the efficacy of acupuncture are invalid.

Study	No. of needles	No. of treatments
Laitinen[98]	2	3
Fox & Melzack[99]	3	2
Emery & Lythgoe[100]	?	3
Edelist et al[101]	4	3
Mendelson et al[102]	4	8

The study by Mendelson et al was a 'crossover study,' meaning that the patients were also treated at another time with four needles on eight occasions as sham treatment.

When we look at the results of studies, all of which were poor, and compare the treatments administered to what the literature indicates, the poor results are no surprise. These studies are very typical. A more comprehensive review of the problem examined 34 head, back, and neck pain controlled clinical trials. All 34 provided inadequate treatment.[103]

In other words, government-sponsored reviews of clinical trials revealed nothing that allows professional researchers to unreservedly endorse acupuncture. However, neither could they ignore the published positive outcomes for pain control and alcohol treatment. Put simply, 'where there's smoke, there's fire.' The US Food and Drug Administration review of acupuncture completed in 1996 drew the following conclusions:

The clinical studies and preclinical animal studies included in the petitions constitute valid scientific evidence in support of the clinical effectiveness of acupuncture needles for the performance of acupuncture treatment. However, reference to a specific disease condition, or therapeutic benefit requires additional valid scientific evidence in the form of well-controlled prospective clinical studies.[106]

Not all researchers are so open-minded. Some have decided that poor study design somehow proves the ineffectiveness of acupuncture. For example, in the conclusion of a recent meta-analysis of acupuncture studies concerning the treatment of chronic pain, Ter Riet and his colleagues state: 'The efficacy of acupuncture in the treatment of chronic pain remains doubtful.'[107] However, another group headed by Patel conducted a meta-analysis of the same literature (but with more stringent inclusion criteria), and concluded that: 'results favourable to acupuncture were obtained significantly more often than chance alone would allow.'[108] There is clearly no consensus among scientists.

Because the research is riddled with inadequate tests and methodological flaws, the issue of effectiveness is difficult to decide. There is

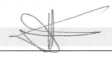

evidence, but most of it is not scientifically compelling. Ter Riet sees the same situation: 'No studies of high quality seem to exist. Therefore, at this moment no definite conclusions on the efficacy of acupuncture in the treatment of chronic pain can be drawn.'[109] However, his bias surfaces in the above-quoted conclusion, where Tier Riet states that it 'remains doubtful.' It is not doubtful; it is simply not known.

Unfortunately for acupuncture, political 'spin' makes scientific bias look mild. The Council Against Health Fraud, a US political health-claim watchdog group, is even more prejudicial when they claim that: 'After more than 20 years in the court of scientific opinion, acupuncture has not been demonstrated effective for any condition.'[110]

We are aware that well-designed research is under way, but at present it is difficult to draw clear scientific conclusions about the efficacy of acupuncture from the published results of controlled clinical trials. Despite these limitations, the scientific evidence is much better than is revealed by the overstated conclusions of skeptics. The recent comprehensive review by the panel of independent experts at the National Institutes of Health makes this clear. This comprehensive review represents the first broad acceptance of evidence for acupuncture for a significant range of medical disorders. Although there is clearly more to be done, we believe that a sufficient body of needle-controlled evidence will eventually exist. As the problems with past research are openly discussed, future research will improve, and acupuncture will finally have 'its day in court.' Then, less expensive, more appropriate and flexible means of understanding the clinical utility of acupuncture will come to the fore. Among these will be the research accomplished in Asia.

ASIAN RESEARCH

There have been many clinical studies performed in China, Japan, and Korea and these do provide considerable information, particularly when combined with studies in Europe and North America. However, it remains difficult for these studies to alter Western opinion. First, Asian studies are only rarely controlled clinical trials. Furthermore, not only are very few of these studies carefully controlled, most are practically unavailable. Few studies published in Asian languages are included or abstracted in any of the mainstream biomedical information systems such as MedLine.[111] Furthermore, although international interaction via the internet is available in China, the price for a single e-mail message has historically exceeded the average monthly salary of a full professor. These barriers have made scientific interchange practically difficult.

Interestingly, the first ever controlled clinical trials of acupuncture were performed in Japan in 1965 and 1966 by Haruto Kinoshita and Sodo Okabe.[112] However, few such studies have been performed there since. In Japan acupuncture is every bit as 'home grown' as is surgery in the West. Because acupuncture is an accepted practice and the Japanese have little experience of dangers associated with it, there has been no impetus to spend the millions required for carefully controlled trials.[113] Even Japan's traditional pharmacotherapy, Kampo, is usually investigated through uncontrolled trials and small practitioner studies. Some 200 formulas were simply 'grandfathered' by long-established use.[114] Unlike pharmaceutical drugs, neither acupuncture nor herbal therapy offer realistic patent potentials. Thus there is no motivation for Asian manufacturers to invest the millions of dollars required to fund research. In addition, the acupuncture community has little understanding of biostatistical methodology.[115]

The situation in China is different, but research there has been equally unable to provide answers suitable for the West. With the blessing (or pressure, as the case may be) of the Chinese Communist Party, socio-political influences have affected study design. Thus many studies performed in China are unacceptable by Western standards, and Chinese work often has a poor reputation among Western scientists. As biostatistics has not been fully adopted in China, very few Chinese studies are adequately controlled, and most use subjective measures (e.g. 'good, better, best') and scientifically meaningless statistics (e.g. counts and averages). Furthermore, placebo treatment is considered unethical and is illegal in the People's Republic of China.[116] As with Japanese work, the data generated by these studies are interesting, useful, and not at all compelling. (See Box 5.4.)

OTHER RESEARCH METHODS

Today, many acupuncturists argue that it is inappropriate to perform placebo- or needle-controlled studies of acupuncture. What they suggest instead is 'normal treatment control' as a form of 'outcome study.' This approach is sometimes known as 'outcomes research,' and is finding favor among researchers, especially those whose concern is health-care finance and

management. At the April 1994 US Food and Drug Administration workshop many researchers were surprised when it was agreed to accept outcomes research. Since that agency's concern is the safety and efficacy of the acupuncture needle, they determined that outcomes research would be a sufficient demonstration that the acupuncture needle was a safe and effective device. They argued that it makes no sense to compare needle controls, and that studies comparing needling with a conventional therapy would meet their needs. This was both heatedly debated and warmly received because it heralded a significant change in the requirements for research in acupuncture. However, full approval for this research approach was not forthcoming.

In standard therapy controlled outcome studies, the effects of acupuncture are compared with a standard treatment (e.g. medication or physical therapy) or a standard procedure

---

Box 5.4 Placebo-controlled clinical research versus outcomes research

There are several arguments commonly cited in acupuncture community in favor of what is loosely called 'outcomes research.' It is most frequently argued that truly double-blinded acupuncture studies are impossible. A second argument concerns the difficulty of designing an appropriate control or truly inactive acupuncture treatment. This is required for even a single-blind study. A third argument concerns the need to individualize acupuncture treatments according to traditional practice, which is contrary to the formulary acupuncture protocols typically tested. A fourth argument states that, because acupuncture has stood the test of time, it is already proven, and thus the strict testing procedures required for drugs are unnecessary. Finally, others note that it is unethical to administer faulty or ineffective treatments to diseased people, and hence outcomes research is the better choice.[117]

But the most important issue is that the study design used in a controlled trial depends on the questions asked. To demonstrate that acupuncture is not a placebo treatment, a placebo or 'sham acupuncture' treatment is required.[118] If you wish to test a traditionally based model of practice to emphasize the unique qualities of that approach, you need to use placebo controls and some form of needle control.[119] On the other hand, if you want to know whether a treatment is cost-effective, relatively safe, and at least as good as the other treatments available, testing acupuncture against a standard therapy is the best research model.[120] As the side-

effects of standard therapies are acknowledged, the cost of biomedical therapies continues to increase. As both government and private health providers face what is often called a crisis of health-care costs, outcomes research is gaining importance.

What is called an outcome study is a clinical trial in which there is no attempt to control for the placebo effect. Instead the study focuses on the effectiveness of the treatment relative to an established treatment. For example, in a study of the treatment of back pain by acupuncture, patients could be randomized into groups that receive either acupuncture, an analgesic medication, or physical therapy. First, the same pretest measurements would be made for each group. Next, appropriate treatments would be administered to each of the groups. Finally, post-test measurements would be made. In these designs acupuncture would be successful if it produced results equal to or better than the analgesic medication and/or physical therapy. In this example, if the post-test to pretest improvement for acupuncture was only equal to the results for the analgesic drug, then further studies might be initiated to learn about the longevity, side-effects, and cost of each form of treatment.

This is an increasingly accepted method of medical research. It is a particularly useful way to measure differences in cost between health-care options. Were it our choice to make, we see these studies as the most practical way of testing acupuncture, given the many problems with placebo-

---

Box 5.4 Placebo-controlled clinical research versus outcomes research *(cont'd)*

controlled trials and acupuncture's history of safe, effective, and inexpensive integration into Asian medical delivery systems. Acupuncture may sometimes be a primary therapy, sometimes an adjunct therapy, sometimes less and sometimes more expensive, and these are all facts that must be known. However, the acceptance of outcomes results will be limited until a critical degree of confidence is achieved in the peer system.[121]

There are always clinical trial examples where standard treatments perform no better than a placebo. Because standard treatments are proven by a volume of studies, not a single successful study, these incidences are not critical. However, it is impossible to know whether or not the standard treatment was no better than placebo in any particular outcome trial. For this and other reasons, many medical school and government researchers who comment on outcomes research feel that it can have little impact on the acceptance of acupuncture as a mainstream medicine.[122] Many medical people feel that a foreign therapy that references mystical ideas such as energy, *yin-yang*, and the five phases is so productive of the placebo effect that nothing short of controlled clinical trials will convince them of its effectiveness. However, this resistance is

increasingly declining as the demand for safe and inexpensive therapies such as acupuncture increases.

Regardless, needle controlled studies remain a 'Catch-22.' If acupuncture is to influence those who govern the future of medicine, it may need to succeed in randomized controlled clinical trials, despite the methodological problems. However, since controlled clinical trials have been uniformly poor and flawed by methodological problems and inadequate treatments, there is little evidence with which to persuade these skeptics. Furthermore, these studies are the most expensive to conduct and, to date, no systematic funding has been available. Until there are more data, or until the scientific community is generally willing to accept outcomes research, the needle-controlled method must be continuously improved.

The acculturation of acupuncture in the West, and more generally in all biomedically dominated societies, is as much a political as a scientific process. The significance of political and socio-cultural trends are as relevant today as they were in the dynasties of ancient China. For a thorough and clear discussion of the difficulties in performing clinical trials of acupuncture see note 123.

(e.g. TENS). No control or sham acupuncture is required. If acupuncture performs as well or better than the standard therapy, or with less side-effects, or at lower cost, it is shown to be an effective treatment. For example, Johansson and his colleagues in Sweden used this approach to study stroke patients. One group received physical and occupational therapy plus acupuncture, and the other group received physical and occupational therapy alone. They found that those who received acupuncture were not only more functional but also were treated for an average of US$26 000 less.[124]

These are very important and useful studies, and, ironically, this is almost certainly the means by which acupuncture will be researched once it becomes generally accepted. This has become increasingly evident with greater mainstream financing of acupuncture treatment and as the relative cost of therapy plays a larger role in planning health care. In studies that directly compare treatments, it is easier to assess the relative costs. The few studies funded by insurance companies have already tended

toward this design. For example, through Group Health in Seattle, Dan Cherkin is using a modified version of this design to test acupuncture for chronic back pain. However, since studies that have compared acupuncture to a standard therapy have also been generally poorly designed,[125] it is not yet clear whether this approach will convince acupuncture's detractors. Some, particularly those who are concerned with health-care policy and management, are interested in the outcomes approach. On the other hand, academic institutions are more conservative and continue to demand needle-controlled trials. The National Institutes of Health have generally funded only studies that involved needle controls. Hence, although change is possible, it appears that it will take time. To paraphrase physicist Max Planck on the reception of new ideas: good ideas do not catch on simply because they are good ideas one has to wait for the proponents of the old ideas to pass away before the new ideas can catch on.

Acupuncture is still flowing in a primarily westward direction from its origins in Asia. It comes with foreign-sounding concepts and from a different world view. The acculturation of acupuncture in the West will almost certainly not occur except on terms that are acceptable to biomedicine. If acupuncture is to make significant inroads into Western cultures, there are few likely options available. At one extreme, it could be completely adapted by becoming biomedicine in essence. This is the direction of the various scientific forms of acupuncture, particularly those that are based on neurological or neurochemical models. In our opinion, it will 'stand and fight,' holding its ground as a viable, independent complement to biomedicine. But to stand and fight it will certainly face a trial by combat on terms chosen by the dominant scientific milieu, with funds begged and borrowed from institutions rooted in that view. As we have just discussed, this has already proven to be an extremely difficult task.

Translation of the subject into terms and procedures acceptable to both camps presents many difficulties, some of which have never been broadly addressed. Although presenting acupuncture in its most popularly acceptable light has helped to garner public and political support, it has also tended to marginalize the field. An acupuncture that is only easily learned techniques and a popular philosophy might be broadly acculturated, but it would very probably diffuse into the lower levels of professional medicine and the general health culture of Western nations. Proving itself just as biomedicine is supposed to have proven itself would put acupuncture on very firm ground, but that task is not easy, if only because the acupuncture community has yet to accomplish funding sources of its own.

Birch has participated in discussions with researchers at the Office of Alternative Medicine at the National Institutes of Health, the US Food and Drug Administration, and Harvard and Yale Medical Schools, as well as Columbia University. He has worked as a board member for both the Society for Acupuncture Research and the National Academy of Acupuncture and Oriental Medicine. Felt has spent 25 years in the complementary medicine field, 12 years in com-

plementary medical publishing, and 8 years as the publicly elected board chairman of an acupuncture school. Because of this long, close relation to the field, we know that it has attracted the support of many intelligent and dedicated people from many fields. They are one of its finest assets, and the field's accomplishments are considerable. However, a source of the financial resources required to meet the challenge of scientific acceptance is as yet unclear, and many significant issues have yet to be addressed. Thus, although we are certain that acupuncture can succeed in fairly constituted clinical trials, the lack of a viable source of resources is probably the single most critical impediment to scientific acceptance of acupuncture.

FOR WHAT CONDITIONS CAN WE SAY ACUPUNCTURE MAY BE A REASONABLE OPTION

Making a determination of what acupuncture can treat based on a strict drug-centered scientific methodology is, as we have discussed, a difficult and frustrating task. It is not easy to make conclusions from the published literature. However, there are many times when physician and patient decisions are more heuristic than scientific, made in the light not of scientific certainty but of current condition, cost, and the results of conventional therapy. Thus, given current data, we offer the following list of conditions that have shown positive results with acupuncture to inform such selection and referral decisions.

What do we mean by 'positive results?' Are these the only conditions for which we recommend that our family, friends, and colleagues visit an acupuncturist? No. Our personal utilization of acupuncture is considerably broader. Our bias is to use it more extensively than this list indicates, and our experience of acupuncture as a family medicine often makes it our first choice of medical care. Then, does this list constitute a 'guarantee of cure?' Again, no. This is a list of conditions that, when specifically tested, showed promising results in published clinical trials.

The list is formed from published sources. You may thus investigate them for yourself. They include the recent Consensus Development Conference indications,[126] the list of conditions presented to the US Food and Drug Administration in 1994,[127] *Acupuncture Efficacy,* a summation of the peer-reviewed literature and from conferences in Germany.[128]

Chronic pain:
- low back pain
- neck pain
- facial pain (including temporomandibular disorder)
- headaches, including migraines
- joint pain, including tennis elbow, carpal tunnel syndrome, knee pain, and also including arthritis, especially osteoarthritis
- fibromyalgia
- myofascial pain
- reflex sympathetic dystrophy.

Acute pain (postoperative dental pain):
- dental pain
- postsurgical pain
- pain of colonoscopy, endoscopy.

Substance abuse:
- alcoholism
- cocaine dependence
- crack dependence
- heroin dependence.

Anti-emesis:
- nausea and vomiting from cancer chemotherapy
- nausea and vomiting postoperatively
- the nausea and vomiting of morning sickness
- motion-induced nausea and vomiting.

Respiratory:
- asthma
- breathlessness
- exercise-induced asthma symptoms.

Neurological:
- sequellae of stroke
- paralysis
- hand paresis
- palsy
- Parkinson's disease.

Urological:
- urgent, frequent urination
- kidney-stone pain
- bladder instability.

Gynecological and obstetric:
- menstrual pain
- induction of labor
- pain of labor
- reduce time of labor
- breech presentation
- menopausal hot flashes
- hormonal irregularity

Gastroenterological:
- gallstones
- diarrhea
- dry mouth.

Psychological:
- depression.

This list can fairly be thought of as including a number of related problems that have not been specifically tested. For example, in conditions such as chronic pain, there are frequently significant psychological–emotional complications. For example, depression and anxiety are commonly found in patients with chronic pain. These two states are also frequent among persons with substance-abuse problems. In all these situations, acupuncture seems to ameliorate the depression and anxiety. Furthermore, knowing some of the mechanisms that can be activated with acupuncture, in particular those based in the release of endorphins, it seems reasonable to suggest that acupuncture may also be helpful for stress and stress-related problems. It is very common to see patients relax considerably during and after their treatment session. Together these factors suggest that acupuncture can be very helpful in the alleviation of these psychological–emotional problems.

Another area where important results have been observed, but not compiled as formal studies, is in the treatment of immune deficiencies. In the substance-abuse population, human immunodeficiency virus (HIV) infection and acquired immune deficiency syndrome (AIDS) are disproportionately common. There are several acupuncture clinics dedicated to AIDS treatment, such as the AIDS Care Project in Boston, and the AIDS and Chinese Medicine Institute in San Francisco. Practitioners in these clinics report that immune-compromised patients receiving acupuncture have fewer secondary infections and less frequent bouts of symptoms such as diarrhea.[129] In many instances, these patients are also prescribed Chinese medicinal formulas in a combination therapy. This appears to enhance the results. The data are anecdotal. Regardless, so many similar experiences are reported from so many different locations, and the costs and risks are so relatively minor that it is ethically untenable to withold the information.

The list of 'indications' or symptoms for which some demonstrable evidence exists continues to grow as more research is performed. The quality of current studies has improved,[130] and although some studies still manifest poor design, we expect to see more and more evidence that acupuncture is safe and effective. Better quality studies have been recently completed or are in process, for example a study completed with the Anesthesia Department of the Brigham and Women's Hospital at Harvard Medical School testing a treatment for chronic neck pain, and there are studies of acupuncture treatment of substance abuse with the Yale and Columbia Medical Schools. The Office of Alternative Medicine funded two studies in 1993, one on unipolar depression and one on attention deficit hyperactive disorder in children. Five further studies were funded in 1994:

- moxibustion in turning babies in breech presentation
- pain of osteoarthritis of the knees
- acute dental pain
- premenstrual syndrome
- sinus infection in HIV-infected individuals.

The Office of Alternative Medicine has funded 13 centers, several of which are looking into acupuncture. Those that include or plan to include acupuncture are listed in Table 5.2.

A National Institute of Health funded study of the efficacy of acupuncture for peripheral neuropathy in HIV-infected patients was recently published.[131] The National Institute on Drug Abuse (NIDA) has also provided funds for studies of acupuncture for cocaine addicts, as has the National Institute on Alcoholism and Alcohol Addiction (NIAAA) for alcohol abusers. There is a 10-unit multicenter study of acupuncture for tension headache planned in the UK.[132] There is also a large HMO-based study of acupuncture and massage for chronic low-back pain at Group Health in Seattle, and a more complicated study using a more complex design being undertaken by the Harvard Center and a local HMO. This study considers the impact on outcomes for acute back pain when patients are permitted to choose acupuncture, massage, chiropractic or standard therapy.

The NIH recently funded a study examining acupuncture for osteoarthritis of the knee at the

Table 5.2 Centers that plan to use acupuncture funded by the Office of Alternative Medicine

Institution	Subject
Bastyr University of Naturopathy, Seattle	HIV infection
Hennepin County Medical Center, Minneapolis	Addiction
Harvard Medical School, Boston	Chronic and internal diseases
University of Maryland, Baltimore	Pain
Kessler Rehabilitation Institute, New Jersey	Rehabilitation of central nervous system damage
Columbia University, New York	Women's health problems
University of California, Davis	Allergy, immunological problems, including asthma
University of Virginia, Charlotteville	Pain
University of Michigan, Ann Arbor	Cardiovascular disease
University of Arizona, Tucson	Pediatric conditions

University of Maryland Center. The NIH also funded studies seeking to improve the methodology of research at the Maryland Center and the Group Health Research Team in Seattle. Birch is a consultant on the Seattle study.

Pilot studies have been conducted on the effectiveness of acupuncture in relapse and rearrest prevention among recently paroled prisoners who have histories of drug abuse. The Institute of Justice and the US Justice Department have expressed interest in these studies. Although it is likely that some of today's studies will evidence the problems we have discussed in this chapter, acupuncture research has clearly entered a period of improvement and innovation.

As we saw at the beginning of this chapter, the list of conditions for which acupuncture is reputed to be helpful is long. Problems of scientific evaluation do not invalidate these claims. However, it is important to distinguish claims that are supported from those that are not. Because the goal of acupuncture is to correct the flow, distribution, and function of qi, the number of symptoms and diseases that can be treated is theoretically limitless. The cumulative anecdotal evidence tends to support long lists of indications, but more research is necessary if acupuncture is to achieve full integration with Western systems of medical care. However, even if we accept only the preceding list of conditions that have shown positive results in clinical trials, the range of application for acupuncture and moxibustion is nonetheless truly impressive. As the problems we have discussed in this chapter are solved, as better clinical research is conducted, and as studies begin to focus on testing traditional models of practice, we feel there will be a proven and significant place for acupuncture and moxibustion in the health-care systems of the world.

NOTES

1 Anon 1998 NIH Consensus development panel on acupuncture. JAMA 280(17):1518–1524

2 Lytle CD 1997 Safety and regulation of acupuncture needles and other devices. Presented at the NIH Consensus development conference on acupuncture. National Institutes of Health, Bethesda, MD, November 3–5

3 See note 2

4 Bensoussan A, Myers SP 1996 Towards a safer-choice. Department of Human Services, Victoria, pp 73–83

5 Norheim AJ, Fonnebo V 1996 Acupuncture adverse effects are more than occasional case reports: results from questionnaires among 1135 randomly selected doctors, and 197 acupuncturists. Complementary Therapies in Medicine 4:8–13

6(a) Kennedy DL, Burke LB, McGinnis T 1995 National postmarketing drug surveillance and reporting to the MedWatch program. Pharmacy Times August
(b) See note 2
(c) A recent report found the incidence of serious adverse events in hospitalized patients to be 6.7%. Lazarus J, Pomeranz BH, Corey PN 1998 Incidence of adverse drug reactions in hospitalized patients. JAMA 279(15):1200–1205

7 See note 2

8 See note 1

9 Gao Wu; 1983 *Zhen Jiu Ju Ying*. Hong Ye Book Shop, Taipei

10 Soulie de Morant G 1994 Chinese acupuncture. Paradigm Publications, Brookline, MA

11 So JTY 1987 Treatment of disease with acupuncture. Paradigm Publications, Brookline, MA

12 See, for example:

(a) Anon 1980 Essentials of Chinese acupuncture. Foreign Language Press, Beijing
(b) Cheng Xinnong (ed) 1987 Chinese acupuncture and moxibustion. Foreign Languages Press, Beijing
(c) O'Connor J, Bensky D 1981 Acupuncture: a comprehensive text. Eastland Press, Seattle, WA

13 Shiroda Bunshi 1986 *Shinkyu Chiryo Kisogaku*, 6th edn. Ido no Nippon Sha, Yokokusa

14 Wu Yan, Fischer W 1997 Practical therapeutics of traditional Chinese medicine. Paradigm Publications, Brookline, MA

15 Porkert M 1987 The difficult task of blending Chinese and Western science: the case of modern interpretations of traditional Chinese medicine. Quoted in: Sivin N 1987 Traditional medicine in contemporary China. Center for Chinese Studies, University of Michigan, Ann Arbor, MI, p 28

16 Wiseman N, Boss K 1990 Glossary of Chinese medical terms and acupuncture points. Paradigm Publications, Brookline, MA, p xxviii

17 The basis of Western medical equivalences is not often discussed in the acupuncture literature. In their introduction, Wu Yan and Fischer present a Chinese view of the matter. See note 14, pp 1–2

18 Zmiewski P 1994 Introduction to the English edition. In: note 10, p vi

19 This is an oversimplification to the extent that the problem is not only one of definition but also of recognition. See the discussion of inter-rater reliability in Chapter 4

20 See note 16, p xxviii

21   Standard 'point book' formats typically include long lists of symptoms, signs, and/or diseases for each acupoint. Although acupuncturists differentiate using traditional principles, and not all the indications are of the same therapeutic rank, naive readers who equate these to the list of claims made for a pharmaceutical easily mislead themselves.

22   Shudo D 1990 Japanese classical acupuncture: introduction to meridian therapy. Eastland Press, Seattle, WA, pp 113–114

23   Wiseman N, Ellis A 1995 Fundamentals of Chinese medicine, revised edn. Paradigm Publications, Brookline, MA, p 174

24   Manaka Y, Itaya K, Birch S 1995 Chasing the dragon's tail. Paradigm Publications, Brookline, MA, p 145

25   So JTY 1985 Book of acupuncture points. Paradigm Publications, Brookline, MA, p viii
   Note: Although beyond the scope of the present discussion, So's biography introduces one of the subtle elements of the difficulties of transmission of acupuncture. Tin Yau So is a Christian minister who began to practice acupuncture full-time in 1939 when his church was forcibly closed after the Japanese invaded China. It was, as was biomedicine for many Western medical missionaries in China, an expression of his faith. In his own words:

   When practicing acupuncture, I always charged my patients very little. My treatments were available to the poor, as well as to the rich. My business grew as my patients referred other patients. This made my patients happy and me happy. God, step by step, guided me to come and work in America in 1973.

   However, Daoism is so commonly linked to acupuncture in Western descriptions that many Westerners assume that acupuncture practice requires a Daoist perspective. While the developmental influences of Daoism and Confucianism cannot be ignored, acupuncture is clinically an expression of practical skills that can, and have been, applied within a variety of religious and secular perspectives.

26   See note 11, pp 314–316

27   See note 10, p 7

28   See note 25, p vi

29   See note 11, p 183

30   Steadman's medical dictionary, 25th edn. Williams & Wilkins, Baltimore, MA, 1990, p 468

31   See 'water swelling' in: Wiseman N, Feng Y 1998 A practical dictionary of Chinese medicine. Paradigm Publications, Brookline, MA, pp 668–669

32   See the Forewords by Chen Ke-Ji and Paul Unschuld in: Wiseman N 1995 English–Chinese Chinese–English dictionary of Chinese medicine. Hunan Science and Technology Press, Hunan, pp 1–3

33   See note 10, p 5

34   World Health Organization 1980 Use of acupuncture in modern health care. *WHO Chronicle* 34:294–301

35   Zhang X. Personal communication

36   See note 34

37   World Health Organization 1985 The role of traditional medicine in primary health care. WHO, Geneva, WPR/RC36/Technical Discussions/s, 12 September

38   World Health Organization 1991 A proposed standard international acupuncture nomenclature; report of a WHO scientific group. WHO, Geneva

39   The meeting to discuss the WHO list followed the National Institutes of Health/US Food and Drug Administration sponsored Workshop on Acupuncture in April 1994

40   See note 37

41   None of the textbooks in common use mention the current role of Traditional Chinese Medicine in the People's Republic of China

42(a) Greenberg RP, Fisher S 1989 Examining antidepressant effectiveness: findings, ambiguities, and some vexing puzzles. In: Fisher S, Greenberg RP (eds) *Limits of biological treatments for psychological disorders.* Lawrence Erlbaum, Hillsdale, NJ
   (b) Greenberg RP, Bornstein RF, Greenberg MD, Fisher S 1992 A meta-analysis of antidepressant outcome under 'blinder' conditions. Journal of Consulting and Clinical Psychology 60(5):664–669

43   Lipman RS 1989 Pharmacotherapy of anxiety disorders. In: Fisher S, Greenberg RP (eds) The limits of biological treatments for psychological disorders. Lawrence Erlbaum, Hillsdale, NJ

44   Moskowitz G, Chalmers TC, Sacks HS, Fagerstrom RM, Smith H 1983 Deficiencies of clinical trials of alcohol withdrawal. Alcoholism: Clinical and Experimental Research 7(1):42–46

45   Chalmers TC, Block JB, Lee S 1972 Controlled studies in clinical cancer research. New England Journal of Medicine 287(2):75–78

46   Blackburn BA, Smith H, Chalmers TC 1982 The inadequate evidence for short hospital stay after hernia or varicose vein stripping surgery. The Mount Sinai Journal of Medicine 49(5):383–390

47   Eisenberg DM, Delbanco TL, Berkey CS, Kaptchuk TJ, Kupelink B, Kuhl J, Chalmers TC 1994 Cognitive techniques for hypertension: are they effective? Annals of Internal Medicine 118(12):964–972

48   See, for example: Sacks HS, Berrier J, Reitman D, Pugano D, Chalmers TC 1992 Meta-analyses of randomized controlled trials. In: Bailar JC, Mosteller F (eds) Medical uses of statistics. NEJM Books, Boston, MA, pp 427–442

49   Lynoe N 1990 Is the effect of alternative treatment only a placebo effect? Scandinavian Journal of Social Medicine 18:149–153

50   Dorland's illustrated medical dictionary, 26th edn. WB Saunders, Philadelphia, PE, 1981

51   Benson H, McCallie DP 1979 Angina pectoris and the placebo effect. *New England Journal of Medicine* 300(25):1424–1429

52   Lewith GT 1993 Every doctor a walking placebo. In: Lewith GT, Aldridge D (eds) Clinical research methodology for complementary therapies. Hodder & Stoughton, London

53   Levine JD, Gordon NC, Fields HL 1978 The mechanism of placebo anesthesia. *Lancet* ii:654–657

54   Parfitt A 1994 Placebo treatments. In: Proceedings of the First Symposium of the Society for Acupuncture Research. Society for Acupuncture Research, Bethesda, Maryland

55   Wickramasekera I 1985 A conditioned response model of the placebo effect. In: White, Tursky, Schwartz (eds) Placebo – theory, research and mechanism. Guilford Press, New York

56   See note 52
57   See note 52
58   See note 52
59   See note 49
60   See note 49
61   See note 52
62   See notes 52 and 54
63   Some reports have used the term 'double-blind' when the studies were in fact modified 'single-blind'. That is, the acupuncturist clearly knew what he or she was doing. See, for example: Gaw AC, Chang LW, Shaw LC 1975 Efficacy of acupuncture on osteoarthritis pain: a double blind controlled study. New England Journal of Medicine 293:375–378
64   McLellan AT, Grossman DS, Blain JD, Hauerkos HW 1993 Acupuncture treatment for drug abuse: a technical review. Journal of Substance Abuse Treatment 10:569–576
65   See: note 12(a), pp 307–308; note 12(b), p 324
66   MacDonald AJR, Macrae KD, Master BR, Rubin AP 1983 Superficial acupuncture in the relief of chronic low back pain. Annals of the Royal Colleges of Surgeons, England 65:44–46
67   In six brochures of ethnic Chinese and American practitioners claiming to practice Traditional Chinese Medicine found at the New England School of Acupuncture in November 1997, five used the term 'painless' to describe treatment
68   See, for example: Ellis A, Wiseman N, Boss K 1988 Fundamentals of Chinese acupuncture. Paradigm Publications, Brookline, MA
69   See 'obtaining qi' in: Wiseman N, Feng Y 1998 A practical dictionary of Chinese medicine. Paradigm Publications, Brookline, MA, p 419
70   This is an oversimplification to the extent that East Asian sources also differ in how needle stimulus is described. In a modern acupuncture text compiled from Chinese sources there is a specfic stimulation technique listed for each of the main channel points. However, descriptions of the sensation itself are less frequent. In Tin Yau So's work, there is a needle stimulus described for virtually every point, but usually only an indication of insertion depth. Clinically, needle technique is determined by the school of thought or training. See notes 25 and 68
71   See, for example:
(a) Gunn CC 1976 Transcutaneous nerve stimulation, needle acupuncture and '*Teh Ch i*' phenomenon. American Journal of Acupuncture 4(4):317–322
(b) Wang KM, Yao S, Xian Y, Hov Z 1985 A study on the receptive field of acupoint and the relationship between characteristics of needling sensation and groups of afferent fibres. Scientics Sinica (Series B) 28(9):963–971
72   See note 69
73   Mendelson G, Selwood TS, Kanz H, Kidson MA, Scott DS 1983 Acupuncture treatment of chronic pain: a double blind placebo controlled study. American Journal of Medicine 74:49–55
74   Vincent CA, Richardson PH 1986 The evaluation of therapeutic acupuncture: concepts and methods. *Pain* 24:1–13
75(a) Margolin A, Thung P, Avants SK, Kosten TR 1992 Effects of sham and real auricular needling: implications for trials of acupuncture for cocaine addiction. American Journal of Chinese Medicine 21:103–111
(b) Margolin A, Avants SK, Chang P, Birch S, Kosten T

1995 A single-blind investigation of four auricular needle puncture configurations. American Journal of Chinese Medicine 23(2):105–114
(c) Margolin A, Avants SK, Birch S, Falk CX, Kleber HD 1997 Methodological investigations for a multisite trial of auricular acupuncture for cocaine addiction. A study of active and control auricular zones. Journal of Substance Abuse Treatment 13(6):471–481
76(a) Vincent CA 1990 Credibility assessment in trials of acupuncture. Complementary Medical Research 4(1):8–11
(b) Vincent CA, Richardson PH, Black JJ, Pither CE 1989 The significance of needle placement site in acupuncture. Journal of Psychosomatic Research 33(4):489–496
77   Birch S, Jamison RN 1998 A controlled trial of Japanese acupuncture for chronic myofascial neck pain: assessment of specific and non-specific effects of treatment. 14:248–255 Clinical Journal of Pain
78   Zaslawski C, Garvey M, Ryan D, Yang CX, Zhang SP 1997 Strategies to maintain the credibility of sham acupuncture as a control treatment in clinical trials. Journal of Alternative and Complementary Medicine 3(3):257–266
79   White AR, Eddleston C, Hardie R, Resch KL, Ernst E 1996 A pilot study of acupuncture for tension headache, using a novel placebo. Acupuncture in Medicine 14(1):11–15
80(a) Le Bars D, Dickenson AH, Besson JM 1979 Diffuse noxious inhibitory controls (DNIC). I: Effects on dorsal horn convergent neurones in the rat. Pain 6:283–304
(b) Le Bars D, Dickenson AH, Besson JM 1979 Diffuse noxious inhibitory controls (DNIC). II: Lack of effect on non-convergent neurones, supraspinal involvement and theoretical implications. Pain 6:305–327
81   Ter Riet G Kleijnen J, Knipschild P 1990 Acupuncture and chronic pain: a criteria-based meta-analysis. Journal of Clinical Epidemiology 43(11):1191–1199
82   Le Bars D, Willer JC, Broucker T de, Villanueva L 1989 Neurophysiological mechanisms involved in the pain-relieving effects of counterirritation and related techniques including acupuncture. In: Pomeranz B, Stux G (eds) Scientific bases of acupuncture. Springer-Verlag, Berlin
83   For specific examples see:
(a) Cheng R, Pomeranz B 1987 Electrotherapy of chronic musculoskeletal pain: comparison of electroacupuncture and acupuncture-like TENS. Clinical Journal of Pain 2:143–149
(b) Johansson K, Lindgren I, Widner H, Wiklung I, Johanssun BB 1993 Can sensory stimulation improve the functional outcome in stroke patients? Neurology 43:2189–2192
(c) Melzack R, Stillwell DM, Fox EJ 1977 Trigger points and acupoints for pain: correlations and implications. Pain 3:3–23
84   Lewith GT, Machin D 1983 On the evaluation of the clinical effects of acupuncture. Pain 16:111–127
85(a) Birch S 1995 Testing the clinical specificity of needle sites in controlled clinical trials of acupuncture. Part I: The importance of validating the 'relevance' of 'true' or 'active' points and 'irrelevance' of 'control' or 'less-active' points – proposal for a justification method. Part II: The problem of 'diffuse noxious inhibitory control' and how to control for it. In: Proceedings of the Second Symposium of the Society for Acupuncture Research. Society for Acupuncture Research, Bethesda, Maryland, pp 274–294
(b) Birch S 1997 An exploration with proposed solutions of the problems and issues in conducting clinical research

in acupuncture. PhD Thesis, Centre for Complementary Health studies, University of Exeter, 1997
(c) See note 77

86 Lewith GT, Machin D 1983 On the evaluation of the clinical effects of acupuncture. Pain 16:111–127

87 Birch S 1997 Issues to consider in determining an adequate treatment in a clinical trial of acupuncture. Complementary Therapies in Medicine 4:172–177

88 Bullock ML, Culliton PD, Olander RL 1989 Controlled trial of acupuncture for severe recidivist alcoholism. *Lancet* June 24:1435–1439

89(a) See notes 85(a), 85(b), and 87

90 Wyon Y, Lindgren R, Lundeberg T, Hammar M 1995 Effects of acupuncture on climacteric vasomotor symptoms, quality of life, and urinary excretion of neuropeptides among postmenopausal women. Menopause 2:3–12

91 See note 87

92(a) See notes 85(a) and 85(b)
(b) Birch S 1997 Testing the claims of traditionally based acupuncture. Complementary Therapies in Medicine 5(3):147–151

93 See note 12(a)

94 See note 12(c)

95 NanJing Seminar Transcripts, London 1985 Journal of Chinese Medicine

96 See note 11

97 Chen RJ, Wang N 1988 Acupuncture case histories. Eastland Press, Seattle, WA

98 Laitinen J 1975 Treatment of cervical syndrome by acupuncture. Scandinavian Journal of Rehabilitation Medicine 232:114–117

99 Fox EJ, Melzack R 1976 Transcutaneous electrical stimulation and acupuncture, a comparison of treatment for low back pain. Pain 2:141–148

100 Emery P, Lythgoe S 1986 The effect of acupuncture on ankylosing spondylitis. British Journal of Rheumatology 25:132–133

101 Edelist G, Gross AE, Langer F 1976 Treatment of low back pain with acupuncture. Canadian Anaesthesia Society Journal 23:303–306

102 Mendelson G, Selwood TS, Kranz H, Loh TS, Kidson MA, Scott DS 1983 Acupuncture treatment of chronic back pain. The American Journal of Medicine 74:49–55

103 See note 85(b)

104 Lytle CD 1993 An overview of acupuncture. US Department of Health and Human Services, Public Health Service, Food and Drug Administration, Center for Devices and Radiological Health Rockville, Maryland

105 See note 64

106 Alpert S 1996 Reclassification order. Quoted from letter included·in: Birch S, Hammerschlag R (eds) Acupuncture efficacy. National Academy of Acupuncture and Oriental Medicine, New York

107 Ter Riet G, Kleijnen J, Knipschild P 1990 Acupuncture and chronic pain: a criteria-based meta-analysis. Journal of Clinical Epidemiology 43(11):1191–1199

108 Patel M, Gutzwiller F, Parravd F, Marazzi A et al 1989 A meta-analysis of acupuncture for chronic pain. International Journal of Epidemiology 18(4):900–906

109 See note 107

110 National Council Against Health Fraud 1991 Acupuncture: the position paper of the National Council Against Health Fraud. The Clinical Journal of Pain 7(2):162–166

111 Tsutani K, Namiki T, Muramatsu S 1993 List of serials in the field of *Toyo-Igaku* indexed in JMEDICINE. Nihon ToyoIgaku Zashi 43(4):63–67

112 See, for example: Shichido T 1996 Clinical evaluation of acupuncture and moxibustion (32). Clinical tests of acupuncture in Japan. Ido no Nippon Magazine 623(8,7):94–102

113 Tsutani K, Shichido T, Sakuma K 1990 When acupuncture met biostatistics. Paper presented at Second World Conference of Acupuncture and Moxibustion, Paris

114 Tsutani K 1993 The evaluation of herbal medicines: an East Asian perspective. In: Lewith GT, Aldridge D (eds) Clinical research methodologies for complementary medicine. Hodder & Stoughton, London

115 Tsutani K. Personal communication

116 Zhang X Personal communication

117(a) Hammerschlag R, Morris MM 1996 Clinical trials comparing acupuncture with biomedical standard care. A criteria-based evaluation of research design and reporting. Journal of Alternative and Complementary Medicine 5:133–140
(b) de la Torre CS 1993 The choice of control groups in invasive clinical trials such as acupuncture. Frontier Perspectives 3(2):33–37

118 See note 77

119 See note 92(b)

120 Hammerschlag R 1997 Acupuncture efficacy: presenting the evidence. Journal of the National Academy of Acupuncture and Oriental Medicine 4(1–2):9–10

121 Temple R 1989 Government viewpoint of clinical trials of cardiovascular drugs. Medical Clinics of North America 73(2):495–509

122 Birch S. Personal interviews

123 Acupuncture 1994 Consumer Reports January:54–59

124 Johansson K, Lindgen I, Widner H, Wiklung I, Johansson BB 1993 Can sensory stimulation improve the functional outcome in stroke patients? Neurology 43:2189–2192

125 See note 117(a)

126 See note 1

127 See special supplement: Journal of Alternative and Complementary Medicine 1996, 2(1)

128 Birch S, Hammerschlag R 1996 Acupuncture efficacy. National Academy of Acupuncture of Oriental Medicine, New York

129 Feldman M. Personal communication

130 Delis K, Morris M 1994 Clinical trials in acupuncture. Proceedings of the First Symposium of the Society for Acupuncture Research. Society for Acupuncture Research, Bethesda, Maryland

131 Schlay JC, Chaloner K, Max MB, Flaws B, Reichelderfer P, Wentworth D, Hillman S, Brizz B, Cohn DL 1998 Acupuncture and amitriptyline for pain due to HIV-related peripheral neuropathy: a randomized trial. JAMA 280(18):1590–1595. This was a large but seriously flawed study, principally because of inadequate treatment and lack of credibility measures.

132 White A. Personal communication

6

Diagnosis and patient assessment: what do acupuncturists do?

We have looked at models of acupuncture from the ancient to the modern, from China to other Asian countries, and westward to Europe and the USA. We have focused on the key traditional concepts. These concepts still provide the basis for most of the acupuncture performed today, because most practitioners in most schools of thought use some variation of these traditional ideas. Patient assessment in acupuncture, as in biomedicine, is the first step toward treatment. It likewise focuses on traditional views.

As we reported in our discussion of *qi*, there are acupuncturists who completely reject traditional concepts, preferring to use empirical methods for biomedical diagnoses. These approaches are less traditional, but are not logically less valid. However, a detailed description of these approaches is unnecessary because Westerners are already familiar with the central concepts. There are also practitioners who accept qi paradigm concepts to some greater or lesser extent but reject traditional methods of practice, particularly in assessment, in favor of new tools or ideas. Typically, these practitioners base their treatments on a specific measurement device. However, keep in mind that devices are not the only modern modification of traditional practice. A claim to have discovered a new pattern or treatment is also a departure from tradition if its claim of clinical validity relies on nontraditional means. Although individual discovery has been as essential to acupuncture as to any other human endeavor, ideas did not become part of the established body of traditional

East Asian medical knowledge only because someone famous promoted them. Ideas were usually accepted only after empirical trial by many clinicians.

Again we see the importance of understanding the historical foundations of acupuncture, in particular its development through schools of practice in economic competition. Apprentice systems allowed for a rough-and-ready inter-rater reliability. Thus naked-sense skills could be reasonably transmitted from person to person and generation to generation, and certain of these skills could be a master's intellectual capital. In this context, evidence of efficacy was successful use by generations of similarly trained practitioners. The so-called 'test of time' required not only survival as a believable concept, but also transmissibility and economic viability. Apprentice knowledge is thus inherently intergenerational to insure, for example, that the identification of a pattern and the outcome of an associated treatment are consistent in many circumstances, for many practitioners.

In this and the next chapter, we describe the most important approaches to patient assessment and treatment. These systems cover a continuum, with emphasis on various traditional ideas; thus you will notice points of seeming contradiction between systems, and even differences in the details of how practitioners use largely identical systems. Although it is impossible to deny that these contradictions could evidence unreliability in Chinese techniques, or in modern systems of training, variation and contradiction have much less importance in Chinese medicine than in biomedical science.

It is fair to say that Chinese medicine does not so much diagnose as identify patterns meant to cue successful treatments. We call this 'pattern identification.' Although the word 'diagnosis' is often used to render the Chinese character *zheng*, it will be easier to understand *zheng* if you set aside the familiar associations of the English word. There are obvious similarities, not the least of which is the use of differential logic. Regardless, the differences are worth preserving.

In biomedicine, diagnoses can be thought of as composing a continuum of probability. The most certain diagnoses are 'exclusionary.' The least certain are 'differential.' An exclusionary diagnosis is one where all other possibilities are eliminated by a finding. The perfect exclusionary diagnosis is a laboratory test that unfailingly identifies a disease. In practice a particular bacterium, a specific gene, or the presence of a certain biochemical *is* the disease. However, diagnostic criteria can also be compound; that is, based on two or more symptoms or signs. In practice, many diseases are diagnosed by more than one symptom. But clinical findings and diseases are always inextricably linked. For example, 'cholera' is the presence of the microorganism *Vibro cholerae*. Its presence excludes the possibility that nausea, vomiting, and diarrhea in the host are the result of any other cause. Although there are many reasons why someone may suffer from nausea, vomiting, and diarrhea, once *V. cholerae* is identified, the disease is known to be cholera, and physicians will look no further to plan a cure.

This singular exclusivity is the standard to which traditional East Asian pattern recognition is most commonly and unfavorably compared. Indeed, most proponents of traditional systems offer no defense in this regard, concentrating instead on the holism of the traditional system. However, the reliability of laboratory tests is in fact measured by the probability that they are wrong. Their limits are described by a percentage of 'false positives' (those whom a clinical test labels as having a disease but who do not) and 'false negatives' (those who have a disease that the test fails to find). Although a primary characteristic of the biomedical diagnostic process is the isolation of a one-to-one relationship between quantified clinical findings, the pathogen it describes and the drug used to combat that pathogen, it too is a probabilistic process.

Although the degree of error in traditional pattern recognition has never been established, it is logically capable of the same type of statistical accuracy. This is particularly true regarding differential diagnoses. In both traditional East Asian medicine and modern medicine differential diagnoses are a formal reduction of the possibilities until only one alternative remains.[1] The Western and the traditional process are logically identical. It is only the observations that differ. In fact, one Western diagnostician speaking against the decline of differential skills in biomedical education points to the manual used to train Barefoot Doctors to emphasize his argument.[2]

In the differential process a patient's symptoms and signs are compared to the symptoms and signs associated with every pathology that could produce those signs and symptoms. For illustration, the simplest form of differential diagnosis is a comparison between symptoms and test results and the formal description of a disease (Table 6.1). In this much-simplified example, the patient would not be diagnosed as suffering from disease A, because he or she showed symptom 1 but not symptoms 2 or 3, and sign 3 but not 1 or 2. The patient would be diagnosed as suffering from disease C because all three symptoms and all three signs associated with disease C are present. In practice, of course, the information is more complex, there is a greater logical challenge, and real conditions are not always so obvious. In addition, the conditions differentiated are often difficult to treat precisely because their mechanisms are neither simple nor clear.

Traditional acupuncturists follow the same logical process. The logic, the probabilism, and the intellectual demands are the same. The more telling difference is that a traditional acupuncturist uses no quantifiable tests. Even when examining clinical specimens (e.g. urine,

Table 6.1 Differential diagnosis: comparison between symptoms, test results and the formal description of diseases

	Symptom			Sign		
Disease	1	2	3	1	2	3
A	Y	N	N	N	N	Y
B	Y	Y	N	N	Y	Y
C	Y	Y	Y	Y	Y	Y

or the pus that issues from a wound) the information sought is sensory and qualitative: size, shape, color, and odor. A few illustrative urinary symptoms are given in Table 6.2. These are just some of the clinical observations related to urine.[3] These are combined with other observable qualities to differentiate a condition. For example, length of urination combines with color or volume to create distinct labels such as: 'short voidings of reddish urine' or 'short voidings of scant urine.' Each of these is an observationally defined and relative, but nonetheless specific. For example, *xiao bian chi se* (rough voidings of reddish urine) describes scant dark-colored urine that is passed in short inhibited voidings. Even seemingly minor elements of the term are important. In this case *chi*, translated as 'reddish,' implies a repletion pattern and distinguishes this condition from the similar but distinct 'bloody urine.'[4]

In modern Traditional Chinese Medicine (TCM) acupuncture these conditions are associated with patterns, which are in turn associated with 'treatment principles' and acupoints. Although this has not been obviously expressed

Table 6.2 Some urinary symptoms and their associated conditions

Condition	Clinical observations
Pang guang shi re niao xue	Bladder, damp heat, bloody urine
Niao xue	Bloody urine
Bian niao qing li	Clear uninhibited stool and urine
Niao duo	Copious urine
Niao chi	Dark-colored urine
Xiao bian qing chang	Long voidings of clear urine
Xia jiao shi re niao xue	Lower burner, damp-heat, bloody urine
Niao chi	Reddish urine
Xiao bian chi se	Rough voidings of reddish urine
Xiao bian hun zhuo	Turbid urine

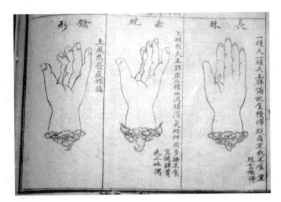

Figure 6.1 Hand patterns from *The Great Compendium of Acupuncture and Moxibustion*. (Courtesy of Paradigm Publications.)

in many English-language beginners' manuals, in Asian literature the differential process is enhanced by weighting signs and symptoms as primary or secondary. A primary pathocondition is necessary to differentiate an associated pattern; a secondary pathocondition may or may not be present. The acupoints used to treat the patterns identified will be selected in conjunction with other factors determined by other clinical observations (e.g. location within the body) and the acupuncturist's assessment of an internal or external cause, as well as an assessment of the individual:

If one treats [all those patients who appear to suffer from one identical illness] with one and the same therapy, one may hit the nature of the illness, but [one's approach] may still be exactly contradicted by the [conditions] of the patient's influences and body.[5]

In other acupuncture systems, signs and symptoms play a greater or lesser role than in TCM. Again, this has historical roots. Not only was observation beyond the range of the human senses technologically impossible during most of Chinese medicine's history, but there was never a perceived need to look beyond the sensory realm. What traditional Chinese practitioners sought was not a critical fact (e.g. the presence of a microbe), but a pattern of natural phenomena that they and their colleagues had seen before. Three of the 'Four Examinations,' the name the Chinese gave to the skills of pattern identification, are purely sensory: looking, listening, and palpating. The fourth, questioning, is a logical process, but it concentrates on gathering information observed with human senses and feelings. In effect, inquiry acquires data of interest to the clinician by examining patients' perceptions.

As we saw when we examined the ideas of vacuity and repletion, this information need not be clinical in the rather narrow sense in which we use this word today. Because patterns did not aim to supply a one-and-only diagnostic key, they not only included a wide range of human responses but also drew upon the expressive abilities of the Chinese language to communicate related images. For example, what we would call 'a hoarse voice' the Chinese called 'broken metal failing to sound.'[6] Because the lungs governed the voice in five-phase theory, the voice belongs to the category of metal, which, as in bells and gongs, is known for its sonorous quality. When lung *qi* is damaged the voice loses its sonority, just as a broken bell fails to ring true. This should not be mistaken as mere literary nicety; it is more than just a poetic way to say 'hoarse voice.' It is an image that clued clinicians' treatment planning. In this case, although the lung governs the movement of *qi*, the kidney governs the absorption of *qi*. Thus treatment depends not only on the lungs, but also on the kidney. The image makes the principle more memorable, and describes a practical clinical relationship.

Furthermore, biomedical diagnoses are absolute and patterns are relative. Diagnosis tries to identify an entity according to specific, absolutely correct criteria that are believed to be valid at any time, at any place and in any human (or even mammalian) population. Traditional patterns identify an individual condition in a particular environment at a particular time. As we noted earlier, there is a strong bedside orientation to traditional clinical observations, and this is reflected in its patterns.

Biomedical diagnoses are exclusive — each names a condition for which there is no other correct identification. Traditional patterns are not exclusive — clinical observations organized by one set of patterns may also be organized by other sets of patterns. The same symptoms and signs that describe one of the organ-centered patterns of Chinese TCM may also be viewed through the five-phase logic of Japanese channel-centered systems. In fact, many of the correspondences beneath *zang fu* images are five phase in origin. Either of these identifications can be correct, if they lead to successful treatment. Both are wrong, if they do not. But neither is inherently right or wrong, and each practitioner's choice between the two, or any other, is influenced by many factors.

Thus, just as in our discussion regarding clinical research, a pattern and a diagnosis are rarely identical. Someone with a single biomedical diagnosis can reflect several different traditional patterns in the course of that disease. One pattern can incorporate what biomedicine describes as more than one disease, and a single acupoint can be useful for a variety of conditions defined by biomedicine. Modern therapies concentrate on attacking a primary causative agent, but acupoint functions were traditionally thought to address a pattern of indications. Thus, while traditional patterns and biomedical diagnoses can be related, these relationships are not formal certainties, but clinical clues — 'Western medical correspondences.' Even when traditional physicians identify what biomedicine labels as a particular disease (e.g. tuberculosis), there are subtle but profound differences created by the traditional emphasis on observation with the naked senses and the treatment clues stored in the language of patterns.

Other differences between pattern recognition and diagnosis are also worth noting. Western diagnostic logic presumes that disease has a material cause, a 'vector.' Thus, there are Western diagnoses for which there are no known treatments. Progressive multiple sclerosis is a current example. Its mechanisms are well understood, but there is as yet no standard therapy. In acupuncture there are patterns which are difficult to treat and patients who cannot be cured, but there is always a treatment. Because a pattern identifies a condition expressed in terms of *qi*, and therapeutic capacities are expressed in the same terms, there is always a treatment available.

Where a disease is, by definition, a patient complaint (disease), everyone reflects some pattern, even people who are healthy in biomedical terms (i.e. those who have no complaint). Thus patterns are also used by an acupuncturist to plan preventive measures, or measures meant to preserve health or improve the quality of life. Systems that emphasize this capacity are sometimes referred to as 'constitutional,' as they encourage a broad view of the individual. Yves Requena's terrain system is a good example of a constitutional system. In his approach, a biomedical history and psychological surveys are combined with channel patterns to produce a composite character type. For each of these types there is an analysis of disease predisposition with preventive and therapeutic measures.

Requena's system is noteworthy because it uses the Berger test, a statistically justified psychological examination, to help bridge the epistemological differences between patterns and diagnoses.[7] As already noted, the foundation of a diagnosis is essentially statistical. It is a test, chemical or otherwise, that uses statistical criteria to say something about a large population from tests administered to a small population. It attempts to describe an aspect of the natural world using norms and standards. A pattern is inherently qualitative, an image of a condition. Traditional patterns do not involve comparisons against statistical norms. Instead they describe how individuals function in their environment. Thus patterns can concern matters such as someone's response to their natural and social surroundings (e.g. the idea of spiritedness, which we discussed in Ch. 3, p. 104). These notions rarely figure in a Western diagnosis, but in psychology and psychiatry various assessment methods are used to create reliable qualitative–quantitative relationships.

However, among these differences there are also significant similarities. From very early on acupuncturists recognized that there were diseases (pathological processes) that were the same in everyone. These are biomedically defined diseases and, in fact, scholars believe they can recognize specific diseases in ancient Chinese writings. Also, material, biological entities were known to be the cause of particular illnesses. For example, Chinese physicians were writing about the smallpox 'spore' long before biomedicine was introduced to China.[8] Terms such as 'flying corpse,' which is today scientized to 'consumption' in translation, nonetheless show that Chinese thinkers understood some diseases to have single, if imperceptible, causes.[9] Furthermore, the characters used to label medical ideas are often borrowed from military language, just as in the West. Ideas such as invasion, defense, and the cutting-off of an enemy's supplies are all used to describe treatment strategies.[10]

There is a Chinese proverb that your life is too precious to waste on a new doctor. So, it is clear that the Chinese understood that some people and ideas succeed more often than others. Neither was their means of guaranteeing validity altogether foreign. When we talk of the 'test of time,' we are talking about what could ironically be called an 'unquantified statistic.' The sense of the test of time is similar and recognizable, but its expression defies reduction to something with which we are easily comfortable or familiar. It is not that traditional pattern identification is entirely and absolutely foreign to Western diagnosis, it is that the practice of traditional medicine developed through human observational skills that are much less emphasized today in the West. Because traditional concepts such as *yin-yang* are rooted in the rhythms and patterns of nature, the medical patterns these ideas describe are logically, linguistically, and clinically descriptions of humans and their natural environment.

These differences do raise issues of scientific validity. These issues were discussed in Chapter 4, and we hope to have shown there that the claims of the traditionalists, pragmatists, and scientists are often culturally derived and not as contradictory as they first appear. It is germane that any society's basis for judging a theory or technique is strongly influenced by socio-cultural, historical, and other nonclinical factors. In the West, among practitioners interested in studying acupuncture there are those for whom its traditional explanations and methods are merely out-of-date metaphysical speculations. There are also those for whom the same methods are a salvation from the horrors of a depersonalized technology. In the East, among those practitioners who study acupuncture there are those for whom it is merely the family trade they follow. In China there are practitioners who were forced to study acupuncture against their will by a government that restricts personal choice. There are also Chinese who see traditional practices as a return to a former cultural greatness and a protection from the invading culture of the West. There are some for whom these practices are only occasionally useful methods of treatment in need of scientific rehabilitation from their metaphysical roots. There are entire Asian populations for whom *yin-yang* and the five phases are as foreign as to any Westerner.[11] In fact, explanatory models and methods of practice change with individual perspective. Although this can make pattern identification look chaotic and fragmented, it is really a remarkably adaptable skill that has survived despite the biases of the cultures in which it has been applied.

HEALTH, DISEASE, AND CAUSES OF DISEASE IN THE TRADITIONAL MODEL

Modern biomedicine has made admirable advances in defining pathologies and describing physiological conditions. The discovery of bacteria and then viruses revolutionized medicine for the entire planet. Unraveling of the genetic code evolves our understanding of disease. Even with the rise of organisms that resist drugs, stubborn, ill-defined diseases continue to yield to analysis. So the question naturally arises: Why do we need another approach? Why do we need an old and unscientific approach? If a patient presents with tendonitis of the elbow, why do we need to talk about *jing luo, zang fu, qi, yin-yang,* and the five phases? If even some acupuncturists think only of tendonitis, why preserve these older ideas?

Because there are those who have considerable investment in rejecting traditional concepts and those who have considerable investment in rejecting modern concepts, no answer will satisfy everyone. However, we can observe that the source of this problem is how we think. Not only is pattern identification technically different from biomedical diagnosis, the 'one right way' approach that typifies Western thought has never been typical of Chinese problem-solving.[12] So, the question could have been: Why not have another way to look at human health problems? After all, there are still plenty of people with tennis elbow.

For Westerners, there can only be one right answer. This is an outgrowth of our religious faiths. Because most of us have been raised to believe in one God, typically a jealous God, our culture takes a monotheistic view of nature. Truth is singular. As a consequence, this belief permeates our thinking. In science, it determines what we believe to be proof. The need to eliminate competing ideas leaving a single defensible explanation is the core of the scientific method.[13] Likewise, in commerce, law, and politics we believe that truth is that which is without contradiction.

Chinese culture, on the other hand, allowed competing theories to coexist. There was no need to prove one idea true and all others false. As Paul Unschuld states it:

The unique feature of the Chinese situation ... is the continuous tendency towards a syncretism of all ideas that exist (within accepted limits). Somehow a way was always found in China to reconcile opposing views and to build bridges.[14]

We are so attuned to one-and-only answers that descriptions that compete with our own are difficult for us to absorb. As we saw in our discussion of modern intellectual history (see Ch. 2, p. 75), this is not a quality exclusive to acupuncture's skeptics; those who advance ideas about acupuncture also express the opinion that because their approach is correct other approaches must do harm. To Westerners, one answer must be right and all others must be wrong. Traditional acupuncture patterns, couched in their metaphoric language and developed without the pressure to reconcile contradictory ideas, just do not fit.

Chinese thinkers, proceeding from the views of reality inherent in Daoism, Confucianism, and Buddhism, were unpossessed of our Western certainty of an absolute and singular truth. Instead, their first principle was change. Although they perceived the universe as orderly, balanced by the complementary oppositions of *yin* and *yang*, they expected to perceive order through faithful observation. The universe was not a complex of God's natural laws to be mastered, but a changing panorama to be observed. Although each of China's three philosophical pillars saw humankind's relation to the universe in different ways, none proposed that humans were able to capture a single, ineffable, and permanent truth. Although acupuncture's principles developed in a long sequence of intellectual climates, each responding to Chinese culture's changing needs, none of those climates featured the hard immutability inherent in Western notions of natural law.

Understanding the Chinese cultural milieu is by no means an academic nicety of no interest to clinicians, because the Chinese concept of pattern identification is not easy to absorb and apply. It is an individual process that recognizes consistent patterns in human health and illness. It posits symptoms and diseases that are utterly familiar as well as conditions never conceived of in the West. It uses words that are part of everyday language, but attributes to them qualities that are not only new or foreign but which are also possessed of unique technical definitions that must be painstakingly learned. You do not need to look at much Chinese printing to understand that red is not always red.[15] We cannot eliminate the difficulties inherent in learning and using traditional medical information, however we can suggest learning aids that facilitate understanding.

First, try to set familiar English words aside. Think not just of 'diagnosis,' but also of 'pattern identification.' This will not only diminish the force of the expectations attached to the English word, but also provide a linguistic hook on which to hang traditional ideas. Beware when you think you understand Chinese medicine in nice-sounding, familiar words. If a notion is comfortable, without a twinge of unfamiliarity, it is probably less than entirely traditional. For example, it takes very little additional effort to accommodate to the idea of a vacuity rather than to the more Western idea of deficiency. However, that effort pays dividends because the image has more room for traditional qualities that do not fit the more familiar English term. For example, imbalances in bodily shape or proportion, expressions of personality, interior weaknesses behind or beneath superficial expressions, particularly those that have morphological or topological expressions, individual rather than normative comparisons, and constitutional traits are all very difficult to fit within the normative expectations of 'deficiency.'

Furthermore, try not to think of patterns as the reality labels of biomedicine. Instead, think of them as images in the language you would use to describe the experience of seeing, hearing, feeling, and responding to people and events. Patterns feature the commonalities that were memorable to practitioners who saw many patients. This is why experienced acupuncturists often concern themselves with what novices think are insignificant nuances and details. Finally, think of a pattern as a relative means to an end, a step in determining what treatment will work, and not as a description of some permanent reality.

In biomedicine a diagnosis is a scientific label for a fact that is believed to have an objective, statistically insured reality. In acupuncture a pattern is a way to identify conditions for which treatments have worked in the past. It is a method for discriminating the acupoints and techniques to use, not a means for categorizing a fixed and universal reality. The assumption that a pattern label (e.g. spleen vacuity) implies an objective entity or condition only leads to confusion.

Virtually no scientific work has been done to verify whether or not traditional patterns identify some aspect of nature, some measurable phenomenon. In the absence of such research, it is unwise to say that any traditional pattern refers to something objective or measurable, or is

directly equal to a biomedical diagnosis. Furthermore, this is both practically unnecessary and clinically limiting. Because acupuncturists gather their data with the unaided senses, often learning as apprentices through the guidance of a more experienced clinician, the real problem was, and is, knowing what can be done to help the patient. That knowledge was assumed to lie in the experience of preceding generations, not in a one-and-only description of presumed reality. Because more than one pattern can be related to a single disease, or more than one disease to a single pattern, too close a relationship can limit the clinical options considered.

The key fact of pattern identification is that in acupuncture every pattern, no matter how individual, has a matching treatment. In biomedicine this is not the case. To be scientific a biomedical diagnosis must be an objective description and label. Therapeutic intervention does not necessarily follow. In fact, in acupuncture practice it is a common experience to meet patients who have seen several biomedical specialists. They have a clear and much confirmed diagnosis, an array of objective measurements and probable outcomes, but no therapy. Indeed, no therapy may exist. In traditional acupuncture there is always a matching treatment. Indeed, those treatments are so neatly matched to a pattern description that there is often an acupoint or combination of acupoints for each of the major and minor aspects of a patient's condition. Where the biomedical physician has the role of describing and labeling a condition, the acupuncturist's role is more direct. He or she may identify a problem in ways that are not exclusive; the pattern may not be as precise as an exclusionary biomedical diagnosis, but it does lead to something that can be done. This is not to say that acupuncturists can cure every problem, only that there is a starting point for therapy, and from that starting point some degree of relief can often be achieved.

In modern terms patterns are organizing models, methods of ordering information. But the words 'organizing model' ought not be prefaced with 'mere' or some other word meant to diminish the idea relative to the greater specificity and objectivity of science. It is different from, but neither inferior to nor easy to replace with, a biomedical skill or concept. For example, today one of the most significant medical problems is the increasing prevalence of chronic disease for which pharmaceuticals are not ideal. Equally common are patients presenting with multiple problems that cannot be identified as a single disease, or which are identifiable as having several different sources. Organizing models, traditional acupuncture patterns, have the potential to make sense of these complex, chronic conditions, while simultaneously providing the possibility of effective treatment.

In clinics where acupuncture is available, when a patient presents with multiple symptoms but no diagnosis, there is always an acupuncture treatment possible. In biomedicine, when patients present with multiple problems for which there is no linking diagnosis, there may be no one therapy, and there can be problems of unwanted interactions between the separate medications prescribed for each of the problems. In these cases acupuncture also frequently provides a viable strategy. Indeed, in the view of experienced practitioners, acupuncture often appeals to patients precisely because its patterns resolve for them the fractured feeling produced when many biomedical specialists are consulted.

This feature of acupuncture, pattern identification, is a direct result of its concentration on organizing observations rather than on discovering a single cause or target of attack. For example, spleen *qi* vacuity as understood in the modern Chinese *ba gang bian zheng* system, or a lung vacuity as described by a modern Japanese *keiraku chiryo* practitioner, both associate many sets of multiple symptoms. In *Fundamentals of Chinese Medicine*, a direct translation of a Chinese medical textbook, the problems associated with spleen *qi* vacuity are described as underlying many digestive disorders, including the Western medical correspondences of chronic gastritis, cholecystic disease, nutritional disturbances, and more general problems such as asthenia and prolapse.[16] The pattern specifically includes problems such as diarrhea, thin stool, and abdominal discomfort.

In *Introduction to Meridian Therapy*, Denmei Shudo describes how lung vacuity can include symptoms described in classic texts as upper back and shoulder pain, respiratory problems, throat problems, fever, and chills. He goes on to list the following symptoms based on modern practice: yawning, flushing, dryness of the throat, sweating on exposure to wind–cold, heat in the palms, pain in the shoulders and supraclavicular fossa, shortness of breath, wheezing and coughing, irritability, and frequent urination.[17] Thus successful treatments for several different problems can be achieved with a treatment based on the lung-vacuity pattern. For example, with only minor variations, the *yin-yang* balancing channel therapy cross-syndrome treatment can be applied for symptoms of four major presenting symptoms. When the one basic pattern is used to focus treatment, several biomedical conditions can be improved or cured. This is illustrated for the cross-syndrome pattern in Boxes 6.1 to 6.4.

The fact that traditionally-based acupuncture patterns usually include a broad range of symptoms, as well as physical and psychological traits, makes them suitable for understanding

---

Box 6.1 Cross-syndrome pattern: a 45-year-old man

Main complaint. Right-sided sciatica for the last 7 months. Pain down the back of the leg and numbness of the lower leg. The resulting lack of activity has complicated the condition via a weight gain of 45–50 lb. The patient reports that he is generally quite athletic and that the problem may have started with athletic activities such as rowing and golf. Chiropractic, osteopathy, and biomedical treatments had failed to help. He is mildy depressed as a result of this problem.

Japanese *yin-yang* balancing channel diagnosis and therapy was applied.

- *Examination:* the whole left deep pulse was weaker; the 'cross-syndrome' pattern of abdominal reactions was very clear.
- *Pattern identification:* a liver-related problem known as 'the cross-syndrome.'
- *Treatment:* Yoshio Manaka's three-step treatment process.

patients whose conditions cannot be well defined using biomedical labels. The Chinese concept includes evidence that would not be considered indications of disease in biomedicine. A pattern is a picture that can include any observable trend, whether or not it is considered pathological by the culture, the patient, or practitioner. The key is the picture itself. This is not to say that acupuncturists do not concentrate on patient complaints, only that traditional practitioners' observations are broader than their patients' symptoms.

Box 6.2   Cross-syndrome pattern: a 16-year-old girl

Main complaint. The patient had had her first menses 4 months prior to presentation, but had had no menses since. Because of a significant family history of menstrual problems, prophylactic treatment was sought. She was an athletic student who also had some achiness of the shoulders, a mild scoliosis of the low back, and occasionally sore ankles.

Japanese *yin–yang* channel diagnosis and therapy was applied.

- *Examination:* the cross-syndrome pattern of abdominal reactions was clear, the pulse showed a pattern consistent with lung–liver vacuity.
- *Treatment:* the usual three-step treatment process was embarked upon.

Box 6.3   Cross-syndrome pattern: a 60-year-old man

Main complaints. Osteoarthritis over the last 10 years that has affected many joints. Currently the lumbar spine and tops of both feet are very painful from the arthritis. There are residual and less significant pains in other joints. He also has a minor problem with hypertension, and has had psoriasis on the hands, feet, elbows, and back for over a decade.

Japanese *yin–yang* balancing channel diagnosis and therapy was applied.

- *Examination:* the pulse showed a pattern associated with spleen–liver vacuity; the abdominal region clearly showed a cross-syndrome pattern of reaction; many blood stasis signs (moles, vascular spiders, and pigmentation) were obvious.
- *Diagnosis:* liver-related blood stasis problems, the 'cross-syndrome.'
- *Treatment:* the usual three-step treatment process was commenced.

Box 6.4   Cross-syndrome pattern: a 36-year-old man

Main complaints. Severe inflammation and pain of the right eye, diagnosed as acute nongranulomatous iritis. The problem had developed one week before. He had severe pain, with referred pain to the right side of the head, photophobia and poor sleep. During the last week he had been using prednisone and scopolamine eyedrops to reduce the inflammation and help open the pupil, but had seen only minor improvements from these medications. When he came for treatment, he was unable to open and use his right eye, had been unable to work, and needed to wear dark glasses because daylight was too painful. He had had the same problem 5 years earlier. At that time he was treated with antibiotics almost continuously, and then with steroids for more than 4 months before the condition cleared. Other than this, he had no significant medical history and was healthy.

Japanese *yin–yang* balancing channel diagnosis and therapy was applied.

- *Examination:* the whole left deep pulse was weak, the cross-syndrome pattern of reactions showed on the abdomen.
- *Diagnosis:* a clear liver-related pattern, the 'cross-syndrome.'
- *Treatment:* the ion-pumping cords were used in combination with some local treatment for the eye.

SYMPTOMS IN ACUPUNCTURE

Symptoms, patient-reported manifestations and signs, and practitioner observations do play an important role in pattern identification. If, for example, a patient complains of headaches, the location of the headache can help determine which channel is involved and how the headache may be treated. For example:

- crown – liver channel
- temples – *shao yang* channels (gallbladder and *san jiao*)
- frontal – *yang ming* channels (large intestine and stomach)
- occipital – *tai yang* channels (bladder and small intestine).

If there are other signs and symptoms, the differentiation of the headache and its associated treatment becomes even more precise. This is described in both classical and modern texts. In Chapter 24 of the *Huang Di Nei Jing Ling Shu* (c–100), seven kinds of headache are described.[18] In the Ming dynasty text *Zhen Jiu Da Cheng* (1601), there are references to 17 different headaches.[19] In the modern (1960) Chinese text *Zhen Jiu Zhi Liao Xue*, six types of headache are described.[20] In each text, each category of headache leads to a different treatment.

Although many traditional patterns use the problem location as a clinical clue, the traditional system can also be used to formulate whole-body treatments. Recall the example of tendonitis of the elbow. Practitioners who consider only the biomedical diagnosis tend to treat only the affected elbow and arm. In fact, even without needling, pressure on painful points surrounding the area can have an immediate effect. These formulary treatments (often diminuitively called 'cookbook acupuncture') have long been used and can have excellent results. The traditional ethic that the superior practitioner treats disease before it arises has never meant that symptom-centered treatments are ineffective. Instead, it emphasizes how practitioners should treat preventively.

For example, if a traditional practitioner examined a tendonitis patient and saw more general problems with bending and stretching, he or she would consider pathoconditions associated with the liver organ or channel. Finding these, a strategy for treating internal tendencies that caused or contributed to the

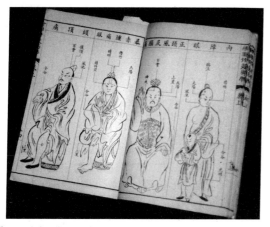

Figure 6.2 'Internal obstruction blindness, center head wind and headache, red and swollen eyes' from *The Study of Acupuncture, Moxibustion and I Jing.* (Courtesy of Paradigm Publications.)

tendonitis would quickly follow. Again, pattern identification involves considering diverse information to uncover the underlying pattern.

Pattern identification also contributes to acupuncture's ability to address future problems and problems that are not part of the Western concept of disease. Health in the traditional model is a positive state. It is that state unique to each individual, where the distribution, circulation, and production of *qi* is balanced and regular. This requires that the channels are relatively balanced, functioning normally, and smoothly circulating *qi*, and that organ functions are relatively effective:

As long as a person's essence and spirits are complete and strong, no external evil will dare to offend [that person].[21]

In a broader sense this also means that *yin-yang* and the five phases are balanced. Any shift away from balance results in illness. This is quite different from the Western definition of health, which is the absence of an objectifiable pathology. It also explains why whole-person observations such as pulse or abdominal palpation, body structure, or personality traits are so highly valued in acupuncture. When two or more of these observations lead to mutually consistent patterns, it is much easier to choose acupoints to treat diverse symptoms.

In the traditional model, health is viewed as the product of many factors. How one lives one's life, habits, environmental factors such as seasonal influences, climate, internal factors such as emotional and mental activity, and the functioning of the organs and tissues, all affect one's health. In *The Second Medical Revolution*, Foss and Rothenberg propose a parallel model for modern medicine,[22] as do others. Yet, these ideas are not the norm of contemporary medical practice. Thus the multifactorial approach to health that acupuncture offers may be one of its more important contributions to the West. This is most easily explained by example.

When a patient presents with very strong symptoms, but is relatively healthy in terms of the traditional pattern perspectives, we expect a quick recovery. This is often what happens when someone attributes a miracle cure to acupuncture. For example, one of Birch's patients presented with arthritis of the hips and spine. The problem had increased during the last 5 years and the patient's activities had become very restricted. Although the symptoms were very strong, progressive, and not very responsive to modern medications, a few simple acupuncture treatments were remarkably successful. Because the patient was very strong and healthy except for his symptoms, he healed quickly.

Conversely, if a patient presents with a minor complaint but their general condition is very poor and there is a pattern of multiple imbalances, the prognosis is poor. These patients take a long time to recover. For example, another of Birch's patients presented with pain in the right hip. It was irritating but not restrictive. She had not had the problem very long and described herself as being 'pretty healthy.' Besides hip pain she had no other complaint. In this case the symptom was relatively mild and seemingly uncomplicated, but the patient responded to treatment slowly because her condition was in fact complicated by a deep underlying vacuity. Although her presenting symptom was mild, the pattern evidenced by her physical and psychological tendencies indicated a vacuity that made it difficult for her to heal. First, she needed treatment to strengthen the underlying weakness.

As these examples show, the idea of a cause of disease is multiple and linked to someone's constitution and general condition. Historically, there are discussions of the 'internal causes' of disease, primarily emotional and mental states. The 'external causes of disease,' known as 'evils' in Chinese, are primarily climatic factors.[23] There are also a few 'miscellaneous' causes of disease. Listed among the internal causes of disease are the 'affects.' Sometimes called 'the seven emotions,' the affects are actually mental and emotional activities: joy, anger, anxiety, thought, sorrow, fear, and fright. If one or more of these affects manifests excessively in intensity or frequency, the circulation of *qi* and its associated organ functions will be disrupted. As we saw in Chapter 3, specific organs are

associated with specific affects (Table 6.3).[24] Practically, the associations frequently appear to be valid in clinical practice.

Why should pensiveness or mentation tend to weaken the spleen, or why should anger depress liver function? Again, these are analogies to the concepts of the qi paradigm, not disease vectors in the Western sense. When organ function and/or its associated *qi* circulation is disrupted, pathoconditions begin to manifest. Thus, ideally, to remain healthy one must harmonize one's thoughts and emotions, to hold to none too long and to moderate all. Not surprisingly, this is another expression of the moderation and self-discipline ideals found in Asian philosophy, particularly Confucianism, but also in Buddhist and Daoist thought. The meditative, visual, and martial arts, for example, all express this concept.

Listed among the external causes of disease are six specific environmental or climatic evils: wind, cold, fire, damp, dryness, and summerheat. In another recognition of material disease vectors, 'pestilential *qi*' was also categorized as an external cause. Susceptibility to each of these comes from overexposure, problems of the associated organs or channels, or a combination of these (Table 6.4).[25] Wind is associated with the liver and the sinews. Thus, a liver problem can cause a sensitivity to wind, which can manifest as aversion to wind or as headaches that follow an exposure to a wind or draft. Cold is typically associated with the kidneys or lungs. Weakness of either leads to a sensitivity to cold; for example, a knee pain or lower back pain that develops or worsens when the temperature drops. The sniffly nose and other respiratory symptoms we call 'catching cold' is

Table 6.3 Organ–affect correspondences

Affect	Injury
Joy	Heart
Anger	Liver
Anxiety	Spleen
Thought	Spleen
Sorrow	Lungs
Fear/fright	Kidney

Table 6.4 The six environmental evils and their corresponding organs

External evil	Injury
Wind	Liver
Cold	Kidneys or lungs
Fire	Heart
Damp	Spleen or kidneys
Dryness	Lungs
Summerheat	Heart

another example. Dampness can both weaken or result from a problem of the spleen or kidney. If these organs become weak, what we call rheumatism can develop. Those who suffer from damp, or cold–damp, experience painful joints every time it rains or is very humid, or damp and cold. Some schools of thought believed that if someone were healthy and balanced, they would resist these external evils and be unaffected. However, for example, once an imbalance of the affects weakens or disrupts the system, susceptibility to the external evils would begin.

Among the neutral factors of disease are dietary irregularity, sexual intemperance, and taxation fatigue, a concept that includes both excessive activity and lack of exercise.[26] Each of these will manifest differently, and can increase susceptibility to both the internal and external causes of disease. Today people propose extending these causes to include destructive lifestyles, smoking, prescription and over-the-counter drugs, improper breathing, and exposure to toxins, powerful electromagnetic fields, radiation, or environmental poisons.

THE NATURE OF DISEASE

According to the traditional model, disease is a disruption of the circulation, distribution, function, or production of *qi*. Such disruptions are defined in terms of the systems that circulate *qi*, the channels, or the systems that produce *qi*, the *zang fu*. These are identified as *yin-yang* and/or five-phase imbalances.

In the traditional framework there was a clear distinction between the underlying issues that gave rise to disease and the actual manifestations of that disease. For example, a migraine headache can manifest as pain along the gallbladder channel (on the right temple and side of the head). Yet, that headache could have been generated by a liver-channel problem. Here, the initial, deepest or 'root,' problem is at the level of the liver channel (in this case a vacuity). It results in an imbalance of the gallbladder channel (a relative repletion described via the *yin-yang*, wood relationship with the liver). This distinction is very important, because it is the difference between the *zhi ben fa* and the *zhi biao fa* (in Japanese, the *honchiho* and the *hyochiho*). These terms are translated as 'root' and 'tips' following their origin in an analogy to plants, which grow from their roots and sprout at their extremities like the leaf buds on trees. Just as the roots are the source and the tips the outward expression, symptoms reflect the condition from which they arise. Thus, in root treatment strategies the symptoms are not the treatment target but the clues to its nature. In the headache example just given, the root problem is the liver-channel vacuity. This would be treated by supplementing the liver channel. The tip is the symptom-control problem, the gallbladder channel repletion. This would be treated by draining the gallbladder channel.

These distinctions are essential to understanding acupuncture practice. Historically, there is as much literature that describes how to treat root problems as there is describing the treatment of symptoms. Although some schools and practitioners argue that only the root approach is 'true acupuncture' (and some claim further that the only 'true' root approach is theirs), symptom control treatment is not only a historically valid approach to practice; it is also the simultaneous development of both approaches that can be found from the earliest books to the present day. As you might expect, this is a subject that is itself a root — the root of heated arguments. The US Office of Alternative Medicine recently become entrapped in this ancient argument when a panel of zealous reviewers rejected a study that did not propose what they considered 'true acupuncture.' The study sought instead to test a standard (and pilot tested) symptom-control treatment. This view is no doubt sensitive to modern expectations, and is hardly new, but it fails to recognize either the historical or modern realities of acupuncture.

The distinction between root and tip is clinically important, but that importance is not due to superiority. This is important, because it is a reality of both Asian and Western practice that most practitioners use a combination of approaches to meet their patients' needs and expectations. In clinical practice the distinction is simple: patients tell you what and where their symptoms are. Thus symptomatic manifestations are obvious. However, it takes diagnostic skill to determine where the deepest source of those symptoms lie. It is in this pursuit, the intellectual skills of pattern identification, by which treatment techniques and points are chosen.

The theories we have discussed certainly play the most significant role in isolating root problems. However, these theories are usually of secondary importance when deciding how to control symptoms. Then, observational skills and treatment experience are often the key. For example, many practitioners will agree which local points are applicable to a particular patient's low-back pain. But their selection of points for treating the underlying issue will be more variable.

This is one of the major practical distinctions between different styles of acupuncture practice. Thus, to characterize any system we can ask: What is the set of theories used to diagnose, label, and treat root problems? Virtually everyone can agree on the nature of symptoms. A headache is one of several headaches, low-back pain is one of several types, and there are acupuncture points that empirical evidence shows to be helpful for many symptoms. But when it comes to how the underlying problems are identified, labeled, and treated, variations arise because this is where a school of practice or an individual practitioner's perspective plays the most significant role.

If a problem is perceived as being primarily at the level of the *zang fu*, it will likely be analyzed via the *ba gang* system (*yin-yang*). If it is primarily perceived as an imbalance of the *jing-luo*, the *keiraku chiryo* system (five phases and *yin-yang*) may be employed. If it is perceived as a problem of the 12 officials, it will likely be considered in the five-phase approach of traditional acupuncture. It is thus in root treatment where cultural and social pressures, and personal beliefs and needs most strongly influence which traditional theories and approaches are used, and even whether traditional concepts or scientific approaches are accepted or rejected.

This distinction also helps to distinguish treatment styles. For example, those who completely reject traditional ideas and methods generally use only symptom-control treatments. They choose treatment points and techniques that are specific to the symptoms. As this empirical approach to practice has a long tradition, and there are innumerable pages describing how to cure this or that problem, these treatments help many people. Other practitioners will select treatment points according to their perception of the underlying problem. This includes those who recognize only scientifically stated diseases, those that depend on a measurement apparatus, and those who use traditional assessments to identify patterns. Most practitioners will add points and techniques specific to symptoms, regardless of the system they use. As Yoshio Manaka puts it, these two approaches are like two wheels on an axle; the cart cannot proceed with only one wheel.[27] This combined approach is what is traditionally recommended, and is the most common approach in clinical practice.

TRADITIONAL METHODS OF CLINICAL EXAMINATION

Traditionally there have been four categories of clinical examination. These are known as The Four Examinations.[28] In each examination type, purely sensory skills are used to gather information:

- visual inspection
- listening and smelling
- inquiry
- palpation.

Although all four methods have been historically recommended, different systems of practice emphasize different information. Here again the theoretical approach chosen by the practitioner determines the development of their clinical skills. Those systems of practice that rely on traditional models of the body often base pattern identification on an inspection of the body's surface. Since the body is viewed as working as an integrated and interconnected whole, a detailed, expert assessment of a single area can be used to assess the person's overall condition. For example, palpation of the radial arteries, inspection of the tongue, and palpation of the abdominal region have each developed into sophisticated whole-body systems.

On the other hand, systems that wholly or partially reject traditional theories tend not to use these approaches very much, if at all. These practitioners look to other assessment methods, such as analysis of a patient's medical history or an instrumented measurement. Each practitioner or school adapts their method of practice to a theoretical framework. Some who are dedicated to a traditional model feel it is the 'one true way;' they thus work exclusively with one traditional model and its allied methods. People trained in biomedicine tend to work with a more empirical approach, but this is by no means a hard-and-fast rule. Those with a background in massage tend to be body oriented, and osteopaths tend to focus on osteopathic methods.

The traditional model adopted affects the methods of pattern identification employed, as certain methods have long been emphasized in particular models. These emphases frequently persist in modern practice. For example, traditional practitioners whose focus is the use of natural drugs tend to use acupuncture only for superficial conditions or pain. They believe that deep treatment is the strength of medicinals. Before looking at these variations, it is useful to study the major clinical observations.

In each observation method the information sought is that correlating with qi paradigm ideas — organ problems, channel problems, or general *yin-yang* and five phase imbalances. In the tables of *yin-yang* and five-phase correspondences there is a rich assortment of corresponding signs, manifestations, and somatic and mental–emotional states. These are often easy to interpret directly. For instance, to determine if heat is present, a practitioner will look for signs of hyperactivity: flushed appearance, reddened tongue, heated emotions, and a faster than normal pulse. To determine if cold is present, the practitioner will look for signs of hypoactivity: pale complexion, pale tongue, a flattened affect, and a slower than normal pulse. If the wood phase and its corresponding liver channel is vacuous, one will find problems of tight musculature (the liver controls the sinews), problems of the nails, blue-green complexion, greasy odor, a shouting quality to the voice, irritability, aversion to wind, and eye problems. Specific patterns of weakness in the radial pulses or pressure reactions on specific areas of the abdomen will further indicate a liver problem.

Visual inspection[29]

Observing the color of the patient's skin, especially on the face and forearm, is usually helpful in the five-phase perspective. There are five major skin hues or colors, each with organ–channel correspondences: green–blue (wood–liver), red (fire–heart), yellow (earth–spleen), white (metal–lung), and black (water–kidney). The overall complexion, including the presence of skin texture changes, pigmentation variances, and various degrees of moistness, are examined as a clue to the patient's general condition. Observing the tone of the musculature and body size and shape also yields useful general information. Observation of the patient's demeanor provides an image of their condition, and helps assess the state of their spirit.

Tongue inspection is probably the most systematized method of visual inspection.[30] It yields information that is very helpful in determining a patient's condition in terms of *yin-yang*. The size of the tongue body, its tonus, and its color are important, as is the tongue coating texture, thickness, and color. The commonly agreed organ correspondences of the tongue are shown in Figure 6.3. When a visible sign is found in a particular region it indicates a problem of the corresponding organ. These correspondences relate directly to principles of the qi paradigm. The general size and color of the tongue body indicates the general strength of the patient (*xu*, vacuity; or *shi*, repletion). If the patient is hot, the tongue will be red colored; if cold, pale colored. The tongue coating yields further but similar information. If the coating is greasy, it indicates dampness; if it is yellow, it indicates heat. (See Box 6.5.)

Listening and smelling[31]

The presence of a distinct body odor can be very useful when formulating a diagnosis, especially in the five-phase system. The five odors are: burnt or scorched (heart), sweet (spleen), raw flesh (lungs), rancid (kidney), and greasy (liver). In the *ba gang* framework, the odor of breath or excreta is significant, but these five-phase odor correspondences are not typically used. Some practitioners use the presence of odor as an indication of the problem's severity. In the US and UK Traditional acupuncture schools, olfactory discrim-ination is trained to a high degree and provides more refined information.

Auditory inspection generally means listening to the overall strength of the voice and discriminating its tone in the five-phase framework. A strong voice indicates repletion, a feeble voice indicates vacuity. The five tones are: shouting (liver), laughing (heart), singing (spleen), weeping (lungs), and groaning (kidney).

Box 6.5 Tongue inspection

The following descriptions are from the *Zhong Yi Xue Ji Chu.*

Tongue body signs
Enlarged tongue: is one that is large, with dental impressions on the side; it indicates *qi* vacuity or dampness.
Shrunken tongue: is one that is thin and small; it indicates *yin* vacuity or dual *qi* and *yin* vacuity.
Fissured tongue: shows cracks or fissures, generally down the middle of the tongue; it indicates dryness or fluid vacuity.
Red speckles and prickles on the tip or sides of the tongue: indicates external heat problems.
Smooth tongue: is free of moisture and coating; this is a 'mirror tongue,' indicating severe *yin*-fluid depletion.
Stiff tongue: is rigid and inhibits speech, indicating more serious problems with the central nervous system.
Limp tongue: is soft and floppy; it generally indicates heat or *yin*-fluid depletion.
Trembling tongue: is generally associated with internal heat or rising *yang.*
Pale tongue: indicates vacuity of *qi* and blood.
Abnormally red or crimson tongue: indicates heat.
Purple tongue: indicates blood stasis.

Tongue coating signs
Excessively moist coat: indicates dampness.
Thick coat: blots out the tongue and indicates a more powerful problem. A thin coating through which the tongue can still be seen indicates a weaker problem.
Slimy coat: indicates phlegm, damp, or digestate accumulations.
'Peeled tongue': the tongue is irregularly covered by areas without a coat; it generally indicates *yin*-fluid insufficiency or stomach *qi* vacuity.
White coat: is generally associated with cold.
Black coat: most commonly indicates a strong external problem.
Yellow coat: is generally associated with heat.

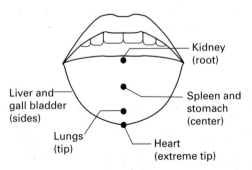

Figure 6.3 Areas of the tongue and corresponding organs.

Inquiry[32]

Taking a detailed medical history is important in every style of practice. Reviewing the condition of major anatomo-physiological systems in the body (e.g. respiratory, cardiovascular, urogenital) is important to both biomedical physicians and practitioners of TCM but different schools of thought also have unique lines of inquiry. In the *ba gang bian zheng*, or eight-principle *yin-yang* school, the questions asked help discriminate between hot and cold, internal–external, and yin-yang. For example, it is important to ask patients whether they feel hot or cold, or whether hot or cold environments, drinks, or flavors make them feel generally better or tend to improve a particular symptom. Asking about sweating patterns, thirst and volume and color of urine is also useful (Table 6.5).

The discriminations suggested by these questions can be very useful in eight-principle pattern identification. Frequently, from a five-phase assessment, this information is irrelevant.

Rather, questions related to correspondence sets are more important, for example: Which taste do you prefer? Do you have any particular dreams? Which season do you prefer? (Table 6.6). On the other hand, this information is often irrelevant for the recognition of an eight-principle pattern. Each approach seeks the information most relevant to the patterns its treatments require. Since acupoints are described in a language matched to that of pattern identification, each system of practice emphasizes a somewhat different, but related, set of symptoms and signs. Reviewing the tables of *yin-yang* and five-phase correspondences will give you an idea of the many probable lines of questioning.

Palpation[33]

The primary techniques of palpation are: radial pulse palpation; body pulse palpation; abdominal palpation; palpation of the back; and palpation of the channels and limbs. Different styles of practice vary tremendously with regard to the relative importance of palpation. In some schools of thought, radial pulse palpation yields information that is so critical to pattern identification that almost nothing else counts. In other systems, palpation is almost completely ignored. Likewise, palpation of the abdominal and thoracic regions is the basis of pattern identification for certain schools, but in others these regions are barely touched. As we noted earlier, some of these differences are rooted in culture and history, but palpation, especially of the radial pulses and abdomen, is so commonly used that it is more the rule than the exception.

Table 6.5 Signs found on inquiry and possible interpretations: eight-principle system

Sign	Possible interpretation
Feel hot	*Yang* repletion or *yin* vacuity
Feel cold	*Yin* repletion or *yang* vacuity
Spontaneous sweating	*Qi* or *yang* vacuity
Night sweating	*Yin* vacuity
Absence of thirst	Cold pattern
Excessive thirst	Heat pattern
Scant dark urine	Heat condition
Profuse colorless urine	Cold condition
Night urination	*Yang* vacuity

Table 6.6 Examples of information sought in the five-phase system

Correspondence set	Wood	Fire	Earth	Metal	Water
Season	Spring	Summer	Long summer	Fall	Winter
Tastes	Sour	Bitter	Sweet	Spicy	Salty
Dreams	Battles	Flames	No food	White things	Boats

Radial pulse palpation

Since the late Han dynasty, radial pulse palpation has been a significant component of acupuncture practice, and many specialized texts have been written on the subject. There are two basic methods of palpating the radial arteries. The first compares the relative strength of the pulsation at three positions on each radial artery: the *cun*, *guan*, and *chi*, the distal, anterior face, and proximal sides of the radial styloid process, respectively. The second looks at the particular tactile quality or 'feel' of these pulsations.[34] These methods can be used separately or in combination. For examining specific positions on the artery, there are two systems of interpretation in common use. In the first, the 12 channels are reflected, one each at two depths in each of the six finger positions. In the second approach the primary organs are reflected, one or two in each of three positions on each wrist. Systems of practice that focus on assessing the channels tend to use the former (Fig. 6.4(a)), and systems that focus on assessing the condition of the organs tend to use the latter (Fig. 6.4(b)).

Pulse-takers look for a variation of strength in one position relative to the others. This indicates a problem with the channel or organ that corresponds to that position. In Worsley's Traditional Acupuncture system, for example, each pulse position is read as either relatively normal, relatively weak (vacuous), or relatively strong (replete) in comparison to the others. Thus, if the second left deep pulse is relatively weak, the liver channel is considered vacuous. If the first right surface position is too strong, the large intestine channel is thought to be replete. In this system the 12 pulse positions are described as a series of plus or minus measures.

In the Japanese *keiraku chiryo* system, general patterns of weakness at the consecutive positions of the deepest pulses are organized as four primary vacuity patterns. These patterns are thought to account for 98% of all cases.[35] These are based on a close reading of the classical acupuncture text, the *Nan Jing*, as interpreted pragmatically through clinical experience. These four primary patterns involve the following findings:

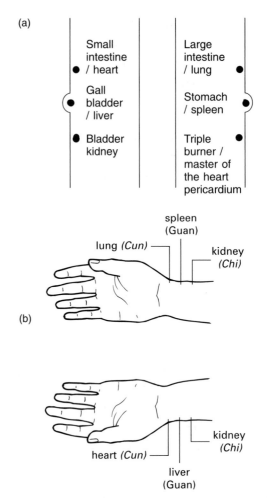

Figure 6.4 (a) Pulse–channel correspondences. (b) Pulse–organ correspondences.

- relative weakness in the first and second right deep pulses (lung vacuity)
- relative weakness in the second right and first left deep pulses (spleen vacuity)
- relative weakness in the second and third left deep pulses (liver vacuity)
- relative weakness in the first right and third left deep pulses (kidney vacuity).

These are represented diagrammatically in Figure 6.5.

When using an approach that examines the individual pulse qualities, practitioners attempt to relate the tactile pattern they feel to one of 24–28 qualities that have been historically

Lung vacuity

heart	○	● lung
liver	○	● spleen
kidney	○	○

Spleen vacuity

heart	●	○ lung
liver	○	● spleen
kidney	○	○

Liver vacuity

heart	○	○ lung
liver	●	○ spleen
kidney	●	○

Kidney vacuity

heart	○	● lung
liver	○	○ spleen
kidney	●	○

Figure 6.5 Pulse pattern correspondences.

described. There is a pattern for each position, and each pattern describes the sensation felt beneath the fingers. Each has a characteristic feel and interpretation (Box 6.6). The following are a few of the more common types:[36]

- Floating: felt with only light pressure, signifies an exterior pattern.
- Deep: felt only with strong pressure, signifies an interior pattern.
- String-like: feels like a plucked guitar string, signifies a liver pattern.
- Slippery: feels like pearls rolling in a basin, a dampness sign.
- Full: feels strong, bounding, a sign of repletion.
- Empty: wide and soft, a sign of vacuity.

Each quality can be felt singly, in all positions, or in one or more position. Thus there are myriad possible combinations. A particular quality may also be found in combination with other qualities. For example, where the whole pulse is slow, deep, and soft, indicating an interior cold vacuity, one position could exhibit the slipperyness that indicates damp. It would not be unusual for an advanced examiner to describe the right *cun* pulse as floating and hard, the right *guan* pulse as string-like, the right *chi* pulse as weak and

---

Box 6.6   Pulse qualities

The following descriptions are based on the modern Chinese textbook *Zhong Yi Xue Ji Chu*, translated by Nigel Wiseman and Andy Ellis as *The Fundamentals of Chinese Medicine*. These pulse quality descriptions are an integral part of the traditional Chinese medical acupuncture system, the *ba gang* system.

Floating pulse: is felt superficially and described as 'like a cork floating on water;' it usually indicates an external problem.

Scattered pulse: is a floating, large forceless pulse without foundation; it indicates dissipation of *qi* and blood.

Scallion-stalk pulse: is floating and empty in the middle, like a scallion-stalk; it indicates heavy blood loss.

Sunken pulse: is distinct only with heavier pressure at the deep level; it indicates problems at the interior of the body.

Hidden pulse: is deeper than the deep pulse and

only apparent with stronger pressure; it indicates problems of *yang qi* and coldness.

Weak pulse: is deep without force; it indicates vacuity of *qi* and blood.

Bound pulse: is deep and strong and feels as though 'tied to the bone;' it indicates cold pain.

Slow pulse: has three or less beats per respiration; it indicates cold or *yang* vacuity.

Moderate pulse: is slower than the normal pulse but not as slow as the slow pulse; it does not generally indicate morbidity.

Rapid pulse: has six beats per respiration; it generally indicates heat.

Racing pulse: has seven or more beats per respiration; it indicates heat with vacuity.

Slippery pulse: is felt like 'pearls rolling in a dish;' it indicates the presence of phlegm or damp and is also seen in pregnancy.

Stirred pulse: is a rapid, short and slippery pulse; it indicates external problems, and is also seen in pregnancy.

Box 6.6 Pulse qualities *(cont'd)*

Rough pulse: sometimes called a choppy or dry pulse, tends to be fine and not smooth, like 'a knife scraping bamboo;' it indicates blood stasis or dual vacuity of *qi* and blood.

String-like pulse: is long and taut, feeling like a guitar or violin string; it generally indicates problems of the liver and/or gallbladder, and can indicate pain.

Tight pulse: is a wiry forceful pulse; it indicates cold and pain.

Drumskin pulse: sometimes called a leather pulse, it is wiry but empty in the middle; it indicates blood loss.

Soggy pulse: is thin floating and forceless; it indicates vacuity of *qi* and blood with dampness.

Faint pulse: is very fine, weak and almost indistinct; it indicates *qi* and blood vacuity.

Scattered pulse: is large, weak, and forceless; it indicates a critical vacuity.

Surging pulse: is broad and large, and more forceful on rising than falling; it indicates heat and/or repletion.

Replete pulse: is broad, large, and forceful on rising and falling; it indicates the presence of a strong external evil.

Large pulse: is broad and large; indicates heat and/or repletion.

Vacuous pulse: it is a general term for forceless pulses.

Knotted pulse: is felt as a slow irregularly interrupted pulse; it indicates *qi*, blood, or phlegm-related problems.

Skipping pulse: is felt as a rapid irregularly interrupted pulse; indicates *qi*, blood, or phlegm-related problems.

Regularly interrupted pulse: is felt to have relatively regular pauses; it indicates *qi*, blood, or phlegm-related problems.

Long pulse: is a pulse felt beyond the third (*chi*) position of the arteries; it is not usually a sign of morbidity.

Short pulse: is a pulse felt only at the middle (*guan*) position of the arteries; it indicates dual problems of the *qi* and blood.

---

slightly sinking, the left *cun* pulse as slightly tight and slippery, the left *guan* pulse as string-like, and the left *chi* pulse as weak and empty. Generally, the focus of a pulse examination is the dominant quality, but this is a system that can become quite complex in clinical application.

Other body pulses

Before radial artery pulse-taking was systematized, Asian doctors used numerous other arteries. For instance, they used the carotid artery and various arteries on the head, face, arms, feet, and legs. Today, some still palpate these locations. In Japan there is a specialist *Keiraku chiryo* school, the *Jingei Myakukai*, that focuses on comparisons of the radial and carotid pulses. However, worldwide, the dominant system of pulse diagnosis is palpation of the radial arteries.

Pulse-taking often seems mysterious or mystical. Western sinology has never prioritized Chinese clinical literature, and it has thus been Chinese-speaking clinicians who have translated or composed most training texts. Without rigorous translation or published glossaries, so many subjectively chosen English words have been used to describe pulse qualities and patterns that comparing the various English language

descriptions makes them appear chaotic. To those familiar with the quantified measures of Western science, pulse diagnosis is difficult to accept because it is hard to see how it could be a reliable diagnostic technique. However, a more practical comparison can help relieve this dissonance. If you think of pulse-taking as a skill, not as an intellectual exercise, and compare it to similar Western skills, it is easier to understand (Fig. 6.6).

Consider, for example, the tactile sensitivity of musicians or tactile artists like potters or sculptors. Through training and repeated

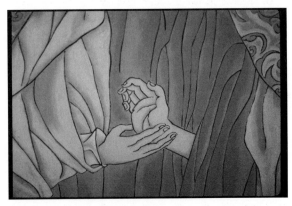

Figure 6.6 Detail of pulse palpation in painting. (Courtesy of Paradigm Publications.)

practice guided by a teacher, musicians learn to control the many, many positions and degrees of finger pressure that make their musical performances expressive but consistent. To accomplish this they must become intuitively aware of the tension, vibration, and relative position of their fingers. This trained sensitivity is what a pulse-taker must also accomplish. In fact, compared to the extensive tonal variety possible on the finger board of a violin, pulse-taking is the more believable skill. If you saw only a catalog of violinists' fingering techniques, or read several violinists' prose descriptions of how it feels to finger a particular note, you would likely conclude that it was impossible to play the violin consistently. Yet, one violinist can follow the performance of another.

This is very much the case with the pulse literature. Because traditional medical literature was so often produced as a supplement to apprentice training, the literary descriptions are difficult to appreciate without hands-on instruction. Consistency and reliability are created by practice, not by literary description. This is so much the case that professional translators who can read a pulse text without so much as a glance at a dictionary may nonetheless spend hours examining and interviewing expert clinicans before undertaking that translation. The meaning of the words is not so much the expression of any one practitioner, or the preference of any one writer, but the common body of technique and training. Even purely intellectual skills such as those of the Western sciences could not be reliably translated if not made rigorous by set terms and accompanied by formulas and procedures to guarantee practical consistency.

In the case of pulse palpation, training was a matter of repeated comparison to a living standard, typically, the master with whom a group of apprentices trained. Acupuncturists achieved reliability just as musicians achieve consistency — through systems of formal practice and comparison. Like needle technique and practitioner-sensed *de qi*, pulse-taking is difficult to teach in the classroom settings that have become the norm in modern Asia. In part because of the diminishment of these approaches in the development of TCM, formal practice systems now play a lesser role than in the past, and play almost no role in modern Western acupuncture education. However, these methods nonetheless persist. For example, in the Toyohari school the intellectual content of pulse-taking is relatively small, there being 'only' the four basic patterns we discussed above. However, the reliability component is very large. Through life-long practice, students compare their pulse readings with those of their fellows and teachers. Their teachers compare their pulse readings not only with those of their students, but also with those of other teachers and their masters. The masters practice with both students and teachers in an interlocking pattern of informal reliability checks.

Abdominal palpation[37]

Abdominal palpation was also somewhat systematized as early as the late Han dynasty. In this information-gathering skill each channel or organ is assessed by palpating a reflex point or area on the abdomen and chest (Fig. 6.7a). These include acupoints traditionally known as the *mu* or *bo* points in Chinese and Japanese, respectively. Each of the five phases and their related primary *zang* also have a reflex on the abdomen. All are centered around the navel (Fig. 6.7b). Each of the extraordinary vessel pairs also has associated reflex areas (Fig. 6.7c).

The practice of palpation has varied according to social factors. Where Confucian tradition is strong, methods of body palpation are not much used because it is considered inappropriate to expose the body, especially for women. One Chinese story describes the prohibition against touching the Emperor's concubines as forcing one creative physician to develop an elaborate system of threads by which he examined their pulses. While attending eunuchs held the threads, the physician is said to have palpated the womens' pulses at a distance. Whether or not this particular story is true or a myth, many historical references describe these methods, a clear sign of their importance. In Japan, where a casually constructed bamboo curtain can still be sufficient to separate the men's side from the women's side of a hot spring, one simply does not 'see' someone in any state of undress, and thus palpation is very common.

There are different systems of interpretation. Again, as with pulse relationships, the aim is to select appropriate acupoints, not to label a universal condition. Figure 6.7 shows two examples of the possible variations. Today, abdominal and chest palpation are frequently used in approaches based on the channels or five phases. The logic of these systems is direct. A

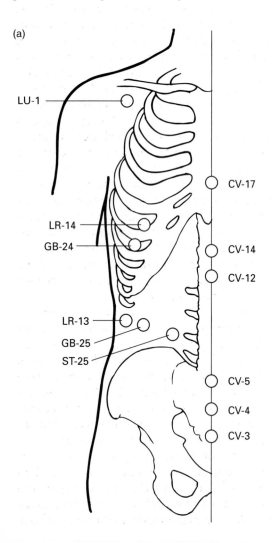

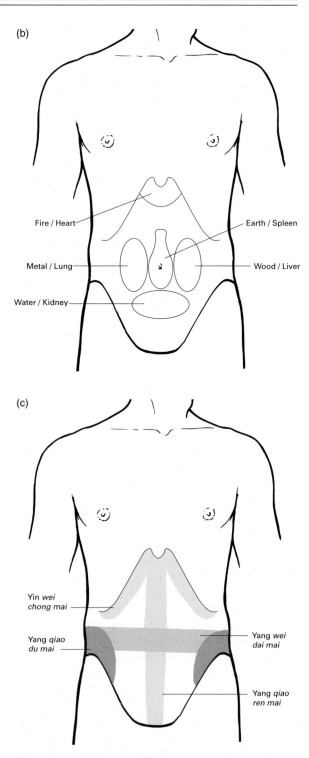

Figure 6.7 Abdominal region correspondences: (a) *mu* points; (b) five phases/organs; (c) extraordinary vessels. (Courtesy of Paradigm Publications.)

reaction in a particular area or at a particular acupoint indicates a problem with the corresponding entity or function. The reactions most often sought are tenseness, hardness, softness, weakness, warmth or coolness, soreness, pressure pain, tickling, or any aversion reaction. But anything that can be observed with the naked senses will also be considered: spider nevi (patterns of visible veins), skin blemishes, moles, sweating patterns, patterns of tension, and the sounds produced by tapping the abdomen. Each of these findings can provide useful information for an appropriately skilled acupuncturist. For example, if the area below the navel is very soft, weak, and somewhat cool to the touch, everything associated with the water phase in general, and kidney vacuity in particular, will be considered as a potential treatment target. In other words, these are the water and kidney reflex areas, and the signs discovered there indicate vacuity. Similarly, stiffness and pressure pain in the subcostal regions (beneath the ribs) indicates a problem of the *yin wei–chong mai* extraordinary vessel pair. Pressure pain with stiffness at *ju que* (CV-14) can indicate a problem of the heart organ or channel, because this is the traditional *mu xue* or 'alarm point,' for the heart.

In the West, hands-on medicine is generally less prestigious than the cerebral skills of a physician. This is also a Chinese bias, as is reflected by the higher pay and prestige afforded the more literary skills of herbalists. However, this is less the case in Japan, where diagnosis without questioning is considered a sign of experience and mastery. Again, like pulse-taking, abdominal palpation is a skill where reliability and consistency are achieved by traditional methods. Because the sensations sought are often confirmed by patients' reports, and the essential observations are organized as complementary pairs of common human sensory experiences (painful and comfortable, loose and tight, hot and cold, shallow and deep) patients are better able to participate in the assessment process. This, combined with the human interaction it provides, makes it popular with many Western patients.

General palpation

Palpation findings from other areas of the body such as the neck, back, and limbs as well as the channels and acupoints are commonly used in pattern identification.[38] Depending on the system, palpation of these areas is of greater or lesser significance in determining treatment. These can be primary indications or simply a means of confirming a pattern indicated by other signs.

ASSESSMENT SYNTHESIS

When traditional methods and concepts are used, the process of choosing an appropriate pattern requires synthesizing information as well as applying differential logic. Relevant information gathered through each examination is searched for obvious patterns, and for a predominance of signs related to a particular pattern. Again, this is an exercise, the success of which bringing not a 'right answer' but an appropriate treatment. It is a theory expressed in terms of acupoints and techniques, and a prediction of positive changes in a patient's condition that will be refined by the results of the treatment applied. Because patterns are not an attempt to label reality but a means of organizing treatment, a patient assessed by acupuncturists from different schools of practice may be given different diagnostic labels. However, each of those labels will provide an image of the patient in the language which that school uses to formulate treatment plans.

Treatment plans may involve a variety of point selections and stimulation methods, but each is a theory that attempts to predict what action will relieve the pattern to be addressed. Among adept acupuncturists, treatment variability, like the variability of pattern identification itself, will be within relatively narrow limits. Because the differences between different schools are typically specializations or refinements of qi paradigm concepts, the assessment of two experienced practitioners from two different schools will differ according to the information emphasized by their respective schools. Among practitioners of the same school, a high degree of consistency is by no means rare.[39] In Toyohari study groups, for example, teachers and their several students routinely arrive at identical radial pulse assessments.

Because the general concepts are so broad, it is also not uncommon to find practitioners using patterns from more than one system. However, this appears to be more frequently the case in the West than in Asia, where specialization is more common and apprenticeships are more generally available. Blending is most common in the USA. As Dan Kenner says 'Caucasian practitioners are incorrigibly eclectic.'[40] Practitioners in the USA also combine acupuncture with other medical systems, such as herbal medicine (East Asian and Western), homeopathy, osteopathy, massage, dietary therapy, lifestyle counseling, and psychotherapy. Such extensive eclecticism is rare in Asia. But in today's alternative medical marketplaces, it is possible to find practitioners of very varied approaches, some of whom follow no tradition but continuously synthesize. This eclecticism is impossible to describe, because it varies with every practitioner who attempts it.

Because it is very difficult to categorize the results of this blending, it is very difficult to know whether these cross-cultural syntheses are successful. One of the most heated debates on the internet discussion groups for holistic medical topics is any argument between various eclectics and traditionalists. Some acupuncturists believe these adaptations dilute acupuncture, while others believe they extend it. It is fair to say only that there is no generally acceptable evidence for either side of the debate. Dan Bensky, a respected acupuncture writer and educator, states it best: 'In any given patient at any particular time, there is a wide variety of appropriate treatments.'[41] How wide that variety may be and whether or not it includes cross-cultural hybrids remains for time and consistent research to tell.

Although it is not at present possible to express these limits, we can look at the process of pattern identification within established systems. From this you can gain a sense of the scope of traditional acupuncture practice. To that end in the following pages we have summarized the information-gathering techniques of several systems and describe how a single case is assessed and treated in three of the more common approaches.

The TCM acupuncture *ba gang* system applies eight-principle discrimination and organ pattern identification through the traditional four examinations, the archetypes of naked-sense data gathering. As we saw in Chapter 2, the modern system matured during China's mid-20th century health-care crisis when philosophies rooted in China's feudal and imperial past were highly suspect. Thus it de-emphasizes specialized correspondence systems and concentrates on information gathered through questioning. Using a set of detailed questions that are thought better to objectify observations relevant to *ba gang* patterns, patients are questioned in loosely structured interviews.[42] There are general medical history questions, general biological systems questions and specific *ba gang* questions. This information is complemented by a pulse-quality assessment, tongue inspection, and other visual examinations. Data are organized into patterns according to the *ba gang* and *zang fu* theories. There are over 100 patterns, and countless combinations.

Because this kind of complexity still requires considerable clinical practice to master, a 'syndrome concept' has also been developed in China. This adaptation permits the streamlining of clinical training and promotes acupuncture's integration with biomedicine. This is an extension of the *ba gang* system, of which Chinese doctors are very proud. As Shi Dian-bang of the China Academy of Traditional Chinese Medicine in Beijing states: 'The study of syndromes in close relation to clinical practice has obtained great progress.'[43] This concept is a further systematization of the basic *ba gang* approach. In this approach each major biomedical disease or symptom is organized into syndromes, each of which is related to the commonly seen *ba gang* patterns that might have given rise to the corresponding symptom or disease. Some examples of symptom and disease syndromes from the Shanghai College of TCM text *Zhen Jiu Zhi Liao Xue* are given in Table 6.7.[44]

Table 6.7 Some disease syndromes given in *Zhen Jiu Zhi Liao Xue*

Symptom	No.	Syndrome patterns
Headache	6	Wind *qi*; heat inversion; damp phlegm; liver *yang*; *qi* vacuity; gallbladder fire damp heat
Low-back pain	4	Wind damp; kidney *yin* vacuity; kidney *yang* vacuity; blood stasis
Painful menstruation	4	*Qi* stagnation; blood stasis; blood vacuity; cold blood
Stroke	5	Exuberant fire; *qi* vacuity; damp phlegm; wind *yang*; *yang* vacuity
Cough	5	Wind cold; wind heat; damp turbidity; summerheat wind; wind dryness

This approach not only simplifies and focuses the *ba gang* system, it also allows traditional diagnoses to be used in parallel with biomedical diagnoses. It is a practical clinical adaptation of the research model where standard therapies provide the control. As we have noted, there are both research and clinical problems in comparing or combining Chinese traditional patterns with biomedical diagnoses, yet, as Shi Dian-bang states, this innovation appears to have aided the teaching, utilization, and spread of traditional Chinese medicine in China and elsewhere in Asia.

Other acupuncture practitioners use the same data-gathering methods but sort and analyze the resulting information only within the scope of traditional patterns. This does not mean that biomedical information is ignored. For example, American practitioner Bill Prensky, who studied primarily with Ju Gim Shek and James Tin Yau So before the *ba gang* system arrived in the West, places somewhat greater emphasis on palpation, including abdominal palpation and channel palpation. He also uses 'any and all methods available including laboratory tests such as standard blood and stool analysis'[45] to obtain a thorough biomedical assessment.

Older Chinese practitioners, such as James Tin Yau So, who trained before acupuncture was standardized and institutionalized as part of TCM, tend to be very pragmatic. In the era in which he worked, acupuncturists more regularly handled what would now be called 'critical care,' for example, endemic diseases such as tuberculosis and life-threatening illnesses such as cancer.[46] His pattern discrimination does not depend on blood tests or biomedical techniques, but concentrates instead on directly observable signs and symptoms. The indicators on which he concentrates (bleeding, pain, and vomiting) are not logically manipulated, but are considered directly in terms of hot and cold, location, *yin* and *yang*. Tin Yau So's assessment of a patient also includes traditional methods, but he uses the information gathered to relate each patient, not to general patterns, but to other patients that he, his teachers, or students have treated successfully. In a very real sense the patient is the pattern. Thus he focuses on highly specific point locations and techniques, particularly the exact quality, direction, and strength of the needle stimulus.

It is of course impossible to categorically state what acupuncture was before the modern era. Surely it was no one thing. However, Tin Yau So's 'grand-teacher,' Cheng Tan An, was one of China's most famous clinicians. His treatments live on formally in TCM as well as in the clinical repertoire of his students. As their approach depends for its function, transmission, and training on hands-on skills rooted in sensory observations, it seems possible that this approach gives us an idea of how much of acupuncture was performed historically.

The Japanese *keiraku chiryo* system also uses the traditional four examinations, but it primarily relies on radial pulse palpation. For these acupuncturists a very important pulse discrimination is the strength at each of the six positions. The assessment of pulse quality is for many a secondary factor. It relies further on abdominal palpation, channel palpation, and questioning. As with the *ba gang* system, the questions tend to elicit either a general medical history or information of the greatest significance to *keiraku chiryo* practitioners. In the broader system of *keiraku chiryo*, for example, that described by Denmei Shudo, palpation tends to be light, but pressure is the key. Light pressure is used to find diagnostic points, and heavier pressure is used to identify symptomatic treatment points known as 'indurations.' In the *Toyohari* system of *keiraku chiryo*, palpation is based on tactile qualities rather than on response to pressure. Touch is used to explore both the tonus of the underlying muscles and the texture of the skin.

The basic *keiraku chiryo* approach recognizes four primary patterns (*sho*) and a number of secondary patterns that can accompany these basic four. The following is a list of typical subsidiary patterns associated with one of the four basic patterns, lung vacuity:[47]

- stomach repletion
- large-intestine repletion
- liver repletion
- gallbladder vacuity
- heart repletion
- small-intestine vacuity
- triple-warmer vacuity.

In this system, typical symptoms for each primary pattern are known, but as each primary pattern can be related to symptoms from as many as six channels, symptoms play a lesser role in treatment planning. In fact the system seeks to assess a patient's *qi* in the most direct manner possible. A quote from Dan Kenner's *keiraku chiryo* teacher, Tamotsu Mii, captures the flavor of this training:

You are not here to become an acupuncture scientist. You are not here to learn theory. If it is theory that you are interested in, go read a book. This training is for your intuition, and to develop your touch and observation skills. Your brain will never heal anyone.[48]

The Traditional Acupuncture approach from England places great emphasis on discriminating the strength of the six pulse positions, the odors, the tones of voice, the facial colors, and the emotional state of the patient, the full gamut of the four examinations. As its founder, Jack Worsley, states:

The Doctor of Acupuncture must strive to see his patient not as he is at the time of examination but as he would be if he were whole and perfect in body, mind, and spirit with every possibility of his 'unique being' realized.[49]

Physician acupuncturist Peter Eckman describes the Traditional Acupuncture system as a blend of Chinese, Korean, and especially Japanese acupuncture combined with British Naturopathic philosophy, carefully structured to attend to the issues to which Western patients attend, especially psychological and emotional concerns.[50] It uses the traditional analogy to 'officials,' positions in China's traditional Confucian bureaucracy, to characterize the 12 channels and 12 organs. This produces a typology of character types. From its Japanese influences, it incorporates an emphasis on examining the relative strength of the 12 pulse positions, abdominal palpation, and Akabane's channel-balancing method. The latter involves applying indirect heat at the terminal acupoints of each channel (24 points, all of which are located on the fingers and toes), while measuring the speed of the patient's response. Treatment is targeted to those channels the right and left branches of which show the greatest disparity in response time. This system, like *keiraku chiryo*, depends on strongly developed sense perceptions and intuition.

As an aside, there is an *Akabanekai*, or Akabane-method association in Japan, the members of which concentrate exclusively on the application and development of this method. This clearly illustrates how the same technique can be used to greater and lesser extents in different circumstances and systems (Fig. 6.8).

Yin-yang channel balancing therapy emphasizes abdominal and chest palpation, and, to a lesser degree, visual inspection and questioning. Here, the Japanese emphasis on palpation is key. This method aims to assess physical structure (i.e. to focus on body structure through palpation), interpreting these findings as manifestations of *qi*, blood, and channel disturbances. It is from this view that the problems which have contributed to the patient's condition, such as psycho-emotional or external factors, are assessed. Birch uses his teacher Yoshio Manaka's development of this system in his daily practice.

In this approach, patterns primarily derive from the relative balance of the 12 channels as expressed through an examination of the extraordinary vessels. Secondary consideration is given to patterns associated with, for example, polar channel pairs, and the three *yin*–three *yang* channel sets. The extraordinary vessel pairs and the polar channel pairs are as follows:

Extraordinary vessels

- *yin qiao–ren mai*
- *yin wei–chong mai*
- *yang qiao–du mai*
- *yang wei–dai mai*
- the 'cross-syndrome' (a combination of *yin wei–chong mai* and *yang wei–dai mai*).

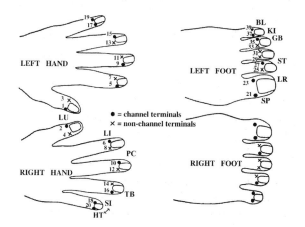

Figure 6.8 Akabane measurement pattern used in the Manaka Itaya Meridian Imbalance Diagram Methodology.

Polar channels

- liver–small intestine
- heart–gallbladder
- kidney–large intestine
- bladder–lung
- spleen–*san jiao*
- stomach–pericardium.

Miki Shima, a San Francisco acupuncturist, uses a variation of *yin-yang* balancing developed by his teacher, Tadashi Irie of Osaka.[51] In this model, one discriminates between patterns associated with the extraordinary vessels, the three *yin*–three *yang* sets of primary channels:

- *yang ming*: stomach–large intestine
- *tai yin*: spleen–lung
- *tai yang*: bladder–small intestine
- *shao yin*: heart–kidney
- *shao yang*: triple burner–gallbladder
- *jue yin*: liver–pericardium.

Patterns of the 'channel divergences,' a secondary channel system, are also considered.

The system of Medical Acupuncture that originated in France with Maurice Mussat and was further developed in the USA by Joseph Helms and his colleagues described as:

A Cartesian filtration of Jesuit-appropriated Han and Ming texts organized for clinical expression by French physicians influenced by Southeast Asian Chinese practitioners and exposed to the rigors of contemporary scientific logic. A European hybrid.[52]

This definition is as precise as it is terse. 'Cartesian' and 'Jesuit-appropriated' remind you of the importance of methods and assumptions in selection and translation. Here, the terms identify the filters that have influenced translation and transmission. 'Han' and 'Ming' describe time periods we explored in Chapter 1, thus the theoretical and clinical emphasis. The reference to physicians and their Chinese and Vietnamese colleagues in France, as well as the reference to scientific logic, relates this system to the line of investigation and acculturation that began with Soulie de Morant in France.

This system emphasizes channel patterns, in particular the three *yin*–three *yang* pairs of primary channels, the extraordinary vessels, and channel divergences. Diagnostic data are gathered through a comprehensive medical history, palpation of the pulses and the abdomen, channels, and acupoints. Other traditional practices, including visual, auditory, and questioning methods, are also used. As the biomedically trained practitioners who use this approach bring their own specialized biomedical knowledge to their treatment rooms, they create individual blends of the Eastern and Western approaches.

It is interesting to contrast this integration of biomedicine and traditional acupuncture with the Chinese syndrome-based integration we described earlier. The indigenous Western development is strongly individual; each practitioner applies his or her biomedical knowledge as they use the traditional methods. In the Chinese integration, biomedical information is used to redefine the traditional approach. Where TCM concentrates on symptom assessments gathered through questioning and organized into organ patterns, American Medical Acupuncture concentrates on channel patterns assessed through touch and organized through qualitative relationships such as correspondence sets and concepts of *qi* circulation. In our opinion, this is an excellent example of acupuncture responding to cultural needs. In China, a socialized system of public health has emphasized the integration of acupuncture into biomedically dominated institutions where acupuncturists are subordinate to physicians. In the USA, a privately financed and delivered biomedical system is adapting to meet the population's desire for more individual treatment. Where the former emphasizes integration, the latter emphasizes individualization. Although this is not an all-encompassing trend, it is nonetheless a good example of the robust adaptability of traditional acupuncture.

Another approach to acupuncture that arrived in the USA from France is the 'terrain acupuncture' described by Yves Requena in his several books and papers.[53] 'Terrain' is a land, ground, or substrate from which all other characteristics derive. The name implies the characterology

that the system develops. Like Medical Acupuncture, it is an inheritor of not only the *qi* circulation model brought to France by George Soulie de Morant, but also of Soulie de Morant's emphasis on clinical confirmation. Like Medical Acupuncture, it absorbs biomedical skills and knowledge; however, in Requena's development the central relationship of patterns is to medical history, particularly childhood illnesses, and character traits as measured by a statistically standardized psychological survey. *Qi* circulation patterns are primary. The terrain patterns are named for the three *yin*, three *yang* channel pairs (e.g. *yang ming*, stomach–large intestine) and related psychological predispositions, potentials for particular illnesses, and successful treatments.

Another US development is the detoxification acupuncture system refined by the National Acupuncture Detoxification Association, spearheaded by Mike Smith, Pat Culliton, David Eisen, Ana Oliveira, and their colleagues. It focuses on first 'detoxing' the patient through the acute initial phases of withdrawal from abused substances such as cocaine, heroin, and alcohol, and then using acupuncture to help prevent relapse. Using a straightforward acupuncture based on symptoms in conjunction with counseling, the patient is moved from the acute withdrawal phase and into relapse prevention. Many methods are used, based largely on the experience of the acupuncturist, but auricular acupuncture applied in a supportive group setting is primary. Because the system deals with a narrow but incredibly complex problem, it is concerned with a single dominant pattern. Addicts are commonly found to have severe yin vacuity.[54] Although this is only one of many TCM patterns, the traditional notion of this pattern has been expanded to incorporate the patient's entire psychosocial environment. The breakdown of someone's supportive and nurturing environment is seen as a manifestation of *yin* vacuity — the vacuum of nurture and support which leads to, or contributes to, addiction. This model is another excellent example of the adaptation of acupuncture to the needs of a new environment.

Illustrative example

On examination, a patient that presented with her physician's diagnoses of cystitis, dysmenorrhea, and chronic low-back pain, was found to exhibit the following signs and symptoms:

Visual. Yellowish coloration around the eyes; a thin, tightly muscled frame; thin, red tongue body with a yellow coat at the rear of the tongue; the presence of pigmentation in the interscapular region with moles on the sides of the neck and abdomen; vascular spiders visible in the left costal region over the liver.

Olfactory and auditory. A slightly sickly-sweet body odor; a song-like, lilting tone of voice.

Questioning. This individual dislikes hot weather; her low-back pain is better when pressure is applied; her hands generally feel very warm. There is a feeling of tiredness and heat in the late afternoon; she is generally very pensive and easily irritated; urine flow is urgent, painful, inhibited, and very yellow in color. Her menstrual flow is heavy, with some pain and clotting; sometimes she sweats at night.

Palpation. The second right deep pulse is the weakest, the second and third left deep pulses are also quite weak; the pulse is overall deep, thin and fast; the abdomen exhibits stiffness in the right subcostal region and above the navel. There is pressure pain and stiffness in the areas immediately to either side of the navel and in the area about 2 inches to the left of the navel, extending below the level of the navel (Fig. 6.9).

1. In the Chinese *ba gang*, or eight-principle, system, this patient would be diagnosed as having kidney yin vacuity with damp heat in the lower burner. The thin body frame, red, thin tongue and the deep, thin, fast pulse, dislike of hot weather, hot hands, late afternoon fatigue and heat, and problems with night sweating all indicate *yin* vacuity. Cystitis and low back pain that improves with pressure establish that the vacuity is related to the kidney. The urgent, painful, inhibited, yellow urine and yellow coat at the back of the tongue indicate damp heat in the lower burner.

2. In the Japanese *keiraku chiryo* system, this patient would be related to the primary pattern of liver vacuity with a secondary vacuity of the spleen. The weakness of second and third left deep pulses and the right subcostal and left side of the navel abdominal reactions indicate the liver vacuity. Liver vacuity is also indicated by the urogenital and menstrual symptoms, the tight musculature, and irritability. The weak second right pulse and the abdominal reactions above and to both sides of the navel as well as the yellowishness around the eyes indicate spleen vacuity.

3. In the Traditional Acupuncture system, this patient would probably be diagnosed with a spleen causative factor. The weakness in the second right deep pulse, the body odor, tone of voice, facial color, and general pensiveness all indicate the spleen.

4. In the Japanese *yin-yang* channel-balancing system, this patient would probably be categorized as a cross-syndrome type, with primary

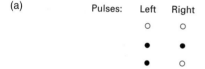

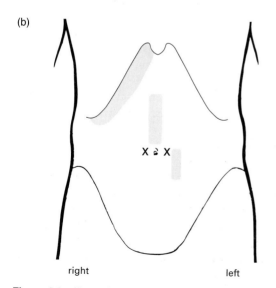

Figure 6.9 Illustrative example: (a) pulse pattern; (b) abdominal pattern.

problems of liver and blood stasis. The right subcostal and left side of navel reactions, presence of pigmentation, moles and vascular spiders, tight musculature, irritability, and dysmenorrhea indicate both the involvement of the liver and blood stasis.

Each of these practice approaches yields different patterns, and practitioners would use different treatment points and techniques to accomplish root treatment. The scientific ramifications of this variety were discussed in Chapter 4. However, the critical point is that practitioners from each school of thought obtain positive results for patients like this one. In the Western 'one right way' mind set, that statement is simply ludicrous. A skeptic would argue that the diagnoses have nothing to do with the therapeutic outcome, since they are entirely inconsistent. We would remind such a skeptic that traditional patterns are keys to the selection of a treatment, and not an attempt to describe an objective entity or reality. But, as true as this may be, it does not logically address the issue of treatment differences, particularly the idea that each treatment could produce a positive outcome.

In summary then, although some Western thinkers might accept our explanation that the assessment differences are not significant because they reference a treatment selection, the idea that the treatments in each system are different yet each produce favorable results is harder to accept. Indeed, this is possibly the paradox that most contributes to Western rejections of traditional pattern recognition. Put simply, without an acceptable rationale for these variances, the obvious Western conclusion will be that traditional patterns are inconsistent, and thus unreliable and unfit for medical use.

However, we think that there are three reasonable explanations for this variety. The first has to do with the nature of the theoretical systems that ground these various approaches. The second takes into account the probability that it is the symptom-control treatments used, or their components, that are common to each system. The third proposes that the results do indeed differ, but that the lack of standard, systematic reporting and assessment procedures hides those differences. These distinctions are, of course, far more interactive in practice than in didactic writing. In any circumstance, any combination of these logical elements could be involved.

If you look at the theoretical basis from which each of these four approaches derive, you find that each system takes advantage of *yin-yang* and five-phase principles. These, as we saw in Chapter 3, describe an integrated system. A change in any one aspect can initiate change throughout the whole. We propose that each diagnostic approach represents a map that is overlaid on the complex, dynamic system of the human somatopsychic being. Each assessment grid yields a somewhat different treatment strategy that takes advantage of the same underlying relationships.

Look, for example, at what each system prioritizes. The view of a TCM acupuncturist is one of linked bodily functions. Thus, the critical diagnostic data are physiological. *Yin* vacuity, in our example case, is determined by signs and symptoms that reflect functions: thin body frame, red, thin tongue, deep, thin, fast pulse, dislike of hot weather, hot hands, late afternoon fatigue and heat, and night sweating. Kidney vacuity is determined by signs of organ-system malfunction (cystitis and low-back pain that improves with pressure), as is damp heat in the lower warmer (urgent, painful, inhibited, yellow urine, yellow coat at the back of the tongue).

Traditional Chinese medical acupuncturists see the human through a map like those that describe trade and economic interchange. Indeed, as we saw in our review of history, such analogies are common in Chinese medical language. Functions generally governed by areas of influence associated with each of the viscera and bowels follow one another, depend on one another, and relate to one another in an extended image. Disease is the malfunction of these relationships expressed by the quality of the results — stagnation, counterflow, inhibition.

On the other hand, with some differences in emphasis, the Japanese and English systems prioritize a global view of the body's inter-relations. In *keiraku chiryo*, the patient is seen as a set of qualitative interrelations. The liver vacuity pattern identification depended on the weakness of the second and third left deep pulses. These assess the relative quality of the circulation of *qi* and blood. The right subcostal and left side of the navel abdominal reactions indicated liver vacuity, because they are a reflection of tensions and imbalances of the body's structure, as is the tight musculature and irritability. The urogenital and menstrual symptoms are also considered, but with less emphasis, even though these were the patient's primary emphasis. To the *keiraku chiryo* practitioner the determining relationship is not the one where the symptoms were expressed. Instead it is the pattern to which the bodily phenomena are most closely related. The secondary spleen vacuity was similarly indicated by the weak second right pulse and the abdominal reactions above and to both sides of the navel, as well as the yellowishness around the eyes. Again, the physical body is perceived as a reflection of its interrelationships.

The map of the human being through which these practitioners perceive their patients does include a functional ecology; however, it primarily posits humans to be a complex, balanced system of relationships. The being they explore with their hands and minds is compared to an ideal of that being, one that is symmetrically balanced. The leg that is shorter, the pulse that is stronger, weaker, or qualitatively out of synchronization, the twists and bends of sinew, are viewed as the most important expressions of the whole system's condition.

Looking at these differences it becomes clearer that they are not contradictory but alternative. Each emphasizes a set of treatment skills, those best developed by that school of practice. This is easily understood. Regardless of how people are looked at as whole systems, it is difficult to point to one factor and say 'that and that alone is the cause of this person's disease.' In the biomedical approach, this is an ideal. What is sought is the bacterium that causes the infection, the biochemical that is out of range,

the determining gene. But, in fact and in practice, biomedicine is not so simplistic. Indeed, among its most powerful accomplishments is its ability to describe biological complexity. For example, our urinary functions work properly only when a set of biological conditions are within certain limits and tolerances. Fluids must pass through the stomach and intestines properly, and digestion must produce an appropriate quantity and quality of fluids without encouraging the growth of pathological organisms. The kidneys' work must be sufficient if the blood pressure is to be within effective limits. If any one of these limits, or any combination, is out of range, problems can arise. If in this example digestion is improved, or fluid absorption modified, or pathogens eliminated, or circulation increased, a urinary problem can be ameliorated.

When taking into account emotional states, interaction with climate and environment, diet, behavior, activity, posture, and so forth, the picture becomes much more complex. Indeed, the idea of a singular cause is very difficult to accept when the human is viewed as a system. This brings to mind the deathbed confession so often attributed to Lavoisier: 'The germ is nothing, the terrain is everything.' In other words, the sickness is not the germ but the condition of the person in which a microbial population has taken hold. In traditional acupuncture models, many things can contribute to each person's disease, and this is where the general classification systems and correspondence sets of *yin-yang*, the five phases, channels, organs, and *qi* make their greatest contribution. They allow operation within a complex, multidimensional image.

If, as thinkers like Yoshio Manaka propose, stimulating acupoints signals change in this interrelated chain, there will be more than one treatment that is sufficient for clinical success. There can be several successful strategies for any condition. Acupuncture treatments do not succeed or fail based on a single selection of acupoints, but are modified according to patient responses during a course of treatment. Thus the critical factor for the application of traditional patterns is that the image they create is matched with a compatible concept of what acupoints do.

The treatments themselves take advantage of self-regulatory mechanisms inherent in the whole system. Each system of practice, if appropriately applied, can create change. Each approach requires different skills and techniques, yet, if the appropriate skills and techniques are applied, good results can be obtained. This multiplicity of approaches in acupuncture is something like the many routes to the top of the mountain. None are 'right,' all have the potential of reaching the top.

One way to illustrate this is to look at the acupoints that would be chosen for our sample case by practitioners of representative systems. In traditional Chinese medical acupuncture (TCM) the treatment regimen outlined in Table 6.8 would not be uncommon.[55] KI-3 is chosen to enrich kidney *yin*, abate vacuity heat, and invigorate original *yang*.[56] The symptoms for which it is indicated are irregular menses, urinary frequency, and lower back pain. It is the source (*yuan*) point of the kidney channel, and is thus a member of a point class the effects of which are particularly directed to the viscera. BL-52 supplements the kidney and boosts essence, disinhibits urine, and abducts damp. It is indicated here for the inhibited urination and signs of dampness. SP-9 warms and moves the central burner (spleen and stomach) and transforms damp. It is directed toward the inhibited urine. BL-28 regulates the bladder and disinhibits the lumbus. It is used here to disinhibit urinary function and lumbar stiffness. BL-40 clears the blood and discharges heat, soothes the sinews, and frees the connecting vessels. Indicated here for the lumbar pain, this point was traditionally used for night sweating. CV-4 banks the kidney and secures the root, supplements *qi* and returns yang. CV-4 is a powerful point known for safeguarding health. Although there are many, many indications associated with CV-4, the most pertinent here are the urinary and menstrual problems. In this treatment, CV-4 is the acupoint most directed to the traditional concept of *qi* circulation. It is the intersection of the spleen, liver, and kidney channels with the controller vessel. This traditional Chinese medical acupuncture treatment is perfectly consistent not only with its pattern but also the symptoms. The points chosen directly address either an organ function or a particular symptom. It is, so to speak, a repair for the organ functions that fail to perform as desired.

In *keiraku chiryo*, the therapy might be as outlined in Table 6.9.[57] LR-8 is the supplementation point of the liver, the uniting (*he*) point of the channel.[58] It is selected principally because it is one of the two primary points to supplement liver vacuity based on five-phase logic first described by the Korean Sa'am in the 16th century. It has also been traditionally indicated

Table 6.8 Traditional Chinese medicine treatment regimen for the illustrative case

Acupoint	Technique	Insertion depth	Stimulus
Bilateral KI-3	Supplement	0.3 *cun* (7.5 mm)	*De qi*
Bilateral BL-52	Supplement	0.7–1.0 *cun* (17.5–25 mm)	*De qi*
Bilateral SP-9	Drain	0.5–1.0 *cun* (12.5–25 mm)	*De qi*
Bilateral BL-28	Drain	0.5–1.0 *cun* (12.5–25 mm)	*De qi*
Bilateral BL-40	Drain	0.5–1.5 *cun* (12.5–37.5 mm)	*De qi*
Bilateral CV-4	Supplement	0.5–1.5 *cun* (12.5–37.5 mm)	*De qi*

Table 6.9 *Keiraku chiryo* therapy for the illustrative case

Acupoint	Technique	Insertion depth (mm)	Stimulus
Bilateral LR-8	Supplement	1–2	None
Bilateral KI-10	Supplement	1–2	None
Bilateral SP-3	Supplement	1–2	None
Bilateral CV-4	Supplement	2–4	None to very light
Bilateral BL-18	Supplement	1–2	None
Bilateral BL-23	Supplement	1–4	None to very light

for difficult urination. KI-10 is selected primarily because it is the second primary point recommended by Sa'am and has long been applied for liver vacuity. It also affects the lower burner (kidney, bladder), and has been traditionally indicated for difficult urination and urinary urgency. SP-3 is the stream (*shu*), earth point and source (*yuan*) point of the spleen channel, and thus strengthens the spleen. CV-4, as noted above, is a powerful point, chosen here for its effect on *qi* circulation. BL-18 is the associated-*shu* point of the liver, its use here is relative to the liver vacuity pattern. Associated-*shu* points are unique in that when the *qi* of an organ is insufficient, these points directly supplement that *qi*. BL-23 is the associated-*shu* point of the kidney. It is used to reinforce the effects of BL-18 and is also indicated for the urinary problems, nutritional weakness, and irregular menses. Again, the treatment is absolutely consistent with the pattern. However, the acupoints have been selected not so much for their ability to relieve symptoms, but for their traditional channel and

five-phase role in *qi* circulation. The primary goal of this treatment is to harmonize the imbalances found through the examination of the body and pulse.

In Manaka's channel balancing system treatment might be as shown in Table 6.10.[59] PC-6, SP-4, TB-5, and GB-41 are used here as they are the master and coupled points of the extraordinary vessels that address the cross-syndrome pattern. These points also have indications, but are used here because the extraordinary vessels can alter the structure of the body and the distribution of *qi*, and thus redress channel imbalances. In this case, they globally address the liver-related pattern. BL-18 is the associated-*shu* point of the liver, affecting both the liver organ and channel. BL-23 is the associated-*shu* point of the kidney, reinforcing the effect of BL-18 and affecting the urinary symptoms. BL-28 is the associated-*shu* point of the bladder, and is used for the urinary symptoms. Again, the treatment and the pattern are absolutely consistent. Like the *keiraku chiryo* treatment, acupoints are not chosen relative to

Table 6.10 Manaka's channel-balancing system treatment for the illustrative case

Acupoint	Technique	Insertion depth	Stimulus
Right PC-6	Ion pumping	2 mm	None
Right SP-4	Ion pumping	2 mm	None
Left TB-5	Ion pumping	2 mm	None
Left GB-41	Ion pumping	2 mm	None
Bilateral BL-18	Heated needle	1 cm	Light, warmth
Bilateral BL-23	Heated needle	1.5 cm	Light, warmth
Bilateral BL-28	Heated needle	1.5 cm	Light, warmth

their ability to alter symptoms or functions, but to redress the imbalances reflected by the body's structure and pulses. The channel-balancing treatment is very similar to the *keiraku chiryo* treatment in intent. Although only two of the five points are identical, the *shu* points are similarly used and the four master-coupled points are aimed at the same imbalances as the five-phase acupoints. The ion-pumping treatment addresses the same channel imbalances as does the five-phase treatment; however, it does so by influencing the body's structure through the extraordinary vessels.

Before we conclude this section, let us return once more to Tables 6.8 to 6.10 and emphasize the stimulus columns. The term 'stimulus' refers to the subjective sensation the patient should experience at each point. The *qi*-circulation centered treatments use very light stimulus, while traditional Chinese medical acupuncture uses a much stronger stimulus. For example, according to modern Chinese sources, the stimulus for BL-28 is 'distension and numbness, sometimes spreading to the buttocks.'[60] In the circulation-centered treatments, the strongest stimulus is only a light sensation or warmth. This is a factor that must also be considered. As discussed earlier, light stimulus may influence different mechanisms than heavier needling, which is known to initiate a chain of neurological and neurochemical actions. Light, shallow needling may have no direct influence on these neurological mechanisms, instead initiating change by affecting the body's information-processing mechanisms.

Summary

By now you have probably thought: Is one of these methods quicker or better than another? We do not know, and neither does anyone else. Although everyone naturally believes that their system is superior, there is no evidence on which to base comparisons. This question is tremendously complex; it is related to how different approaches can each achieve positive results. However, there are also very difficult practical problems with information gathering

that have yet to be resolved. Most at-scale medical comparisons require a central data repository that can process information statistically. Not only is there no central repository of information for acupuncture, until recently almost none of the Western acupuncture literature was written so that it could be cross-referenced to anything else. Because so few of the extant training texts maintain a relationship between the English and the Chinese, even if data-collection mechanisms were available, it is unlikely that practitioners' clinical records would be consistent enough for meaningful analysis. Until these problems are addressed, system-to-system comparisons will remain subjective.

However, it is nonetheless clear that there is a broad consistency of treatment. As we have noted, theoretical models of how the body works are mostly relevant to root treatment. In most styles of practice, and those outlined here being no exception, there are also symptom-control treatments. Often, several different sets of acupoints will be used during a therapeutic course. For example, in the experience-centered acupuncture of Tin Yao So, urinary problems, similar to those of the sample case presented above are treated by SP-6, SP-9, BL-22, BL-23, BL-27, BL-28, CV-4, CV-6, and ST-28, in other words, many of the same points.[61] Although this further complicates the question of what works best, because the relief of symptoms could logically have nothing to do with the root treatment, it does show that there is a reasonable consistency between systems.

What we feel the preceding examples show is that system-to-system consistency appears only when you examine an entire course of treatment and the logic behind the selection of acupoints and techniques. Note too that, because root treatments are created to enhance the body's ability to heal itself, rather than to relieve particular symptoms, it is possible that different symptom-control treatments work better with one root treatment than another. Since root-treatment effects would be more likely notable over the longer term, and because they are aimed at deeper, more structural and functional processes within the body, it is not at all unlikely that a considerable variety of approaches could be effective.

Although it is impossible to reduce traditional pattern recognition to some single, clear conclusion, it is possible to say that, even with a considerable theoretical variety, thousands of possible treatments, and multiple views of humans in their environment, traditional methods of pattern recognition are capable of consistent repeatability — at least among acupuncturists of similar training. Practically, for patients the best system is probably the one used by the most experienced acupuncturist available. It is expertise and experience that combine with treatment approach and technique to determine the outcome of any particular treatment.

DIAGNOSIS IN SYSTEMS THAT REJECT OR PARTIALLY ACCEPT THE TRADITIONAL MODELS

New approaches have developed simultaneously with the adaptation of traditional systems. There are practitioners who accept no discussion of *qi*, *yin-yang*, five phases, channels, or *zang fu* as relevant to clinical practice. Typically, practitioners who hold this opinion use either no clear theoretical model, or use empirical knowledge about the acupuncture points as the only basis for their treatment plans. They may also work from a scientific model. In these approaches to acupuncture it is the biomedical disease entity or a patient's description of their symptoms that becomes the operative diagnosis. For example, a patient who presents with low-back pain and accompanying sciatica due to nerve impingement from disc degeneration would be treated with acupoints with a reputation for treating lumbar pain and sciatica. The effort is to stimulate acupoints with techniques that have worked for the condition at hand. This is seen in the work of practitioners such as Tung of China[62] and Mori of Japan.[63]

In more scientifically oriented systems, points are treated according to anatomical knowledge of trigger points, motor points, muscle attachments, nerve routes, and neuromotor functions. Practitioners such as Ulett in the USA,[64] Gunn in Canada,[65] and Baldry[66] and White[67] in the UK use these approaches. Again, what is common to these approaches is reliance on the disease entity as the key to treatment. The biomedical diagnosis is considered sufficient. Variation in selection of points depends on the framework chosen by a specific practitioner. One may gain experience with trigger points while another works with motor points, but both consider pressure sensitivity as diagnostic. The more sensitive points are frequently also those treated.

There are a number of different but related systems that rely on Western theoretical models. Each of these uses a biomedical diagnosis as a starting point, but then reinterprets that diagnosis in terms of a particular model. These models use scientific terms and concepts, but the reinterpretations are unique and are as yet not generally accepted by the biomedical community. For example, there are systems based on the idea that autonomic nervous system imbalance causes disease. Several competing models of this theory are active in Japan. There is also the method of neural therapy of Huneke of Germany and the neurological models of Mann from England and Bischko from Germany. These are all examples of thinkers who have rejected traditional methods in favor of their own unique approaches.

There are also practitioners who accept some or many traditional concepts and principles, but who nonetheless reject traditional diagnostic techniques (e.g. pulse and body palpation, and questions asked in the context of the five phases and *yin-yang*). Many of these practitioners accept the existence of the channels with their several classes of acupuncture points, but attempt to objectify diagnosis and acupoint selection. The middle ground typically taken in these systems is the use of an instrument to quantify a diagnostic measure. The most common measurement is electrodermal. Several relatively popular machines have been created by German and Japanese practitioners. Among the most commonly used are Voll's Dermatron, Schimmel's Vegatest, Nakatani's Neurometer, and Motoyama's AMI. In the USA there are micro-current instruments, such as Rossen's Microstim system.

The basic principle of these instruments is simple. As early as 1950, researchers found that acupuncture points and channels had lower electrical resistance than the surrounding skin, and this finding led to the the invention of the devices just mentioned, among others. These measurements are made by applying a small electric current through a reference electrode and measuring the current that returns through the acupuncture point tested. Knowing the current applied and the current returned, the resistance of the point can be calculated. The therapeutic theory to which these findings are applied is that acupoints will have a particularly low resistance if there is a problem in the traditionally associated channel. By measuring a series of points related to all the channels, a diagnosis of which channels have the greatest problem is formed. Treatments are then applied to those channels. The basic circuit used in such instruments is shown in Figure 6.10. Each instrument based on this idea applies a slightly different current to different reference areas, and uses different points as indicators of channel condition. This technology was discussed in greater detail in Chapter 4.

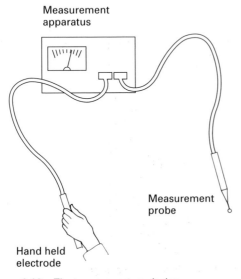

Measurement apparatus

Measurement probe

Hand held electrode

Figure 6.10 Electro acupuncture device.

The *Ryodoraku* system invented by Yoshio Nakatani[68] and applied by his colleagues Masayoshi Hyodo[69] and Hirohisa Oda[70] uses electrical measurements of the source (*yuan*) acupoints to assess the condition of the channel system and, more generally, the autonomic nervous system. Based on a computer analysis of the readings obtained with the neurometer device, treatments are designed to correct the imbalances measured. This is combined with the needling of acupoints indicated for the patient's symptoms.

Reinhold Voll's 'electro acupuncture according to Voll' (EAV) involves the use of similar electrical measurements made at the terminal acupoints of the channels. The patient is then treated using acupuncture, homeopathy, or a combination of the two. In Voll's system the channels are not traditional, and are seen as predictive of Western pathologies, not traditional patterns. This system was developed in the 1950s and is quite popular in Europe, but less so in the USA.[71]

There are a number of other means used to objectify patient assessment, some of which are instrumented and some of which are not. An example of a noninstrumented approach is the 'bi-digital O-ring test' developed by Yoshiaki Omura.[72] This is a kinesiological (muscle strength) test that Omura has researched and used to map channels, points, and pathologies. The bi-digital O-ring indicates a problem at a diagnostic acupoint if the finger muscles lose strength when that point is touched.

Another instrument-assisted diagnostic method is the use of sphygmamometers to measure the radial pulses. Researchers in China, Taiwan, Japan, and the USA have built instruments that can measure pressure waves in the radial artery.[73] The theory is that if radial pulse diagnosis is as useful as the literature implies, pressure-sensitive devices can measure what is otherwise subjectively assessed by practitioners. Treatment is based on the measurement results. Various devices have been built. Most who use this form of instrument see it as an adjunct to their diagnostic process, rather than as a sole means of making the diagnosis.

Another area where diagnosis has been instrumented is visual inspection of the tongue. Chinese researchers have developed the 'tongue colorometer,' which uses sensitive light meters to assess the condition and color of the tongue.[74]

There are also systems of acupuncture that neither accept nor reject traditional methods, but rather propose original theories and methods. One such system is the French system of auriculotherapy, developed by Nogier.[75] Initially this system was a simple correspondence system where ear acupoints and areas corresponded to all the major body systems and parts (Fig. 6.11). This system has grown in complexity, presenting new theories of the body and auricular correspondence. Now, instead of a single map with a one-to-one correspondence between a body area and a

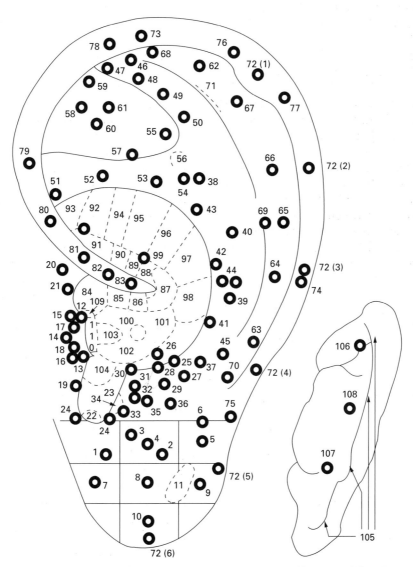

Figure 6.11 Ear point correspondences from Chinese charts. (Courtesy of Paradigm Publications.)

1 tooth extraction anesthesia	2 upper jaw	3 lower jaw
4 tongue	5 upper chin	6 lower chin
7 tooth extraction anesthesia	8 eye	9 inner-ear
10 tonsils	11 cheek	12 apex of tragus
13 adrenal	14 external nose	15 throat
16 internal nose	17 thirst point	18 hunger point
19 high blood pressure	20 outer ear	21 heart organ
22 internal secretion	23 ovary	24 eye 1 and 2
25 brain stem	26 toothache	27 throat and teeth
28 brain point (pituitary)	29 occiput	30 parotid gland
31 stop wheezing point	32 testicles	33 forehead
34 subcortex	35 *tai yang*	36 vertex
37 cervical vertebrae	38 sacral vertebrae	39 thoracic vertebrae
40 lumbar vertebrae	41 neck	42 chest
43 abdomen	44 breast	45 thyroid
46 foot	47 heel	48 ankle
49 knee joint	50 sacroiliac joint	51 sympathetic
52 sciatic nerve	53 kidney	54 lumbar pain point
55 *shen men*	56 pelvic cavity	57 hip joint
58 uterus	59 high blood pressure	60 asthma point
61 hepatitis point	62 finger	63 clavicle
64 shoulder joint	65 shoulder	66 elbow
67 arm	68 appendix 1	69 appendix 2
70 appendix 3	71 urticaria point	72 helix 1–4
73 tonsil 1	74 tonsil 2	75 tonsil 3
76 liver *yang* point	77 liver *yang* point	78 auricular apex
79 external genitalia	80 urethra	81 rectum
82 diaphragm	83 point zero	84 mouth
85 esophagus	86 stomach cardiac orifice	87 stomach
88 duodenum	89 small intestine	90 appendix 4
91 large intestine	92 bladder	93 prostate gland
94 ureter	95 kidney	96 pancreas (left), gallbladder (right)
97 liver	98 spleen	99 ascites
100 heart	101 lung	102 bronchii
103 trachea	104 *san jiao*	105 lower blood pressure groove
106 upper back	107 low back	108 mid back
109 low abdomen	110 upper abdomen	

Figure 6.11 (cont'd)

part of the ear, there are four overlying maps, each relating to different embryological origins and each activated by different stimuli.

The method of diagnosis that has developed along with this system involves palpating the radial artery while a small stimulus or signal source is applied to the ear. This initiates a vascular autonomic signal (VAS), which is a strong pressure wave felt in the artery. The appearance of this wave is correlated with the ear zone stimulated and the nature of the stimulus applied. This information is used to devise a treatment plan. This system proposes that problems in the body result from primary imbalances of the autonomic nervous system.

Thus it strives to restore a proper balance between the sympathetic and parasympathetic aspects. This can be both an exclusive and a combination therapy. For example, Dan Kenner of Santa Rosa, California, uses Nogier scanning in conjunction with the methods of his Japanese training to help clarify difficult cases.

This review of the diagnostic processes employed by practitioners of different traditions illustrates the basic theoretical models that have developed. As we have seen, these are the means by which acupoints and stimulus techniques are chosen. In the next chapter we describe the treatment tools and principles used in each system, and give case illustrations.

NOTES

1   Abstracted from: Sapiro JD 1990 The art and science of bedside diagnosis. Urban and Swarzenberg, Baltimore, MD, pp 534–537
2   See note 1, p 533
3   Wiseman N 1998 A practical dictionary of Chinese medicine. Paradigm Publications, Brookline, MA, p 642
4   See note 3, p 509
5   Unschuld PU 1990 Forgotten traditions of ancient Chinese medicine. Paradigm Publications, Brookline, MA, p 113
6   See note 3, p 51
7   Requena Y 1989 Character and health. The relationship of acupuncture and psychology. Paradigm Publications, Brookline, MA, pp 153–164
8   See note 5, p 336
9   Soulie de Morant G 1994 Chinese acupuncture. Paradigm Publications, Brookline, MA, p 585
10   Unschuld PU 1987 Traditional Chinese medicine; some historical and epistemological reflections. Social Science and Medicine 24(12):1023–1029
11   Unschuld PU 1998 Chinese medicine. Paradigm Publications, Brookline, MA, p 87
12(a) See note 10
    (b) Unschuld PU 1992 Epistemological issues and changing legitimation: traditional Chinese medicine in the twentieth century. In: Leslie C, Young A (eds) Paths to Asian medical knowledge. University of California Press, Berkeley, CA
13   See note 12
14   Unschuld PU 1985 Medicine in China: a history of ideas. University of California Press, Berkeley, CA, p 57
15   Much direct mail, periodical, and book printing is done in Asia for reasons of cost or quality. However, because Asians perceive colour differently than Westerners, Western art directors need to supervise color printing to ensure that it satisfies Western tastes.
16   Wiseman N, Ellis A 1985 Fundamentals of Chinese medicine. Paradigm Publications, Brookline, MA, pp 218 ff
17   Shudo D 1990 Japanese classical acupuncture: introduction to meridian therapy. Eastland Press, Seattle, WA, pp 113 ff
18   *Huang Di Nei Jing Ling Shu Yi Jie*. Chinese Republic Publishing Company, Taipei, 1978, pp 235 ff
19   Yang Ji-zhou 1982 *Zhen Jiu Da Cheng*. Da Zhong Guo Tu Shu, Taipei, 1982, p 120
20   Shanghai College of Traditional Chinese Medicine. *Zhen Jiu Zhi Liao Xue*; Hong Kong, Shao Hua Cultural Service, Hong Kong, pp 90–93
21   See note 5, p 130
22   Foss L, Rothenberg K 1987 The second medical revolution. Shambhala, Boston, MA
23   Data abstracted from note 16, p 77
24   See note 16, p 82
25   See note 16, pp 77–82 and note 17, pp 25–28
26   See note 16, p 83
27   Manaka Y, Itaya K, Birch S 1995 Chasing the dragon's tail. Paradigm Publications, Brookline, MA, p 156
28   See note 16, p 89
29   Abstracted from note 16, pp 89–105 and note 17, pp 36–37
30   Abstracted from note 16, pp 95–101
31   Abstracted from note 16, pp 105–107 and note 17, pp 37–39

32   Abstracted from note 16, pp 107–116 and note 17, pp 39–44
33   Abstracted from note 16, pp 116–124 note 17, pp 44–106 and note 27, pp 131–143
34   For a complete list, see: note 16, pp 125–136
35   Okabe S 1988 Keiraku chiryo shomei to rinsho no myaku no hikaku. Nihon Shinkyu Chiryo Gakkai Shi 14(1):9–24. Cited in Shiohara K, Giula MF 1900 The arterial pulse analyzer as a potential replacement for manual pulse palpation in Oriental medicine. Unpublished manuscript
36   See note 16, pp 125–136
37   For a description of basic abdominal patterns, see: Matsumoto K, Birch S 1988 Hara diagnosis: reflections on the sea. Paradigm Publications, Brookline, MA, pp 249–268
38   See note 16, pp 122–124
39   If you observe, for example, internet correspondents discussing cases this becomes clear. However, there is as yet not much formal proof, such as that obtained in inter-rater studies. One example of inter-rater agreement can be found in Birch S. Preliminary investigations of inter-rater reliability of traditionally based acupuncture diagnostic assessments (submitted).
40   Kenner D. Personal communication
41   Bensky D. Personal communication
42   Chinese patients carry a case record with them to hospitals that serve both in and outpatient populations. These records are kept by the patient, updated by each practitioner, and are an on-going medical history that is available to any physician whom the patient chooses to consult.
43   Shi Dian-bang 1991 Development and prospect of traditional Chinese medicine at the contemporary era. In: International congress on traditional medicine. State Administration of Traditional Chinese Medicine, Beijing
44   Shanghai College of Traditional Chinese Medicine n.d. Zhen Jiu Zhi Liao Xue, pp 25–30, 48–51, 90–93, 100–102, 139–141
45   Prensky B. Personal communication
46   So JTY. Personal communication
47   Fukushima K. Clinical lecture in Tokyo, July 1990
48   Kenner D. Personal communication
49   Worsley JR 1973 Is acupuncture for you? College of Traditional Chinese Acupuncture, Leamington Spa, p 3
50(a) Eckman P 1996 In the footsteps of the yellow emperor. Cypress Book Company
    (b) Eckman P 1992 Lecture. Oxford, November
51   Shima M. Personal communication
52   Helms J. Personal communication
53   See, for example: Requena Y 1986 Terrains and pathology in acupuncture. Paradigm Publications, Brookline, MA
54   Smith M. Personal communication
55   This is a simplified example drawn from TCM literature and confirmed in interviews with working practitioners. It is illustrative rather than exhaustive
56   The functions and indications quoted are from the acupoint sections in: Ellis A, Wiseman N, Boss K 1991 *Fundamentals of Chinese acupuncture*, rev edn. Paradigm Publications, Brookline, MA
57   This is a simplified example drawn from *keiraku chiryo*

literature and confirmed in interviews with working practitioners. It is illustrative rather than exhaustive

58 The traditional associations of the acupoints quoted are from: note 56, pp 412–446

59 This treatment example is based on examples in note 27

60 See note 56, pp 213–214

61 So TY 1987 A complete course in acupuncture. Vol 2: *Treatment of disease with acupuncture*. Paradigm Publications, Brookline, MA, p 232

62 Paldan D (transl), Lee M (rev) 1993 Tung's acupuncture by Dr. Ching-Chang Tung. Blue Poppy Press, Boulder, CO

63 Mori H 1979 Shinkyu no tameno Shindan to Chiryo. Ido no Nippon Sha, Yokosuka

64 Ulett G 1992 Beyond yin and yang. WH Green, St Louis, MI

65 (a) Gunn CC 1988 Reprints on pain, acupuncture and related subjects. Vancouver
(b) Gunn CC 1996 The Gunn approach to the treatment of chronic pain. Churchill Livingstone, Edinburgh

66 Baldry PE 1989 Acupuncture, trigger points and musculoskeletal pain. Churchill Livingstone, Edinburgh

67 Filshie J, White A 1998 Medical acupuncture. Churchill Livingstone, Edinburgh

68 Nakatani Y, Yamashita K 1977 *Ryodoraku* acupuncture. Ryodoraku Research Institute, Tokyo

69 Hyodo M 1975 *Ryodoraku* treatment. *Ryodoraku*, Autonomic Nerve System Society, Osaka

70 Oda H 1989 *Ryodoraku* textbook. Naniwasha, Osaka

71 Kenyon JN 1983 Modern techniques of acupuncture, vol 1. Thorsons, Wellingborough

72 See e.g. Omura Y 1986 Practice of 'bi-digital O-ring test'. Ido no Nippon Sha, Yokosuka

73(a) Broffman M, McCulloch M 1986 Instrument assisted pulse evaluation in the acupuncture practice. American Journal of Acupuncture 14(3):255–259
(b) Fu Cong-yuan 1988 Achievements of research on pulse-taking with integrated traditional Chinese and Western medicine. Chinese Journal of Integrated Medicine 8(special issue 2):108–112

74 Chen Ze-lin 1988 Development of research on tongue diagnosis. Chinese Journal of Integrated Medicine 8(special issue 2):104–108

75 Nogier PFM 1983 From auriculotherapy to auriculomedicine. Maisonneuve, Saint-Ruffine

7

Treatment

In Chapter 6 we saw how different schools of practice, each with different emphases and preferences, handle pattern recognition. We have discussed practitioners who rigorously apply traditional theories, and practitioners who reject traditional theories in whole or in part, concentrating instead on biomedical diagnoses or symptoms alone. We have noted that still others depend upon a diagnostic device. As you saw in the treatment plans we used to illustrate pattern identification, there is diversity in acupoint selection, there are techniques that do not involve needling, each with a long history, and there are many techniques that have evolved in modern practice, all of which can be said to be acupuncture. What is common to all is some degree of acupoint stimulation.

Although there is a broad consistency in point selection at the symptomatic level, differences in the rationale for root treatment come from the theoretical and diagnostic framework employed. As we have seen, a practitioner of the *ba gang bian zheng* school will select different treatment points and techniques than will someone schooled in the methods of *keiraku chiryo*. This is because the means for categorizing acupoints is determined by the frame of reference in which humans are viewed. As goes the latter, so goes the former. Treatment is consistent with pattern recognition because the two partake of the same assumptions.

When the *ba gang* system describes a condition like *yang* vacuity, or an exterior wind evil, there are matching acupoint function descriptions. For example, there are acupoints labeled as 'enriching kidney yin' (e.g. *tai xi*, KI-3),[1] or 'coursing the channels' (e.g. *feng men*, BL-12),[2] and 'harmonizing the stomach' (e.g. *xian gu*, ST-43)[3] or 'transforming damp' (e.g. *yin ling quan*, SP-9).[4] These are ordered via a top-down logic. Therefore, it is these acupoint qualities, rather than the specific acupoint selections and combinations, that we emphasize in the case stories, given later in this chapter.

Clinically observed conditions are matched to acupoint functions through general treatment principles such as 'supplementing vacuity.' But, although there is an entire set of points that supplement vacuity, certain acupoints are related to specific organs or functions. Thus, clinical experience is categorized and specified. These relationships are often expressed in the Chinese acupoint names and indications; for example, an indication that uses the Chinese term translated as 'fortify,' immediately reminds Chinese-speaking acupuncturists of its relationship to the spleen. These relationships serve Chinese speakers as memory aids and keys to consistency.

In the *keiraku chiryo* system, patterns such as 'lung vacuity' or 'liver vacuity' identify *qi* circulation related states where channels are vacuous or replete according to the engendering cycle of the five phases. Therefore, five-phase points on the lung and spleen channels (e.g. *tai yuan*, LU-9, and *tai bai*, SP-3, for lung vacuity) or liver and kidney channels (*qu quan*, LV-8, and *yin gu*, KI-10, for liver vacuity) are selected for their ability to supplement channel vacuity,[5] as are the needling techniques applied, the stimulation sought, and sometimes even the time of treatment. Here too acupoint names and indications codify the relationships. Although the channel-centered perspective leads to a difference in how acupoints are applied, that difference is not exclusive to *keiraku chiryo*, but part of the general multiplicity of perspectives available. Thus, there is a rich intellectual environment for point selection.

CULTURAL INFLUENCES ON ACUPUNCTURE TREATMENT

However, nonclinical factors such as culture, history, and economic need also contribute to this multiplicity. For example, China's population is predominantly occupied in rural and laboring occupations, and thus the techniques used in modern Chinese practice are suitable for the problems of a physically active population treated in a public health environment. In Japan, where most of the population lives and works in cities, techniques have evolved to suit an increasingly sedentary urban society treated by private physicians. The main technical difference is that modern Chinese practice centers on heavier needling techniques, whereas lighter techniques have become the trademark of Japanese practice. As discussed in earlier chapters, 'heavier needling techniques' means using thicker needles that are more deeply inserted and manipulated to produce a stronger sensation. 'Lighter needling techniques' means using thinner needles that are more shallowly inserted and handled so as to produce little or no sensation.

As a general observation, the more industrialized and urbanized the country and the wealthier the economy, the lighter the treatment techniques. Historically, this was true even within China's socioeconomic hierarchy. Classical acupuncturists were taught that laborers' more corporeal and external complaints were better served by stronger needling and that nobles or intellectuals were to be treated with more delicate stimuli. In addition, the depth and technique of insertion were varied in accordance with the patient and the disease.[6] This was the case until the mid-20th century.[7] It is also clear that each needling technique is believed to work in its country of origin. What is not clear is the degree of cultural interchangeability. We do not know, for example, whether using techniques from China in Japan would, on the whole, be well received. We can guess that there are limits, because many of our colleagues who undertook studies in China describe how they were criticized by patients and teachers for using techniques that were too light. On the other hand, Birch and others have had the opposite experience in Japan. There patients and teachers object if the techniques used are too heavy.

In addition to these cultural influences, treatment techniques are tied to the theoretical framework within which they developed. Some techniques are thus more suitable in one treatment style than another. Different schools are often very explicit about these details (Box 7.1). Teachers in the *ba gang bian zheng* tradition inform their students that they must obtain *de qi* for treatment to

succeed. Patients must experience aching, numbness, distension, tingling, fullness, or some pain. On the other hand, *keiraku chiryo* teaches the opposite. The patient does not have to feel anything, and should not be made in any way uncomfortable. As we have noted before, it is possible that these different stimulus levels actually elicit different bodily responses.

Box 7.1 Comparison of names and metaphors of basic Chinese and Japanese needling techniques

The following labels, metaphors and descriptions are extracted from the *Fundamentals of Chinese Acupuncture* by Ellis et al,[8] *Acupuncture and Moxibustion* by Auteroche et al,[9] *Acupuncture Science* by Jayasuriya,[10] *Meridian Therapy* by Fukushima,[11] and *Introduction to Meridian Therapy* by Shudo.[12]

In most texts of the Chinese *ba gang* system of traditional Chinese medical acupuncture it is stated that one must obtain the *qi*, or get *de qi*, if the treatment is to be effective. The *de qi* phenomenon typically describes something that the patient feels as a result of the needling: 'Obtaining the *qi* (*de qi*) refers to the sensation produced when a point is needled. The sensation can be described as soreness, aching, distension, heaviness, numbness, or tingling, depending on the point in question and the condition of the patient.

When the *qi* arrives the patient can feel a sudden tightness that resembles the feeling of a fish biting a fishing line. This sudden tightness has traditionally been said to be the *qi*, but is now assumed to be the muscle into which the needle is inserted, grasping the needle as it contracts around the needle. However, *de qi* may also be felt by the acupuncturist, as a sense of tightening felt through the needle due to local muscle spasm. It has been shown by several researchers in China that this sensation is not felt when a muscle is denervated such as in paraplegia.

Various manipulations of the needle are used once it is inserted and one frequently finds expressions such as: 'lifting and thrusting,' 'cranking and shaking,' 'blocking,' and 'cocking the cross-bow.' Depending on what is to be achieved by the needle manipulation there are a number of metaphoric names given to commonly used Chinese techniques: 'burning mountain fire method,' 'penetrating heaven cooling method,' 'green dragon swings his tail method,' 'white tiger shakes his head method,' and the 'dragon and tiger come to blows method.'

As you can see from these names and metaphors, they suggest aggressiveness, power, and strength. To learn these Chinese needling techniques, it is recommended that 'the student begin practicing the insertion techniques on a tightly bound pad of paper, a ball of cotton cloth, or a tightly bound piece of sponge rubber.' Practice on these hard, somewhat

dense objects is used to learn the insertion and manipulation required in these techniques.

These ideas and metaphors contrast strongly with the names and metaphors found in the Japanese *keiraku chiryo*, channel-therapy approaches. In this system, there is great stress on practitioners feeling the *qi*, rather than the patient's response. This idea is based on the *Nan Jing*:

> He who knows how to needle relies on his left hand and he who does not know how to needle relies on his right.

> As soon as the arrival of the *qi* (felt by the left hand) resembles the (proper pulsation of *qi* in the channels) insert the needle.

When needling, the left hand holds the needle at the point and the right hand advances and manipulates the needle. Thus this idea highlights the difference between having the left hand feel the arrival of *qi* instead of having the right hand feel the grasping of the needle, or attending to the patient's description of *de qi* sensations.

In contrast to obtaining the *qi* (*de qi*), which is felt by the patient, the arrival of the *qi* is something that the practitioner feels. The extremely delicate changes that an experienced practitioner learns to sense are known as 'needle subtleness,' and the 'arrival of *qi*' is felt as a sensation of warmth in the thumb of the left hand which is supporting the needle.

The descriptions are of very subtle phenomena. Understandably, one finds metaphors that strongly reinforce this idea: Japanese writers say that one should needle 'as if walking over thin ice,' or as if 'peering into the abyss.' One should grip the handle of the needle 'as if gripping the tail of a sleeping tiger.' The acupuncturist of great skill is 'like one who is able to haul a ton of stones with a single lotus thread' and is able to 'needle a sleeping cat without waking it.' There are further metaphoric descriptions that reinforce this idea: one should 'advance the needle until it meets resistance like a needle pressed into a spider's web.' In the *Toyohari* system there is one technique called the *jin* (dust) technique, applied like 'brushing dust off of a table.' There are also various non-insertion techniques (*sesshokushin*, 'contact' or

---

Box 7.1 Comparison of names and metaphors of basic Chinese and Japanese needling techniques *(cont'd)*

'touching' needling) commonly found in the *keiraku chiryo* system.

In one school students practice needling a piece of fruit (such as an apple, orange, or lemon) that is floating in a bowl of water filled to the brim. Any pressure on the fruit spills water from the bowl and

students must learn to insert a needle without spilling any water. Another method of practice is to insert a needle into an inflated balloon without bursting it. The images of the metaphors and descriptions are completely different from the Chinese ones, stressing instead ideas of subtlety, lightness, and passivity.

In this chapter we explore this range of methods and techniques as applied in case stories, and the different rationales for point selection each exemplifies. This exploration includes actual cases provided by people who practice these approaches, some in Asian cultures. The case histories are not presented in a way that would meet the standards of technical detail, history-taking, and follow-up required of professional documentation. Instead, they have been edited to demonstrate how pattern recognition is used to formulate treatments. We have not used 'textbook' cases, as these are already edited. As we have discussed, pattern identification is a means of selecting treatments from the range of treatment options with which a practitioner is familiar. Thus, in each of these cases the cultural, educational, and clinical experiences vary, as do the theories of practice. As the theories vary, so do the methods of information gathering, pattern recognition, and treatment.

The evidence we have at this time does not show that any one method is more effective than any other, because appropriate comparative studies are lacking. Thus, these cases simply exemplify principles. The clinical approaches do not represent standards or exclusive answers. There are limits to any practitioner's knowledge, and thus the decisions of the clinicians whose treatment we present reflect a variety of factors. Clinicians' experience tends to be bound by their training, interest, and the nature of the patient population they serve. Historically, even the most famous clinicians have contributed in an area of specialty. Theoretical richness, the need to acquire clinical experience, and the time required to develop physical and sensorial skills all limit each practitioner's view. Thus none of the techniques presented here are the only way in which a particular problem might be addressed.

For example, a Traditional Chinese Medicine (TCM) practitioner, taught that without achieving *de qi* his or her treatment will fail, is very unlikely to have learned, applied, or observed shallower needling. Similarly, *keiraku chiryo* practitioners believe that, without the needling characteristic of their system, treatment cannot work. Some have gone so far as to suggest that *ba gang* needling be used as a 'placebo' for clinical trials, and we often find shallow painless needling used as the sham acupuncture in trials of TCM treatments. Although this clearly shows why heated interschool rivalry is no stranger in acupuncture research, it is probable that every approach has limits and that each depends in some significant way on the techniques applied. Acupoint functions are probably best thought of as including the particular needling depths, specific techniques, and needling tools by which they were determined.

In practice, practitioners who are well educated have a depth of knowledge and experience, and limit themselves to systems developed in their own milieu, through the training and experience of their teachers and peers, and, of course, their personal preferences and opportunities. This is not dissimilar to the situation in Western medicine. In addition to personal limits, there are social and political limits to any practitioner's choices in treatment. Today, even the country or region in which one lives or trains has an impact on practice skills. Complex historical and social pressures mold what is and is not available, acceptable, or expected. For example, based on politics and misinformation, a number of established Japanese, German, and other techniques and devices have been banned in California. Practitioners there can no longer study or observe those systems.

In any practice demanding aquired human skills a narrowed clinical scope is not inherently bad. As Tin Yau So is fond of saying: 'Use only one kitchen knife and it will always be sharp,'[13] an expression of the fact that pattern identification and treatment are human skills which, like music or athletics, must be constantly practiced. A 'jack of all trades,' as the expression goes, may have mastered none. In this sense, limitations to a practitioner's theoretical perspective are a means of quality control. Traditionally, one was considered to have mastered a skill, or to be qualified to teach, only when able to repeat a teacher's performance, or to train apprentices, with accuracy.

These limitations of perspective not only curtail the availability of ideas and techniques, but also tend to increase the individuality of approach. Together, these factors further encourage diversity. Historically, this diversity has been dealt with economically and politically. Whether it was the emperor's order to create a point-standardizing bronze statue, or the selection of certain books by today's examination boards, political process has constrained diversity and required uniformity. Since most traditional physicians worked in 'sink or swim' competition for patients and apprentices, economic survival has also provided a constant check on diversity. In Meiji Japan, the strains of modernization led to a restriction and narrowing of the scope of acupuncture. In modern China, faced with incredible public health and economic problems after the Second World War, acupuncture was made uniform and institutionalized. Now, with economic reform, there is again a blooming of different treatment approaches in China, just as there was in Japan when the Meiji restrictions were loosened.

Today, there is a similar impetus toward uniformity in the West. Generally taking the modern Chinese model as a standard, uniformity of approach has been a practical component of the effort to win greater recognition and acceptability for acupuncture. The creation of today's educational, licensing, and practitioner establishment without the aid of public funding or political support is a visionary accomplishment very few believed possible even only 20 years ago. However, although we doubt anyone knows with certainty what the most useful future strategy might be, it does seem certain that change will continue.

Acupuncture has often blossomed after it has been limited. As in modern Japan and China, the richness of its intellectual tools, the potentials of its clinical skills, and the force of human creativity have always met the challenge of the times. Thus it seems reasonable to suggest that the Western acculturation of acupuncture will follow a similarly changing course.

In this chapter we have tried to explore a broad range of treatment methods and techniques that exist in the field.[14] Each represents, in one sense, the cultural or social adaptation of particular practitioners or schools of thought that we have discussed throughout this book. In another sense, all these approaches represent the creative genius of hands-on doers.

THE TOOLS OF THE TRADE

The term for acupuncture is *zhen jiu* (*shinkyu* in Japanese), more accurately, 'needling and moxibustion.' In China at different times this has meant either two separate practices (needling and moxibustion) or the two intertwined methods known today as 'acumoxa therapy.' There is a similar historical interweaving in Japan, but today both are separately licensed. Moxibustion appears to be one of the oldest forms of therapy devised in China. As you may remember from our review of history, some of the oldest acupuncture-related texts contained information about moxibustion.

Moxibustion involves placing small variously shaped pieces of the processed mugwort plant ('moxa,' after the Japanese *mogusha*) on the body surface. These are ignited so that the heat of the burning herb stimulates the acupoint. There are over 10 different methods of application in common use today. Historically, there have been more than 50 different moxibustion methods.[15] Several treatises were entirely devoted

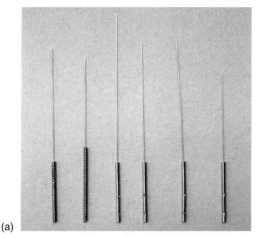

(a)

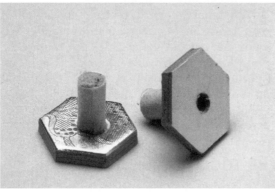

(b)

Figure 7.1 (a) Acupuncture needles and (b) Commercially prepared moxa. (Courtesy of Paradigm Publications.)

to moxibustion therapy. Moxibustion is commonly used directly on the skin or indirectly on an intervening media. Some of the variants are:

Direct moxa:

- the cone is placed directly on the skin
- the cone can have various shapes, densities, and sizes
- varying degrees of heat can be felt by the patient
- blisters and small scars are sometimes formed (though with decreasing frequency in modern practice).

Indirect moxa:

- the moxa cone is placed on top of a slice of ginger or garlic, or a mound of salt or bean paste

- the moxa is wrapped into a cigar-shaped stick, ignited, and held over the body
- varying degrees of heat are applied.

Moxibustion is used by many as a way of adding heat when patterns of coldness are found and as a way of supplementing vacuity. It is mostly used in combination with needling, but can be used alone, as is seen in Japan where there are moxibustion specialists. Based on the idea that moxibustion heats points or areas of the body, some practitioners prefer to use infrared heat lamps instead of actually burning moxa. A moxa cone and styles of moxibustion are illustrated in Figure 7.2.

In the earliest literature, there are references to using *bian zhen*, or stone needles, to treat disease. Too little is known to make any supposition about stone needles, but whatever the case may have been, the original materials would have been replaced by metal needles as soon as metal technology developed. The earliest application for metal needles appears to have been bloodletting, since it is the primary method of therapy described in the *Huang Di Nei Jing Su Wen*.[16] This technique uses a special needle, the *feng zhen* (in Japanese *hōshin*) which has three sharp edges. This needle was only one of the nine needles described in the 'needle classic,' *Huang Di Nei Jing Ling Shu*, each of which had different dimensions and uses (Fig. 7.3). These nine needles are the:

- *chan zhen (zanshin)* arrow-headed needle
- *yuan zhen (enshin)* round-headed needle
- *shi zhen (teishin)*, blunt needle
- *feng zhen (hōshin)*, sharp/three-edged needle
- *pi zhen (hishin)*, sword-shaped needle
- *yuan li zhen (enrishin)*, round sharp needle
- *hao zhen (gōshin)*, filiform needle
- *chang zhen (chōshin)*, long needle
- *da zhen (taishin)*, large needle.

The names in the above list are the Chinese, Japanese (in parentheses), and English names, respectively.

Each of these needles has evolved over the centuries, and each is used in modern practice in some form. By far the most commonly used needle is the *hao zhen*, or filiform needle. It is

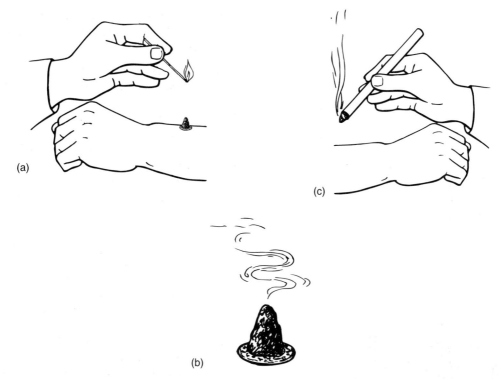

Figure 7.2 Moxibustion techniques: (a) direct moxibustion with a moxa cone; (b) indirect moxibustion – a layer of vegetable tissue (e.g. ginger or garlic) or salt is placed between the moxa cone and the skin; (c) indirect moxibustion with a cylindrical moxa stick.

easy to understand why. It is the thinnest and sharpest of all the needles, and therefore is easier to use. Its insertion is less painful for the patient, and would have historically been less likely to introduce infection. It is the form of needle that can be most inexpensively made from mass-produced wire by industrial equipment. Because disposable needles are an ideal response to societies' concern to control the spread of diseases such as hepatitis and the human immunodeficiency virus (HIV), less costly mass production is a significant advantage.

Several interesting factors have influenced the form of modern acupuncture needles. First, the oldest metal needles in existence were made of silver and gold, but today, the metal most commonly used is stainless steel. As just noted, it is cheaper, sturdier, easier to manufacture, and holds its qualities when sterilized by all clinical or industrial methods. Despite the dominance of stainless steel, needles made of silver and gold are still regularly used, as are needles made of zinc and copper. Less commonly, metals such as molybdenum and cobalt are also used. Each metal has different electrical and chemical properties and several systems of practice take advantage of these.

Second, two of the nine needles were blunt. The *yuan zhen* (round-headed needle) and the *shi zhen* (blunt needle) were used without insertion; that is, they never penetrated the skin. Instead, they were rubbed and pressed on the acupoints. The *chan zhen* (arrow-headed needle) has also evolved so that its modern form is no longer inserted. The *feng zhen*, which was used for bloodletting, and the *pi zhen*, which was used for lancing boils, were essentially surgical instruments designed for shallow incisions, a reminder that acupuncture was traditionally a bedside medicine. The remaining four needles were inserted in the manner most commonly encountered today.

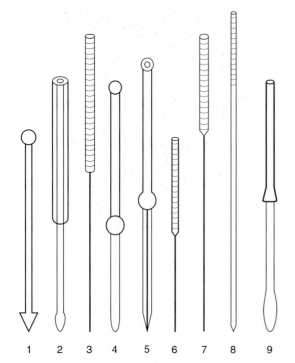

Figure 7.3 The nine needles from the Zhen Jiu Da Cheng (+1601)

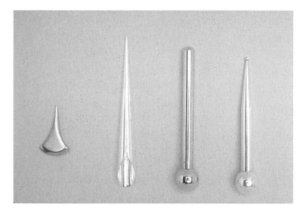

Figure 7.4 Examples of *shonishin* equipment. (Courtesy of Paradigm Publications.)

The original nine needles reflected the medical practices of their era. That included not just acupuncture as we know it but also minor surgery and therapies that did not require needle insertion. Non-insertion acupuncture survives in modern practice, especially in Japan, where the three specialized needles, the *enshin, teishin*, and *zanshin*, have evolved along with refined non-insertion techniques. Although these specialized tools are also used for adults, they have most notably developed in pediatric practice. Other specialized tools that are applied by rubbing, tapping, or pressing are also used to treat children, a practice known as *shonishin* or 'children's needle therapy.' In certain areas of Japan, it is extremely popular and is the parents' first choice for children's conditions. Some *shonishin* equipment is shown in Figure 7.4.

Many practitioners in Japan, especially tacitly gifted blind practitioners, have learned to obtain therapeutic effects without insertion for adults as well as children. These techniques are taught through various *keiraku chiryo* associations. There are thus traditions of practice in acupuncture where needles are pressed, touched to the skin, or held close to the skin surface. Recognizing this, some Japanese practitioners refer to 'East Asian needle therapy' rather than 'acupuncture.' Various forms of finger pressure, manipulation, and massage are also used to stimulate acupoints. In all of Asia traditions of manual therapy are on going.

Of course, the most common form of practice is acupuncture, where needles of different widths (commonly 0.12–0.30 mm) are inserted to different depths (commonly 1–2 mm to several centimeters). Different schools of thought employ different gauge needles inserted to different depths. Once at the points to be treated, or once inserted, many different techniques of stimulation are applied, again according to the system of practice, the needs of the patient and the anatomical detail of the particular acupoint. The various needle types are shown in Figures 7.5 a–c and 7.6.

Today the gauge of needles and depths of insertion used in China in the *ba gang* tradition are entirely different from those used in the *keiraku chiryo* tradition of Japan. In *ba gang* so-called 'number 6' (0.26 mm) or 'number 8' (0.30 mm) needles are typically used. The average depth of insertion is about 14 mm. In the *keiraku chiryo* tradition, so-called 'number 0' (0.14 mm) to 'number 2' (0.18 mm) needles are used, with an average depth of insertion of only 1–2 mm. Within the practices applied in each system, both techniques appear to work.

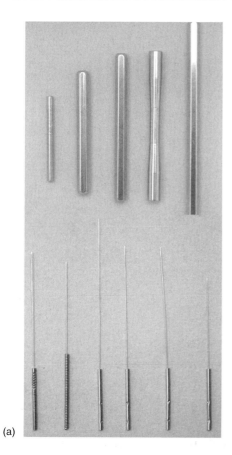

(a)

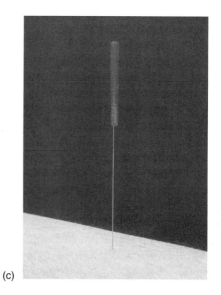

(c)

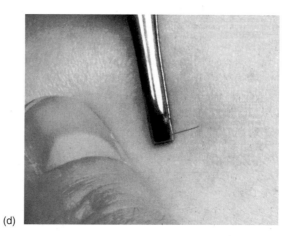

(d)

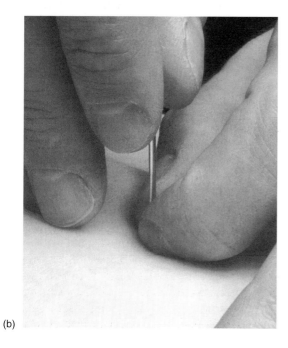

(b)

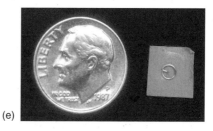

(e)

Figure 7.5 (a) Acupuncture needles and insertion tubes. (b) Insertion technique. (c) Standing insertion. (d) Intradermal insertion. (e) Press tack needle. (Courtesy of Paradigm Publications.)

NEEDLE TECHNIQUES

Traditionally, one supplements vacuity and drains repletion, not only through the choice of acupoints, but also by the technique applied. Variations of these two techniques have been routinely used for about 2000 years. Supplementation and draining depend to a large extent on manual dexterity and skill. Supplementation and draining techniques coordinate with point and channel selection, and there are several ideas how to accomplish both through five-phase and *yin-yang* principles. There is also 'standing insertion' where the needle is inserted with no thought of supplementation or draining. This is very common and has different manifestations depending on who is using the needle.

Specialized tiny needles have been developed which stimulate points in place for up to a week. Examples of these are: the *enpishin*, or press-tack needles, thought to have developed in China and now used in many countries; and the *hinaishin* or intradermal needles, developed and widely used in Japan, but now commonly used in many other countries. The advantage of these tiny retained needles is that they are very thin and are inserted very shallowly. They provide a mild but continuous stimulation, usually without being felt by the patient. The needle sizes are shown in Figure 7.5 d and e.

Another relatively popular technique is to use the 'plum-blossom needle' (Fig. 7.7) and the 'seven-star hammer,' both of which are commonly used in China. These instruments utilize a number of needles embedded in a small head at the end of a flexible handle. This is used by lightly tapping an acupoint or area. These needles have many uses.

Many other techniques have evolved in the modern era. We know that as early as 1825 electrical experiments and devices were in use in France.[17] In recent years, many electrical machines have been developed for the stimulation of inserted needles. The application of an electrical current to inserted needles adds further stimulation, and has been found to be particularly effective in treating pain. Many 'electro-acupuncture' devices are commercially available. The features that vary between these devices are: the strength of the current applied; the voltage; the frequency and regularity of stimulation; the waveforms (the shape that the rise and fall of the current produces on an oscilloscope); and the number of output channels. There appear to be different biological responses to some of these factors (see Ch. 4).

Electro acupuncture appears to be popular, judging by the number of devices sold. Although there are practitioners who claim that acupuncture is not effective unless electrical stimulation is directed to the needles, on the whole electrical stimulation is used to effect a heavier stimulation than is provided by manual needling. In large clinics it is used to allow practitioners to

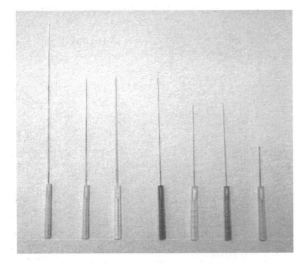

Figure 7.6 Needle sizes. (Courtesy of Paradigm Publications.)

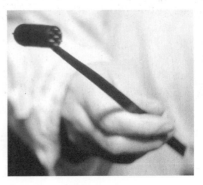

Figure 7.7 Plum-blossom needle. (Courtesy of Paradigm Publications).

attend more patients simultaneously, by relieving them of manual needle manipulation. An electro acupuncture device is shown in Figure 7.8.

There are a number of variants of electrical stimulation. A relatively popular one in Japan invented by Yoshio Manaka is a diode-terminated (one-way) wire called an 'ion-pumping cord.' The reference to ions in the name reflects the first use of ion-pumping cords in the treatment of burns, where Manaka hypothesised that they worked by pumping ions out of burnt tissue where there is a build up of positively charged ions. Thus, this device uses no external electrical current. The cord connects one shallowly inserted needle to another, allowing for a tiny electrical current to flow between the two needles. The patient typically experiences a profound feeling of relaxation, but does not sense the current itself. It is the subtle placement of the needles and the orientation of the diode that generate the effect. The overall effect is powerful, but the stimulation is tiny, particularly because the needles should not be inserted more than 2 mm.[18]

There are also 'micro-current' stimulation devices, some of quite recent invention. These are electro acupuncture devices that deliver only the most minute electrical stimulation to the needles and acupoints. The current levels are significantly smaller than those delivered by earlier electro acupuncture devices. This is a technique that is slowly developing, especially in the West. The Microstim device developed by Joel Rossen is a good example.

Another increasingly popular method is 'two-metal contact therapy,' a technique that has been developed in Japan and Germany during the last few decades. This method uses needles made of different metals at different places but at the same time. The idea is that the different electrovalent properties of two metals will create a minute current between two inserted needles. This is similar to the principle operating in a lead-acid car battery. The metals most commonly used for this technique are copper and zinc, or gold and silver.

In modern practice many other methods of stimulating the acupuncture points have been developed. The use of low-power lasers has become popular in Europe, especially Germany, as well as in China, Japan and more recently, the USA. Microwave radiation has been routinely used in countries of the former USSR, and effects that are frequency-specific have been reported. Colors and sounds have also been used to stimulate points; methods have been developed in Germany, Japan, and the USA. Physician practitioners also inject acupoints with various drugs in dilute solutions. Typically, novocaine, lidocaine, or steroids are used. Injection into the points is also done in China. The same approach is used by some to deactivate or stimulate 'motor' points or 'trigger' points, concepts that have arisen from biomedical practice.

Magnets or magnetic materials were historically used as part of the Chinese *ben cao* or *materia medica* of natural drugs. More recently, mass-produced magnets of varying strengths have been used to stimulate acupoints. This technique is very popular in Japan, where it is nationally advertised for over-the-counter sales, not unlike commercial cold remedies. This approach is also relatively common in China, Europe (particularly France), Canada, and Korea,

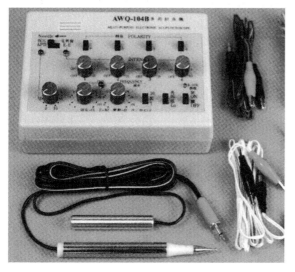

Figure 7.8 Electro acupuncture machine. (Courtesy of Oriental Medical Suppliers, Inc.)

as well as the USA, where products ranging from small tape-backed magnets to magnetic necklaces are popular.

Cupping therapy, the application of suction cups to the body, was originally called 'horn therapy' in China. It also has a long history of use in acupuncture practice. Cupping is often combined with bloodletting, but is also a specialized method of therapy in its own right. There are, for example, specialist practitioners in Japan who are famous for their cupping cures. However, cupping is usually used as an adjunct to acupuncture. Cups and cupping techniques are shown in Figures 7.9 and 7.10. The three traditional forms of cupping use cups placed in one position and left in place according to the indications, cups quickly placed and removed, and cups placed and moved over a body area.

Cupping therapy is thought to stimulate blood circulation, and is therefore indicated for blood stasis. A related technique that serves almost the same function, but without suction, is *gua sha*. This technique is thought to have developed in Southern China. It uses a vigorous rubbing, pressing, or scraping over a congested area following the application of a thick lubricant such as petroleum jelly.

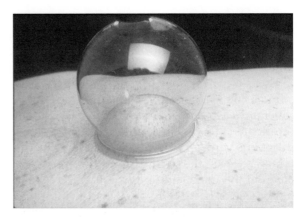

Figure 7.10 Modern vacuum cupping. (Courtesy of Paradigm Publications.)

Aromatic mixtures are often used to stimulate surface circulation. Rubbing is done using ceramic soup spoons, metal lids, smooth pieces of bull horn, and a variety of individually favored tools. Gua sha is not generally applied to specific acupoints but to areas of the body where there are signs of blood stasis visible on the body's surface. These signs include discoloration, vascular spiders, tension in the skin and underlying muscles as well as small string-like warts. This technique is primarily used in Chinese approaches to practice, and has been less popular in the West because of the temporary but unattractive skin coloration it produces.

In China, in recent times, minor surgical techniques have returned to the purview of acupuncture. However, often for legal reasons, these are rarely practiced outside of China. These techniques include: suture embedding therapy, where pieces of suture are placed and left in acupoints; incision therapy, where the superficial tissues are cut and stimulation applied to the underlying tissues; and direct stimulation of the nerve root, where an incision over a nerve root is followed by stimulation. Injection therapies where various fluids are injected into acupoints are also used.

Although we have by no means described every technique employed in the field of acupuncture around the world, the above includes the major techniques used by the major

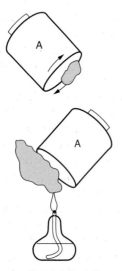

Figure 7.9 Cupping fire. (a) Alcohol swabbed. (b) Ignited and placed on skin.

traditions currently active. In the following section, we present the broad outlines of most of these traditions, and present an organized view of practice as it actually happens. In the first scheme, we discuss the range of theoretical paradigms or belief structures associated with different styles of practice. This will give you a practical sense of how the theoretical and diagnostic information we have discussed is applied in practice. In the second arrangement, we outline the range of sensations that patients typically experience. From this, you can imagine something of the patient's experience in each of the cases we describe. In the third scheme, borrowing an organizational theme from our colleague Dan Kenner, we outline a more theoretical framework based on the research model underlying these practices. Interestingly, there is often a firm correlation between systems in each of these organizational schemes.

THE CONCEPTUAL FRAMEWORK OF ACUPUNCTURE TREATMENT

Again, it is diversity that makes explaining treatment in acupuncture difficult. If we look only at the techniques, only at the models or practice applied, if we listen only to enthusiasts of one system or another, we are almost forced to look at details, forgetting the fundamentals. Acupuncture is built on the basic observations we discussed in Chapters 3 and 6. Treatment applies these understandings to individuals at a particular time, in a particular culture and in a therapeutic setting. To preserve this emphasis we have arranged categories of acupuncture treatment as a continuum. Thus, while the following summary does not mention every method of acupuncture practice, it includes them in the range of the qualities described. By keeping these continua in mind as you examine the cases we present, you will be able to see how different schools of practice choose and apply traditional observations and concepts.

In this first arrangement, practice systems are thought of in terms of the relative predominance of traditional and biomedical ideas.

It is thus also roughly a reflection of historical development:

1. Adherence to and belief in traditional (East Asian) concepts only. Complete rejection of the biomedical (scientific) model.

2. Adherence to and belief in traditional concepts, with a limited utilization of biomedical concepts.

3. An interweaving and mixing of traditional and biomedical concepts.

4. Adherence to and belief in biomedical concepts, with the subsuming of traditional concepts where they can be subsumed.

5. Adherence to and belief in only biomedical concepts, with complete rejection of traditional models.

Virtually every school of acupuncture practice fits somewhere in these five levels. Within each level, there is at least one, and probably more, competing schools of thought, each with different methods of practice, methods of research, and standard concepts. For instance, at level 1 you will find most of the *keiraku chiryo* associations such as the *Toyohari* association. At level 2 or 3 you could place the five-phase Traditional Acupuncture practiced in both the UK and USA, although experts in both systems would identify some differences. The modern Chinese system of TCM acupuncture fits into level 3. Manaka's *yin-yang* balancing approach and Requena's terrains approach fit into level 4, along with the approaches of various biomedical researcher-practitioners such as Nogier and Mussat of France, Mann of the UK, Voll and Bischko of Germany, and Nakatani and Hyodo of Japan. At level 5 are the strict biomedical approaches of researcher-practitioners, such as Ulett of the USA, Gunn of Canada, and Baldry of the UK. There is competition between systems at each level, and between systems at each of the different levels.

The second schema arranges the methods of clinical application according to the heaviness or lightness of the techniques employed; that is, according to the subjective sensations experienced by the patient. In this regard, a useful distinction is made in Japan by referring to *shigeki ryoho*, stimulation therapy, and *qi* therapy, for example *keiraku chiryo* (or channel therapy). This is essentially a distinction of the degree to which the patient experiences a subjective reaction to the therapy and the degree of stimulation applied. The concept of 'stimulation' includes the Chinese concept of *de qi*, where needling is applied until the patient becomes aware of certain feelings (soreness, numbness, pain, or distension). However, it also includes the application of any technique that gives the patient a strong response (e.g. hot moxibustion or electro acupuncture). We have chosen to arrange methods and techniques in five levels following these basic distinctions:

1. The application of extremely delicate techniques and tools. The patient feels no stimulation.
2. The application of delicate techniques and tools where the patient experiences some sensation, but little stimulation.
3. The application of techniques and tools where the patient is clearly aware of the method applied, but where little stimulation is given.
4. The application of techniques and tools where the patient is very aware of the method applied and the stimulation given.
5. The application of techniques and tools where the patient is not only very aware of method but also strongly perceives the stimulation.

Given this five-level framework, essentially a range from no subjective sensation to very strong sensation, common treatment methods could be arranged as follows.

At level 1 we would place the subtler variants of *keiraku chiryo*, such as *Toyohari*, non-insertion and touching–needling techniques, the application of color, 'cold' lasers, or microwave radiation. At level 2 there are light moxibustion, intradermal needles, shallowly and delicately inserted needles, techniques characteristic of Japanese *keiraku chiryo*, US microstimulation approaches, and Korean hand acupuncture. Most forms of light needling, including ion pumping, two-metal contact, most 'micro-system' techniques (e.g. ear acupuncture), warm moxibustion, and Japanese pediatric *shonishin* tech-

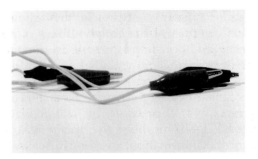

Figure 7.11 Ion pumping cords. (Courtesy of Paradigm Publications.)

niques belong at level 3. At level 4 are the lighter or mild needling techniques of modern Chinese acupuncture. The *de qi* sensation is elicited, and generally deeper needling techniques are applied. Hotter moxa techniques, bloodletting, and cupping also belong at level 4. At level 5 are the heavier *de qi* sensations of normal to strong modern Chinese acupuncture, very hot moxibustion, electro acupuncture, surgical acupuncture analgesia, and very strong cupping.

Because there are no objective standards for measuring needling sensation, any one expert might disagree with where we have placed a specific method or technique in either of these two arrangements. For example, what one practitioner thinks of as 'normal to mild' Chinese needling another may find 'strong.' However, regardless of any particular bias, these basic levels are relatively correct. For example, although a Chinese acupuncturist might feel that normal Chinese needling belongs to a higher level, he or she would not likely think that level to be higher than for electro acupuncture analgesia. Thus these levels can help clarify a number of important distinctions, particularly with regard to the research issues discussed previously (see Chs 4 and 5).

We have also discussed the fact that the great diversity within acupuncture makes it difficult to embrace all approaches and methods in a single model. However, even when this diversity is ignored, each model put forward to explain acupuncture tends to be offered as all-embracing. Thus when the models are put to the test, the results are often limited. To understand this problem, it is useful to look at an arrangement of the field that places different approaches according to the different research methods required by each. Here, again, we are following the schema developed by Dan Kenner.[19] He proposes that there are essentially four types of acupuncture, each of which is informed by a distinctly different theoretical approach. In other words, there are four general forms for which different treatment targets and different treatment techniques apply:

1. Acupuncture analgesia, including any heavy stimulation method intended for pain control.
2. Acupuncture physical therapy, the needling of anatomical structures such as trigger and motor points.
3. Channel acupuncture, including most traditional methods.
4. Homuncular acupuncture, micro-systems such as ear, hand, or nose acupuncture.

These four types parallel the classification of the stimulus used. The strength of the stimulus decreases incrementally from level 1 to level 4. Kenner argues that the first two types are rooted in biomedical knowledge, neuroanatomy, and physiology. Types 3 and 4 are rooted in field and information theory. In other words, those systems of therapy that apply heavier techniques activate mechanisms best described by anatomy and physiology. Those systems that use lighter techniques activate mechanisms that are best described by emerging descriptions of the body's information-processing systems. Systems of practice that involve levels 1 and 2 tend to reject or subsume traditional models, relying instead on biomedical concepts. Systems of practice at levels 3 and 4 tend to rely on traditional models or have parallel models developed in the modern era.

Aside from serving as maps for organizing and labeling methods of acupuncture practice, these categorizations segue with the research issues discussed in Chapters 4 and 5. For example, do the explanatory models that have been developed for acupuncture analgesia or acupuncture physical therapy tell us anything about systems of practice that use much lighter

stimulation? Are there explanatory models for lighter methods of practice that are compatible with traditional theories? Can the research methods appropriate to levels 1 and 2 be used to explore levels 3 and 4, or vice versa? Thus, as we examine cases, it is important to be aware of these technical differences.

CASE HISTORIES

Because our aim is to describe accurately treatments that exemplify the range of acupuncture practiced, the following case descriptions were taken either from formal sources or obtained from practitioners with whom we could conveniently interact. However, we also surveyed clinical textbooks and surveyed working acupuncturists through written responses to a practitioner questionnaire. Thus, the following cases exemplify techniques commonly used by those who have identified themselves as belonging to major schools of thought and practice.[20] This is far from absolute proof of generality, but the cases described here are probably fairly representative.

Boxes 7.2 to 7.7 give descriptions of fictionalized cases that were created in order to illustrate the various mixes of theoretical and technical qualities used in treatment. In these six cases, each of the following qualities is assessed:

- explanatory model of sources
- main pattern identification method
- root treatment logic
- symptom control treatment logic
- source of tools used.

Each of these qualities is rated as follows:

1. only traditional methods and sources
2. mainly traditional, but some modern methods
3. mixed traditional and modern methods
4. mainly modern, but some traditional methods
5. only modern methods and sources.

Similarly, stimulus level is rated as follows:

1. very mild
2. mild
3. moderate
4. strong
5. very strong.

Traditional Chinese medical acupuncture

The *ba gang bian zheng* (TCM) system predominantly uses medium to wide gauge (0.26–0.30 mm) needles, inserted somewhat deeply to obtain *de qi*. Most TCM authorities assert that without *de qi* (stimulation level 4), treatment will be ineffective. These practitioners use direct and indirect moxibustion, electro-acupuncture, cupping, and bloodletting. Practitioners in this system incorporate other techniques to varying degrees, whether or not they fit the *ba gang* system. Examples of these are: microsystems such as ear acupuncture, facial acupuncture, periocular and perinasal acupuncture, scalp acupuncture, foot acupuncture, hand acupuncture, and the 'wrist and ankle system' of Zhang Xin-shu. Also incorporated are suture embedding, acupoint injection, incision, and direct stimulation of the nerve root, although not usually in Western nations. Many practitioners also combine the use of traditional medicines with acupuncture, as has been the trend in China during recent decades. In the TCM cases described below, we have included cases where pharmacotherapy was and was not used.

The following cases were provided by Nigel Wiseman. These cases are illustrative of the *ba gang bian zheng* system as it is used in both the Republic of China and the People's Republic of China, The first two cases are from a Taiwanese physician acupuncturist.

Case 1

Patient: Female, 57 years.

Main complaint: For the last 15 years, frequent common colds with cough and panting especially in hot weather.

Symptoms: Cough that prevents sleep, hasty breathing with copious phlegm, phlegm rale, chest pain associated with coughing, and constipation.

Examination: (Palpation) Slippery floating pulse. (Inspection) White slimy tongue fur, large solid build.

Diagnosis: Phlegm–rheum panting.

Treatment strategy: Transform phlegm to relieve breathing.

Acupoints were selected to: Anesthetize the bronchi, transform phlegm, dissipate depressed *qi*, upbear the clear and downbear the turbid.

Treatment and outcome: On the first visit, a single acupoint was needled bilaterally on the legs. Two days later, the patient returned and reported that the panting was relieved and the stool freed. On this occasion, acupoints at the top of the sternum and two bilateral points on the legs were needled. Two days later there was marked improvement, and on this occasion a single bilateral acupoint on the arms was needled. In the next three treatments the same acupoints were used. After a total of seven sessions, the patient was discharged. Two years later the patient returned with her husband and reported no recurrence since the initial treatments.

Case 2

Patient: Male, 56 years.

Main complaint: Nearly normal vision in the day time, but poor vision or a complete loss of vision at night or in dark places.

Symptoms: Sudden poor, blurred vision in the evening, normal vision in daylight.

Examination: No visible obstruction; blood pressure normal.

Diagnosis: Poor night vision due to lack of nutrition.

Treatment strategy: Enrich the kidney and calm the liver to restore vision.

Acupoints were selected to: Dissipate local *qi* stagnation, enrich kidney water, calm liver *qi*, downbear turbid *qi*, and improve the assimilation of nutrients.

Treatment and outcome: A bilateral acupoint at the inner corner of the eyes, two acupoints on the back, and two on the legs were needled, and moxa was applied to the knuckles of the thumb. The patient was relieved in six treatments using these points, and was completely returned to normal.

The following three *ba gang* cases are from practitioners in the People's Republic of China.

Box 7.2 Brief case: male, 42 years, People's Republic of China

The patient, a hospital administrator, first went to the busy acupuncture clinic at his Beijing hospital for relief of osteoarthritis in his neck, wrists, and knees. He had first chosen to see a rheumatologist, who prescribed anti-inflammatory medication. While the medicine helped, the patient became concerned because his condition improved so little. He decided to go to the acupuncture clinic, because it had a good reputation for treating chronic pain.

The patient was seated in a large room with many other patients. The acupuncturists were moving among all the patients, questioning and then treating each one. Finally, an acupuncturist arrived at the patient's side. She questioned him, looked briefly at his tongue, and quickly felt his wrists. Then, while the patient was sitting in the chair, she quickly inserted needles to points in his hands, wrists, shoulders, occipital region, around the knees, and on the tops of his feet. She asked the patient at each point whether he felt a distinctive sensation, and stopped twirling the needle when he reported feeling *de qi*. While he was still sitting with needles in place, she connected the leads of an electrical stimulator to points on his knees and shoulders, increasing the current intensity until the muscles near the connected needles twitched. Then she ordered blood tests and instructed the patient to see the phlebotomist as soon as the treatment was complete.

After 30 minutes the machine was turned off and the needles removed. The patient felt distinctively better, with less stiffness and pain. He was happy to return daily for the next 9 days.

Explanatory model of sources: 3
Main pattern identification method: 3
Ba gang root treatment logic: 3
Symptom control treatment logic: 3–4
Source of tools used: 3–5
Stimulus level: 4–5
Relative cost to patient: None

The first is from Jiang You Guang, Acupuncture Department Director and Physician of the Chinese Medical Research School, Guang An Gate Hospital.

Case 3

Patient: Male, 65 years.

Main complaint: Five days earlier when arising in the morning the patient, a commune member, felt that the limbs on his left side were feeble and difficult to use, especially the leg. He was unable to get on the ground and walk, sitting up was difficult, and he was unable to grasp objects in his left hand. In addition, he had headache and constipation.

Examination: (Inspection) The patient had a clear spirit. The left side of his nasolabial groove was slightly more shallow than the opposite side. The tongue was straight, but the brachial muscles had increased tension. Grasping strength of the left hand was poor compared to the opposite side. The biceps and triceps muscles of the arm had normal reflexes. The pulse was vacuous and wiry. Blood pressure was 160/100 mmHg. The tongue fur was white and thin. (Palpation) The left side abdominal fullness sign was positive, the left knee was hyperreflexive, and there was clonus in the left ankle. The Achilles tendon reflex was normal, and Babinski's sign was negative.

Diagnosis: Based on these observations the diagnosis made was wind stroke hemiplegia (channel stroke). It ascribes to empty and vacuous connecting vessels that develop *bi* obstructions.

Acupoints were selected to: course wind and free the connecting vessels, all on the left side.

Treatment and outcome: The needling sensation was guided to the tips of the extremities; strong sensation was employed, but the needles were not retained. After 16 days and eight acupuncture treatments, the left-sided hemiplegia was basically ameliorated, and the patient's blood pressure was 130/90 mmHg.

Jiang You Guang's comments regarding technique describe both the treatment logic and technique. Although *bi* is often translated just as 'rheumatism,' it actually refers to a variety of pathoconditions having to do with obstruction.

The above case of wind stroke ascribes to channel stroke, with wind evil creating a *bi* obstruction of the channel *qi*; it is primarily marked by hemiplegia. The principles for treatment are to course and free the channels and connecting vessels. The *Ling Shu* contains the saying: 'The essence of needling is that when *qi* arrives the treatment is effective.' When treating hemiplegia in the clinic, acupuncturists are required to use a needle sensation that produces numbness and distension, and for this sensation to be conducted into the crippled limb. If the stimulation is strong, one can obtain good results.

In Jiang You Guang's detailed treatment record, he refers to stimuli of 'an electric sensation that goes from the shoulder to the upper brachia, lower brachia, and into the tips of the thumb and index finger.' Regarding another point: 'an electrocution feeling extends into the thumb, and the index, middle, and ring fingers.' In other words, his treatment is composed of techniques with stimulus levels 4 to 5 which he considers essential to efficacy.

The following is a case from the acupuncture department of the Tian Jin TCM College Affiliated Hospital.

Case 4

Patient: Female, 46 years.

Main complaint: While sleeping at night, the right shoulder of the patient (a school teacher) was exposed outside the blankets. When getting up the following day she felt pain in the right shoulder. After a month the pain in the right shoulder was more severe, and the shoulder's range of motion had decreased. The pain was particularly bad during the night, and affected her sleep. The patient was unable to comb her hair.

Examination: (Inspection) There was no abnormality in the outer appearance of the right shoulder. (Biomedical) The shoulder's activities were noticeably hindered. The upper arm when raised to the anterior could reach an angle of 60°, posterior extension reached 30°, and lateral abduction reached 45°.

Treatment strategy: Free the channels and quicken the blood.

Acupoints were selected to: Course wind and free the channels.

Treatment and outcome: Acupoints were needled to a depth of 1–2 *cun* with a filiform needle; lifting and thrusting with rotation was applied to one acupoint, and lifting and thrusting with twirling for another. While needling a point on the leg, a sensation of

numbness and distension was directed to the foot and the patient was instructed to move the affected shoulder during insertion. When the pain stopped or was reduced the needle was removed. Fluid injection therapy was also employed. After 1 week of treatment the pain was reduced, the right shoulder could be raised to reach past the head, the patient could manage to comb her own hair, and she was able to sleep at night. After treatment for 1 month the pain was ameliorated.

The comments in the above case note that, due to sleeping in the winter season, cold evil exploited vacuity to enter and invade the shoulder region. *Qi* and blood were obstructed and stagnated by the cold evil, and thus were blocked and not free. This manifested as painful *bi* and disuse ('with flow stoppage there is pain'), and therefore the treatment was primarily to free the channels and quicken the blood.

The following TCM case is from an anthology of case histories published in the People's Republic of China. Dr Shao Jing Ming is the director of the Acupuncture Research Office in the He Nan College of TCM, where he is an Assistant Professor.

Case 5

Patient: Female, 19 years.

Main complaint: The patient had gastroptosis for half a year. The year before she had joined in the work of digging a river and carrying earth. From that time she started to have uncomfortable feelings after eating (distension around her stomach and a sinking sensation). At times there was slight pain. Her dietary intake decreased, and medical treatment had no effect. She was thinner and weaker than before. Almost 2 years earlier at the Number One People's Hospital of Kai Feng Municipality, barium-meal radiographs showed that the stomach had fallen on both sides to 9 cm inferior to the line connecting the iliac crests. This was diagnosed as gastroptosis.

Examination: (Palpation) The pulse reading was deep, moderate, and forceless. The tongue fur was thin and white; the tongue substance was pale red. (Inspection) The patient had a lusterless facial complexion, and when lying flat her upper abdomen was boat shaped.

Diagnosis: The diagnosis was spleen and stomach vacuity and weakness, and downward falling center *qi*. This, combined with the barium-meal X-ray images, conformed to a second-degree gastroptosis.

Treatment strategy: Fortify the spleen, boost *qi*, and upbear the clear.

Acupoints selected for treatment: a fixed formula for gastroptosis and gastrointestinal disorders.

Treatment and outcome: Acupuncture was performed on alternating days. Each time the needles were retained for approximately 20 minutes, with the needles moved 2 or 3 times during the treatment period. On one acupoint the needles were inserted obliquely to a depth of 2.5–3 *cun*. A medium-strong hand stimulation method was employed to make the patient feel a relatively strong sensation of contraction and lifting. After nine treatments the patient's appetite had returned, and there was obvious improvement in the abdominal distension and sinking. After resting for a week, another three acupuncture treatments were performed, and the patient felt that all the symptoms had been ameliorated. A barium-meal X-ray examination on April 13 showed that the position of the stomach had returned to normal. In a follow-up examination half a year later, the patient had robust health, and to that time had no recurrence of the disease.

The acupuncturist made the following comments on the above case.

Gastroptosis is frequently due to a weak constitution, or else the effect of a chronic illness that leads to a decline of the dynamic capacity of the spleen–stomach. This results in downward falling center *qi*. In this particular circumstance the patient's problem developed from doing heavy physical labor. The patient had normal health and did not reach the depths of debilitation, so the acupuncture treatment was able to reap a fine result, with no further relapses of the disease.

This fixed, routine point formula for treating gastroptosis and gastrointestinal disorders promotes peristalsis of the stomach and intestines and assists digestion, speeding up expulsion of air. Because of this, it frequently happens that after acupuncture treatments there is an increase in appetite, abdominal distension and stomach pains are reduced or eliminated, and there is a restraining effect on acidity (pantothenic acid) and belching. Because the points stimulated pertain to the foot *tai yin* spleen channel, needling can accomplish the work of fortifying the spleen, boosting *qi*, and upbearing the clear. One should master the needle direction. Needle obliquely along the epidermis toward the umbilical region, but do not allow the needle point to enter the abdominal cavity; this is in order to avoid damaging the internal organs.

The next case illustrates how traditional Chinese acupuncture is used in the USA by an experienced American acupuncturist. Bill Prensky is one of the original US acupuncturists, and not only does he have one of the longest-standing clinical practices in the USA, but he also introduced the Chinese acupuncturist Tin Yau So, clinical trials, and the development of the first acupuncture center and school in the USA. Bill is presently a Governor of the National Academy of Acupuncture and Oriental Medicine, and Dean of the Mercy College acupuncture program.

Note the stronger emphasis on the psychological aspects of the case, which is both in keeping with Prensky's academic background, general trends in US patient populations, and the circumstances of the patient's complaint. This case is also interesting because it highlights correspondences predicted by theories of systematic correspondence. Both the patient's affect and presenting physical problems correspond to his earlier liver disease.

Case 6

Patient: Male, 26 years.

Main complaint: At the time of presentation, the patient was an otherwise healthy man. At the age of 22 he had contracted infectious hepatitis (type A), during a trip to the coast of Mexico and after eating what was presumably contaminated raw seafood.

The patient was an engineering major at university, with a demanding and high-pressure curriculum. His hepatitis resolved itself normally in about 10 weeks, with seemingly little sequeli, except for a tendency towards more angry outbursts during frustrating situations in school. Because his girlfriend was a psychology major, he was urged to attempt psychological approaches to therapy for his anger, and was treated by psychological counseling for about 6 months. During that time he reported that he 'got in touch with his feelings' and 'learned to anticipate his anger,' becoming 'able to deal with it and channel it in other directions.'

Symptoms: Approximately 4 years after the bout of hepatitis, the patient developed vision problems, with diminished sight and loss of visual acuity.

Examination: (Biomedical) Complete medical evaluation could reveal no obvious cause for the patient's condition; all laboratory and physical examination results were negative. He was able to see, but reported that his vision was dimmed almost to the point of legal blindness. There was no visible retinal pathology, nor was there damage to the optic nerve. His intraocular pressure was normal. (Inquiry) The patient's experiences with his anger and frustration in counseling were explored by his physician, but were given consideration only in arriving at a conclusive diagnosis of 'hysterical (conversion) disorder manifesting as hysterical blindness.' He was advised to seek further psychological therapy. Six months of further counseling and psychotherapy produced no change in his condition. The patient then sought acupuncture and Oriental medicine therapy, on the advice of a new girlfriend who was a student of these subjects. Evaluation of the patient's condition revealed a condition of continued depression of the liver *qi*, with some occasional headaches and a feeling of heaviness in the hypochondrium. The patient's description of his previous state of chronic anger following his hepatitis were explored in the evaluation.

Diagnosis: Depression of liver *qi*.

Treatment strategy: Rectify liver *qi*.

Acupoints were selected to: Rectify liver *qi*.

Treatment and outcome: The treatment plan included both acupuncture and herbal medicines. Almost immediately, within 2 weeks of beginning treatment, the patient reported that he felt much calmer, no longer angry, and that his headaches had disappeared. His abdomen felt more normal and 'cooler.' His vision began to return to normal, and, slowly, over the next 2 months, he reported that his vision was no longer dimmed and that he was able to see at night and to drive at night for the first time since these problems had begun. The patient was discharged from treatment after 3 months of weekly acupuncture, and has reported no return of symptoms after 2 years.

The following case comes from the busy practice of Pat Culliton, a practitioner with more than 15 years' experience who has trained with Korean, Chinese, and American senior teachers. Pat is the Clinical Director of the Alternative Medicine Clinic at the Hennepin County Medical Center in Minneapolis. Although much of her work there focuses on the treatment and rehabilitation of patients with problems of substance abuse, she maintains a private practice using TCM acupuncture.

Case 7

Patient: Female, 47 years.

Main complaints: The patient had suffered interstitial cystitis for 10 years. She suffered from frequent, burning urination, night urination, pelvic pain, insomnia, and fatigue. She had to stay constantly close to a bathroom, was easily irritated, emotionally fragile, and suffered from mild depression. She had been a nurse and lobbyist, a homemaker and mother, but the cystitis had made her unable to work, and had also limited her capacities as a homemaker and mother. She had poor temperature control, easily becoming chilled or hot. She had tried many different medications over the years, with no success.

Box 7.3 Brief case: male, 36 years, USA

The patient, a carpenter from San Francisco, finally went for acupuncture because his friends had been encouraging him to do so. They all knew about his bad back. Over the years his lower back had become worse and worse, and was now 'going out' every few months, leaving him unable to work for as much as a week at a time.

The acupuncturist, a Chinese American in his fifties, felt the patient's wrist as he questioned him and carefully inspected his tongue. The acupuncturist then explained that the problem was related to 'insufficient kidney *yang*,' which was why he also awoke to urinate every night, felt cold easily, and was fatigued so much of the time. To the patient's surprise the acupuncturist also explained that there was 'cold damp wind' stuck in his back. He was told that this was why his back pain worsened in inclement weather.

The patient felt a 'jolt,' a tingling and grabbing sensation that was not really a pain, as the acupuncturist inserted and manipulated the needles. While the patient was lying on the table, the acupuncturist held a lighted 'moxa cigar' near each of the needles in his back as he explained to the patient that we would like him to take some herbs. Did he want to boil them himself, or would he rather take a powdered preparation?

At the end of treatment the patient felt invigorated, warmer, and his lower back felt somehow lighter. He was a little nervous about the odd-looking things in the packets of medicine he was given, but he was reassured that it would help and would not smell or taste too bad. As he was leaving, the patient was asked to bring his insurance information with him when he returned in 3 days.

Explanatory model of sources: 3
Main pattern identification method: 3
Ba gang root treatment logic: 3
Symptom control treatment logic: 3
Source of tools used: 3
Stimulus level: 4
Relative cost to patient: about US $60–90

Examination: (Inspection) red and dry tongue with a white greasy coating. Facial rosacea. (Palpation) Occlusion of the right radial artery from an accident; the left pulse was weak and rapid.

Diagnosis: Damp-heat in the small intestine and liver *yin* vacuity.

Treatment and outcome: The patient was needled at two points on the legs, one or two points on the arms, two points on the lower abdomen, three points in each ear, and, on alternate treatments, two or three points on the back. She was also instructed to apply acupressure to a point above each inner ankle daily. She was treated twice a week for the first 6 weeks, once a week for the next 6 weeks, and then every other week, tapering off. After the first year, the patient attended the clinic once or twice every few months as needed for relief of recurring symptoms.

After 2 weeks of treatment the pain began to improve. After 6 weeks there was improvement of the night urination, frequency, urgency, and burning on urination. This allowed the patient to sleep better, and she was able to regain her energy. She was once again able to participate more fully in family, social, and church functions, all of which helped relieve her depression and emotional debility. Approximately 2 years after beginning treatment, with teary eyes, the patient reported that for the first time she had been able to watch her son perform at a state championship athletic event. She had been unable to do this before because there were no toilet facilities at such events. She had been outside for a total of 6 hours!

At the time of reporting this case, Pat Culliton described what she had most recently heard from her patient. She was teaching in Russia where there were no indoor bathrooms and the living conditions were very austere. She was managing with no problems, something that would have been impossible only a few years before. Although the patient feels that she is not completely cured of the illness, she is able to function at a virtually normal level of activity for the first time in 13 years. She self-administers acupressure to control any symptoms when they arise.

Pat Culliton has experience of a number of similar cases of successful treatment of interstitial cystitis, a disease for which there is very little medical relief. It is extremely debilitating, and thus depressing, for those who suffer it. At this time Pat is collecting more data, and hopes that a grant application to the National Institutes of Health, Washington, DC, will provide her the funds required to test the treatment experimentally. If she is successful, her work will bring relief to many who suffer from this disease.

Traditional Japanese channel therapy

Keiraku chiryo, traditional Japanese channel therapy, is notable for its use of extremely fine, thin needles (0.12–0.14 mm wide) that are inserted to a depth of only 1–2 mm, or are not inserted at all. Because the emphasis is on regulating *qi* and not on stimulating anatomical or physiological functions, the patient rarely feels the needling. There is also a greater emphasis on the training and sensitivity of the practitioner. As Dan Kenner states: 'This training is for your intuition, and to develop your touch and observation skills.'[21] It is the practitioner who must feel the *qi*, so that the change produced by needling may be gauged during treatment. Treatment varies according to the practitioner's skills and beliefs. Practitioners such as Toshio Yanagishita of the *Toyohari* Association rarely, if ever, do symptom-control needling. Their emphasis is almost exclusively on root treatment, which is understood as promoting the balanced flow of *qi* in the channels.

The following case from Denmei Shudo illustrates how the system is used. Shudo is one of Japan's premier acupuncturists, an articulate leader and respected writer whose work has recently been introduced in the USA.[22] The supplementation needling technique involves the use of needles that barely break the skin, being inserted just enough to remain in the acupoint. The other needle techniques involve insertion to a maximum of only a few millimeters. Note, however, the immediate changes in blood pressure that occur without any of the *de qi* reactions normally associated with the release of neurochemicals.

Case 8

Patient: Female, 70 years.
Main complaint: The patient awoke that morning with acute dizziness and nausea.

Symptoms: The patient's blood pressure while prone on the treatment bed was 185/105 mmHg. It appeared that her symptoms were due to an acute elevation of blood pressure.
Examination: (Palpation) The second and third deep left (liver and kidney) radial pulses were weak.
Diagnosis: The patient's pulse indicated a liver vacuity pattern.
Treatment and outcome: With the patient lying on her back with her eyes closed, a needle was inserted to a midline point on the skull just behind the forward hairline. Needles were inserted to the dizziness points in each ear. Supplementation technique was applied to two acupoints on the knees, and to an acupoint near each elbow. The needles were retained in the points. The patient was still dizzy when she opened her eyes. Acupoints in the occipital region were needled and all the needles were retained for another 15 minutes. After this, she reported no further dizziness, even when she opened her eyes. Her blood pressure was taken again, reading 152/90 mmHg. All needles except those in the ear and midline skull points were then removed. The patient was asked to sit up and moxa was applied to a point on each shoulder. The remaining needles were removed and intradermal needles were placed at the dizziness points in the ears. The patient reported no further symptoms. Her blood pressure was taken again, reading 140/90 mmHg.

The patient returned for two more visits; the same treatment was applied. Treatment was then discontinued, as she had no further symptoms and her blood pressure remained steady and closer to normal.

The following case from Birch's practice illustrates the *Toyohari* style of traditional Japanese channel therapy. Note that, with the exception of the use of intradermal needles on the back, no needles were inserted. In the *Toyohari* style of treatment, the basic needling techniques involve the use of very thin silver needles that are held at the skin surface to produce changes in the *qi* system, these changes being observed through changes in the pulse taken at the radial arteries.

The patient, a bank clerk, first went to the large acupuncture center in Tokyo for her menstrual pain and headaches. The center had a tremendous reputation with her friends at work. The 82-year-old blind man who was chief of the center was particularly revered. When the patient arrived at the center she was directed to a changing room where she dressed in loose-fitting treatment clothes. She was then called to a treatment bed in a large open room with many other patients, acupuncturists, and assistants. A young acupuncturist in his thirties introduced himself and began questioning her about her health. He then lightly touched her abdomen, legs, arm, and neck, spending a long time repeatedly examining the pulses at her wrists. When he was finished, he called the elderly blind acupuncturist who questioned both of them, and re-palpated her abdomen and wrist.

After confirming the treatment plan, he left the patient to be treated by the younger apprentice. When the apprentice began treatment, the patient asked him what he was doing, because she did not feel the needles. He explained that what he was doing was *ki* (*qi*) therapy, and that it was best done without actually inserting the needle. She was somewhat confused, but also pleased because she had been afraid of the needles anyway. When he had finished, he called another assistant who burnt moxa on the patient's back, neck, wrists, and ankles, and performed bloodletting and cupping on her upper back. Finally, the senior acupuncturist returned to check the treatment. After scolding his apprentice for not finishing the treatment properly, he joked with the patient and promised that she would feel better before she left. He added his touches to her treatment.

When the treatment was finished, the patient felt very invigorated, mentally clear, and fresh, as if she were waking from a relaxing rest. She dressed and paid for her treatment, scheduling a second visit at the end of the week.

Explanatory model of sources: 1
Main pattern identification method: 1
Keiraku chiryo root treatment logic: 1
Symptom control treatment logic: 1–3
Source of tools used: 1–2
Stimulus level: 1–4
Relative cost to patient: about US $50–100

Case 9

Patient: Male, 7 years.

Main complaint: Severe asthma since the age of 3 years. Since the start of his asthmatic symptoms, the patient had spent up to 8 months of every year on steroid medications, and used an inhaler and a nebulizer to control his symp-

toms. He required several visits to an emergency room and had been hospitalized once. The asthma would typically begin as a cough following a cold or other viral infection, rapidly progressing to a full, acute asthma attack. The symptoms restricted his activities; he could not run normally and thus had difficulty engaging in childhood sports with his friends. He also had seasonal and allergic sensitivities.

Examination: (Inquiry) The patient appeared basically healthy except for his symptoms. He appeared to be very sensitive, which is typical of children in general, and made it known that he did not expect to be needled. He consumed large quantities of cow's milk products but had no clear allergic reaction to them. (Palpation) The radial pulses were generally a little weak and evidenced a liver pattern. The abdomen showed stiffness over both subcostal regions, with some stiffness to the left of the navel, and lack of luster in the lower left quadrant of the abdomen. Examination of his back revealed remarkable tightness and reactivity on the upper back around points traditionally associated with asthma (the so-called 'asthma yu (*shu*) points[9]).' Simply touching the area made him cringe and cry.

Diagnosis: Liver vacuity, probably with secondary lung vacuity with involvement of the *yin wei-chong mai*.

Treatment and outcome: As is always the case when treating children, the first treatment was aimed at making the patient comfortable with the practitioner and helping him understand that it was a safe and painless experience. The *shonishin*, Japanese pediatric acupuncture style acupuncture (see below), and the *Toyohari* systems of acupuncture can be applied without insertion. For a child who is very needle shy, this was obviously the right place to start. A basic *shonishin* treatment was applied (rubbing the limbs and back with an *enshin*, and tapping with a *herabari* on the upper back). Supplementation was then applied using a *teishin* to two points on the left knee, to strengthen the liver vacuity. Tiny press-spheres (small metal pellets) were taped over the sensitive points on the upper back. The first treatment finished with a lengthy discussion of the probable need to reduce and then eliminate the consumption of dairy food. This treatment regimen was followed once a week over a period of 6 weeks, during which the patient also eliminated dairy products from his diet. Despite a cold, he did not progress beyond minor asthma symptoms.

With further treatments he became comfortable enough to allow intradermal needles to be left in the sensitive points on his upper back. He allowed Birch to use thin silver needles in place of the *teishin* to administer the *toyohari* root treatment. As the winter season descended, the patient's worst season, he strayed from his dairy-free diet, triggering a progression of symptoms sufficiently strong that his parents considered using drugs again. At this session cupping was used on the back. The patient's symptoms improved dramatically. After this episode, cupping was used on a regular basis. The patient has received over 30 treatments during the course of a year and has had no major asthma attacks, no need for steroids, and has greatly reduced his use of the inhalant and nebulized medications. He is able to participate in sports and physical activities, and was impressed enough with the acupuncture to choose it as the topic for his school project.

English traditional acupuncture

English traditional acupuncture is a five-phase system. It typically involves the use of 0.12–0.20 mm needles, and both direct and indirect moxibustion. Treatments are aimed at correcting constitutional problems at the levels of the five phases and 12 officials, which are described as functional relationships and their subsystems, left–right channel imbalances determined by Akabane's method, and clearing energy blocks or disturbances, using techniques such as the 'aggressive energy treatment,' the 'internal dragon' and 'external dragon,' and the 'conception vessel-governing vessel' treatment. The basic approach is to identify and clear stagnation, and to transfer *qi* within and between the phases and officials.

The following case comes from senior practitioner Zoe Brenner of Bethesda, Maryland. It shows how the traditional acupuncture system of practice is combined with other methods of practice to suit the needs of each patient. It clearly illustrates an acculturation of this method of practice. Note that the pattern and acupoint indications in this system include features of the patient's personal, familial, and social relationships.

Case 10

Patient: Female, 50 years.

Main complaint: Severe migraines since childhood which were unresponsive to medication. The patient experienced loss of peripheral vision and nausea with migraines that started on the right and settled on the left eye.

Symptoms: The patient was menopausal (no menses for 9 months), but reported only a few hot flashes and some weight gain during the last year. She had minor problems with urination, and seasonal allergies.

Examination: (Inquiry) The patient had been in a serious car accident 3 years prior to presentation. She had undergone reconstructive surgery and a metal plate was inserted in her left cheek. There had been problems in her family, an abusive uncle, which left one of her sisters 'emotionally disabled.' This, combined with a family history of cancer, rendered her the primary caregiver for her family. The patient was softly spoken, frequently apologizing for herself. Her voice had a singing quality and she liked sweets. She was sweet, kind, and overly concerned for others. (Visual and Olfactory) The patient had a fragrant body odor, and a green and yellow face. (Palpation) Both wood pulses had a tight, full quality. Her fire pulses were low, her earth pulses were slippery and full, metal was floating and water low. Stomach and gallbladder abdominal points were reactive and numbness was found on the left stomach channel on the face below the eye. The neck and jaw regions were tight. (Akabane testing) Left–right imbalances were found on the spleen, stomach, gallbladder, kidney, bladder, *san jiao*, pericardium, and lung channels.

Diagnosis: Primary assessment — earth with secondary wood imbalance. The earth was replete, oppressed on the outside (stomach) and vacuous on the inside (spleen). The wood was stagnant and unable to control the earth. Secondary assessment: problems on the stomach and gallbladder channels on the face (result of car-accident injury).

Treatment and outcome: The first treatment concentrated on correcting the Akabane imbalances. At the next visit the patient reported that she had been better and that the migraine she did experience was not as debilitating. At this second visit, treatment was focused on needling one face, one hand, and one foot point. At the next visit the patient reported that almost an entire week had passed without a migraine and that she felt greater emotional stability. At this visit, two arm acupoints were needled to 'pull the stagnation and pressure from earth to metal.' The next visit was 2 weeks later. The patient reported having only one mild headache and less anger. A point on the neck was treated to open the flow of *qi* into and out of her head. A point on the arm was needled to descend the *qi*. The next visit was 10 days later. The patient had not had a headache, but had experienced facial swelling over the metal plate and a release of sadness from crying a few days before. Palpation of the face found numbness and sensitivity at several points. Two facial points were needled, as was one point near the elbow, to 'encourage movement away from her face and towards a letting go.'

The next series of treatments, given on and off during the succeeding few months, had a similar focus. There was some needling of the face and needling to affect earth and wood, and to treat acupoints to 'clear the head and spirit,' and support the idea 'that she has something valuable to contribute to the world.' At the end of this treatment series, the patient was rarely having headaches and was not using any medication. She had a greater range of movement in her jaw. She had also become more confident and independent, and was re-fashioning her family's notion of who she was. Treatment appeared to have been successful in several layers, both at her core and in terms of her symptoms.

> **Box 7.5** Brief case: female, 26 years, USA
>
> The patient, a secretary from South Boston, went for acupuncture because she had been encouraged to by her mother who had obtained much relief of her arthritis. The patient told the practitioner of her headaches and problems with abdominal pain, distension, and cramping, with frequent bouts of diarrhea. Her gastroenterologist had told her that it was irritable bowel syndrome, and advised her to relax more often.
>
> When she first visited the acupuncturist, a young man in his thirties, she was surprised how many sore points he found on her abdomen, back, legs, arms, neck, and shoulders. That he spent so long feeling her wrist pulses seemed odd. After interviewing her and finding even more sore points, he explained her condition as a problem with two channels that started at her feet, running upward. What encouraged her was that his explanations presented her several seemingly unrelated symptoms as being due to this central underlying dysfunction.
>
> When he started treating her, she was very surprised that she felt no pain; indeed, the needles were so shallowly inserted that they seemed only barely to stay in place. Although she meant to ask, she became so relaxed that she forgot to inquire about the wires attached to the needles in her hands and feet, or what it was he used to heat the needles on her back. The needles he placed and taped on her back at the end of treatment were so tiny she could not see them without her glasses.
>
> When the acupuncturist was finished, the patient realized that her headache was gone and that she felt very loose all over. He instructed her to eliminate or reduce certain foods, and asked her to return for another treatment the following week. She paid for her treatment, knowing that her Health Maintenance Organization (HMO) would not cover the treatments, even though her internist thought that acupuncture might be a good idea.
>
> Explanatory model of sources: 4
> Main pattern identification method: 4
> *Yin-yang* channel-balancing root treatment logic: 4
> Symptom control treatment logic: 1–3
> Source of tools used: 1–2
> Stimulus level: 1–4
> Relative cost to patient: about US $50–100

The NADA acupuncture detoxification approach

The 'acupuncture detoxification' auriculo-therapy system, which has undergone significant development in the USA and, more recently, Eastern Europe, is exemplified by the work of Michael Smith of the Lincoln Hospital in Bronx, New York, and Pat Culliton at the Hennepin County

Medical Center, in Minneapolis, Minnesota, as well as many others. It predominantly uses relatively thin needles placed in ear points and, occasionally, a few body points. Mike Smith, and all the members of the National Acupuncture Detox Association (NADA), daily confront one of the world's most intransigent social problems: substance abuse and its complex of associated problems. If there is a 'drug war,' they are the front-line doctors. Some, like Mike Smith, have been there for 20 years. Their success in salvaging the lives of those who are most at risk, the addicts and their dependents, is arguably the most hopeful and productive innovation to emerge from the political uncertainty that surrounds prohibited drugs and the devastation wreaked by alcohol addiction.

The NADA acupuncture protocol developed exactly as we have seen acupuncture develop throughout East Asian history; that is, through the efforts of individuals who have used their practical observational skills and the rich theoretical foundation of acupuncture to confront a problem in the clinic. Their work is then taken up and developed by others in a variety of circumstances, gradually developing the refinement and broad experience required of the 'test of time.' Originally based on the work of Dr Wen of Hong Kong, who applied electrical stimulation to a single lung point,[23] the lack of funds and a nervous and demanding clientele forced continuous adaptation, the method reaching stability a little less than 10 years ago. In acupuncture's language, the protocol treats the complex of signs associated with an insufficiency of the functions associated with the symbol fire. To appreciate this traditional analogy, think of the flickering and unstable flame of a coal fire that has nearly exhausted its fuel. Flames flicker at the surface, fed only by the last gases released from the dying coals. In observational terms, the NADA protocol allows the addict to relax, alleviating not only the effects of withdrawal, but also the many restive behaviors common to addicts.

The NADA program is more that just an acupuncture treatment; acupuncture is the gateway to a whole program. It provides a foundation on which counseling, social and psychological therapy, and groups like Narcotics Anonymous can build. The following case is from Pat Culliton who runs the Alternative Medicine Clinic at the Hennepin County Medical Center, in Minneapolis. Pat is well known for an alcohol recidivism study that she co-authored. This brought considerable attention to the power of the NADA treatment when it was published in the *Lancet* in 1989.[24] This case shows that system's ability to transform the difficult and chaotic life of individuals caught in the trap of drug addiction.

Case 11

Patient: Male, 35 years.

Main complaints: The patient's history of alcohol and cocaine abuse with an inability to maintain sobriety included numerous detox episodes and deteriorating health, and family and social support. He had difficulty holding jobs, was divorced, and had problems with insomnia, decreased libido, gastric complaints, irritability, headaches, exhaustion, and fatigue.

Examination: (Inspection) Dark circles under the eyes; thin red tongue with a yellow coating on the back of the tongue. (Palpation) The pulse was rapid, thin, and wiry.

Diagnosis: A *yin* vacuity pattern typically found in substance-abusing patients; the beginning of signs of *yang* vacuity.

Treatment and outcome: Acupuncture was applied using the NADA detox protocol ear points, supplemented with arm and head points as necessary. Counseling was undertaken when required. The patient was treated with acupuncture daily, five days a week for the first month, and then three days a week for the next year. During this year, the patient remained sober, his family and social situations ameliorated, his health improved, and he was able to begin work and hold a job.

At the end of the year of treatment, the patient was asked if it was possible that he had transferred his alcohol and cocaine addiction to acupuncture, which, although viewed as healthy, was discussed as a potential problem. As a result of this discussion he reduced acupuncture treatment to once a week, and occasionally two to three times a week, for the next year. In the third year of treatment, the patient attended for treatment intermittently, only when it seemed necessary. Now, after 8 years of sobriety, he has his own business, is financially stable, and has achieved a stable family situation.

The patient claims that he was not addicted to acupuncture during the initial year of treatment. Rather, he felt that, after 15 years of heavy drug and alcohol abuse and chaotic living, he was so ill that it took that long to get well. In his own mind it never felt like an addiction, rather a choice for health. He now runs a business employing troubled kids, teaching them commercial painting, skills they use on houses in poor neighborhoods.

Based on current rates for the NADA programs in Minnesota that Pat Culliton helps operate, the total cost of this patient's treatment was approximately $800 — a nominal cost to transform a life totally.

Japanese *yin-yang* channel-balancing therapy

The Japanese *yin-yang* channel-balancing therapy system predominantly uses shallowly inserted needles, polarity applications such as the ion-pumping cords, needles with moxa on the handle, direct moxibustion, blood-letting, intradermal needles in body, ear, and hand acupoints, and simple, often 'at home,' structural adjustments. The following two cases from Birch's practice describe typical treatments employing *yin-yang* channel-balancing therapy.

Case 12

Patient: Male, 48 years.
Main complaints: Chronic low-back pain resulting from a skiing accident 4 years previously. The facette joints of the two lower lumbar vertebrae were crushed. The patient

had chronic stiffness of the lower back, with arthritis at the site of injury. The back pain was worse in cold or damp weather, and when the patient was fatigued. Aside from chronic diverticulitis, which had been corrected with a sigmoidectomy, he was relatively healthy.

Examination: (Palpation) The patient showed a very clear 'cross-syndrome' pattern on the abdomen, with weakness in the second and third deep left and second deep right pulses.

Diagnosis: A clear liver-related pattern.

Treatment and outcome: Manaka's four-step treatment process was employed.

1. One needle was placed in acupoints at each of the wrists and feet. Ion-pumping cords were attached for a few minutes.
2. Needles with moxa on the handles were applied to acupoints on the mid- to lower back.
3. A simple structural exercise (*sotai*) was performed.
4. Tiny intradermal needles were placed, one in the low back and two in the right ear.

The pulse is taken constantly throughout the treatment. It is not a diagnostic tool in the sense that it is used solely to determine the pattern. Rather it is a gauge of treatment, a source of feedback for each technique applied.

The patient returned for five more visits over the next 2 months. At each occasion, much the same treatment was applied. He saw significant improvement of the pain following the first treatment; by the third treatment, he reported being considerably less sensitive to cold and damp weather. By the last treatment, his back stiffness was virtually eliminated, and the pain significantly reduced. During the next 2 years, he returned for four more treatments when he experienced an acute back twinge and an injury to his right knee. At the last visit, 26 months after treatment had started, the patient's back pain remained significantly improved.

The patient described in the next case is typical in the sense that many seek treatment for conditions that fail to respond to biomedical treatment because they are well advanced, organic, or otherwise irremediable problems.

Case 13

Patient: Female, 66 years.

Main complaint: Atrial fibrillation, which had been treated for the last 3 years with various medications, including blood-thinning and diuretic medications. The fibrillation caused a shortness of breath that left the patient unable to function at normal activity levels. She had undergone many tests for the fibrillation, but her physicians had been unable to isolate the problem. The patient had severe chronic low-back problems. She had undergone surgery for a herniated disc 30 years before, and now had osteoarthritis of the lumbar spine and spinal stenosis with low-back and left-leg pain. If she raised her arms above shoulder level, she had increased pain, with weakness of the left leg. The patient also had osteoarthritis of the knees, and had already received a right knee replacement.

The patient's significant history also included probable fused cervical vertebrae, with stiffness and some pain of the neck, and irritable bowel syndrome. She had undergone a total hysterectomy 8 years previously for a precancerous condition. She had retired 5 years earlier and was not happy with retirement.

Examination: (Palpation) The subcostal region of the abdomen was tight and tender on palpation, indicating the *yin wei-chong mai* pattern. The pulse was very irregular and difficult to discern, but the right pulse was generally weaker than the left.

Diagnosis: Given the complexity of the patient's symptoms and the unclear etiology of the heart problem, an initial symptom-oriented treatment was commenced.

Treatment and outcome: A three-step treatment was applied:

1. Needles were applied to each wrist and foot, with ion-pumping cords attached.
2. Needles were shallowly inserted at a few acupoints on the neck, shoulders, and back.
3. Three tiny intradermal needles were inserted on the low back and left ear.

The patient returned the next week reporting that she had experienced less back and leg pain and was more 'nimble'. The same treatment was repeated, with the addition in step 2 of moxibustion applied to the handles of the needles inserted on the patient's back. Bloodletting and cupping were cautiously applied on the lower and upper back.

The patient returned a week later, reporting significant improvements in both the back and leg pain, but no change in the atrial fibrillation. The same or very similar treatment was applied seven times on a once-per-week schedule. During this period the patient continued to increase her activity levels, after which she went on a week-long canoeing trip. She returned from this trip feeling quite well, despite the almost continuous activity and strain, particularly on her lower back. She had sufficient energy, and her back and leg had taken strain without difficulty. However, the fibrillation remained unchanged.

The patient came for treatment seven more times over the next year. During that year, continued biomedical testing finally revealed multiple pulmonary embolisms and an enlarged heart; the condition was quite advanced. Her back and leg pain remained much improved. A year later she returned for treatment of a left-hip bursitis, which had not responded to treatment by physical therapy. A similar acupuncture treatment immediately improved the hip pain. A course of 10, once-a-week treatments was sufficient.

Despite having a chronic nonresponsive cardiovascular disorder which impaired heart function and thus adequate systemic circulation, the patient responded extremely well to acupuncture for the management of complex back and leg problems. She was able to gain more energy, despite advanced organic cardiovascular anomalies.

Medical acupuncture

The French and American medical acupuncture system developed by Mussat in France and further developed by Joseph Helms in the USA predominantly uses 0.30-mm gauge needles with indirect moxibustion or electrical stimulation. Generally, this system tries to use fewer points, in an effort to give the correct inputs. In his book, *Acupuncture Energetics: A Clinical Approach for Physicians,*[25] Helms describes how treatment attempts to create gradients that encourage energy flow in the correct directions and through blocked areas so as to restore more normal energy flows in the body. The needles are described as creating electrical polarity gradients that encourage tiny electrical flows from one needle to another. His work is based on French theoretical explanations of the physics of needles and needling, combined with traditional treatment principles.[26] This model of practice is taught in an educational program that allows physicians to assimilate it quickly and begin integrating it into their primary-care practices (See Box 7.7).

Box 7.6 Brief case: male, 37 years, Germany

The patient, an executive, had suffered problems with his right shoulder for many years. Doctors told him that it was from spending too much time working on his computer and from playing too much tennis. Usually when it bothered him he could quiet it with over-the-counter anti-inflammatory pain killers and ice, a little stretching, and a little massage. This time though, it had not responded. His doctor referred him to a pain clinic in a nearby Munich hospital.

After perusing his medical history and checking his right arm and rotator cuff range of motion, the specialist palpated the painful area, finding sore spots, which he called 'trigger points.' He found these very easily because there were several very tender ones on the shoulder, upper back, and arm. When the specialist inserted needles into the most painful of these points, the patient felt a very heavy throbbing sensation. The physician left the needles for about 10 minutes, and then checked to see if the points felt the same and whether the needles could be moved with less resistance. Most were better, but two were still very stiff and sensitive. He then attached an electrical stimulator to those two needles, and increased the current until the muscles twitched. After a few minutes, he shut off the electrical stimulator and checked the needles again. They were looser and less sensitive, and were removed. The patient felt looser, and his right arm and shoulder mobility had increased. As he left the clinic he was asked to give his insurance information to the office staff and to return in 2 weeks.

Explanatory model of sources: 5
Main pattern-identification method: 5
Trigger points root treatment logic: 5
Symptom control treatment logic: 5
Source of tools used: 3–5
Stimulus level: 4–5
Relative cost to patient: about US $50

Japanese children's needling

The Japanese *shonishin*, or children's needling methods of pediatric acupuncture, predominantly use a variety of noninserted needles/instruments with some light moxibustion and needling. On children under the age of 5 years, treatment rarely involves the use of inserted needles. Rather, rubbing, tapping, or stroking are used to stimulate the body surface. Over the age of 5 years, needles and moxa tend to be used more frequently, but typically with very light, delicate techniques. The following two of Birch's cases illustrate the *shonishin* approach, where treatment was applied very successfully.

Case 14

Patient: Female, 2 years.

Main complaint: During the last year the patient had suffered eight ear infections, repeated colds, two bouts of pneumonia, one of which required hospitalization, and had developed symptoms of cold-induced wheezing asthma. During the warmer months she had had one cold a month, and during the colder months, one a week. She had been treated with numerous courses of antibiotics during this year.

Examination: (Inquiry) The child's mother was quite distressed and frustrated by the chronic recurrent infections and the repeated courses of antibiotic therapy. The *Nan Jing* saying that to 'treat a vacuity in the child, one must supplement the mother' is a specific reference to a five-phase therapeutic strategy. It is also a traditional image analogy, so the difficult circumstances of the case suggested physically involving the mother in the treatment, by having her repeat treatments at home. Not only would this provide greater continuity to treatment, it would also support the mother, thereby helping the child as the mother's sense of helplessness was replaced by the positive feeling of helping in a noticeable way.

Treatment and outcome: Using the Japanese *zanshin* and *enshin shonishin* instruments, a whole-body treatment was applied. This treatment takes about 5 minutes and involves pressing, rubbing, and tapping the body surfaces with these instruments. The mother was taught how to give this treatment so that she could repeat it daily at home. The child had only one cold during the next three and a half months, only returning to the clinic just before Christmas. The chronic cycle of repeated infections seemed to have stopped.

Case 15

Patient: Female, 22 months.

Main complaint: The child was born with cerebral palsy. She had atonic spastic quadriparesis. Generally, her locomotor control, especially of the legs, was poor. She had no flexion contracture of the hips, and had limitations in mobility and range of motion of the legs, and structural problems of the feet due to spasticity. She was unable to push herself into a sitting position, and unable to walk even with support. The child had been receiving physical therapy twice a week for almost a year, craniosacral therapy twice a week, as well as regular speech therapy. Otherwise, the child was quite healthy and evidenced a very strong spirit.

Treatment and outcome: The mother and child flew into Boston from New York for the treatment, at great cost and inconvenience. Because of this, and the fact that Birch was soon to depart for summer-long studies in Japan, the mother was taught to apply regular daily *shonishin* at home.

A 5-minute *shonishin* treatment was applied to all body surfaces, focusing slightly more on the lower back, abdomen, and legs. A gentle source of electrical heat was applied to two key acupoints on the upper and lower spine. The rest of the visit was spent teaching the mother how to repeat the treatment. The mother was instructed to do daily treatments, and was given an electrical heating device and some *shonishin* instruments.

The mother called 2 weeks later to report that she had done the treatment regularly every day, and that her daughter had suddenly started to push herself upward into a sitting position. This was very encouraging, and continued daily treatment was heartily undertaken.

The next telephone follow-up was months later. The mother reported that she was still applying the treatment daily and that her daughter's rate of improvement had continuously increased since the first treatment. She had gained greater use of her legs and had begun walking with limited support. The next telephone follow-up was just less than a year later. The mother reported that her daughter continued to see benefits from the treatments, which she continued to apply daily.

Ryodoraku

As we have seen, the *Ryodoraku* system of acupuncture is based largely on a series of computer-analyzed electrical measurements of the channel system. The diagnosis focuses on the traditional concept of *jing-luo*, or channels, and aims to establish a pattern of imbalance. In interesting contrast to the modern diagnostic approach, the treatment applies traditional point-selection methods. The root treatment focuses on restoring relative balance to the channels (based on the electrical readings of the channels) by treating the supplementation and draining acupoints of the traditionally indicated channels. These two classes of point are so classified because of a strict interpretation of five-phase theory and point categorization as explicated by the mother–child principle first described in Chapter 69 of the *Nan Jing*. The second part of the treatment focuses on empirically demonstrated point combinations that address local problems or symptoms. As we saw in Chapter 4, there are technical challenges with this method of diagnosis, but it is a very interesting blend of traditional and modern methods of practice. It is quite commonly used in Japan and elsewhere around the world. The following case study from Hirosuke Suzuki is an example of how this system is employed.[27]

Case 16

Patient: Female, 46 years.

Main complaints: Chronic hepatitis. The patient had suffered from hepatitis for 3 years, during which time she had been hospitalized three times, for 3 months on the first occasion and for 2 months on each subsequent occasion. She had shown no significant improvement at any time during this 3-year period.

Examination: (Inquiry) The patient was extremely fatigued, with feelings of instability, heavy headedness, palpitations, undefined pain in the epigastrium, lack of appetite, nausea, itchy skin, and joint pain. (Palpation) Palpation of the liver revealed that it was swollen. Pressure pain was found at a number of acupoints on the abdomen, back, shoulders, legs, feet, and arms.

Diagnosis: *Ryodoraku* measurements were made. While most readings were in the range 40–50 µA, the following abnormalities were found: H1 (lung), 80 µA; H4 (small intestine), 75 µA; H5 (*san jiao*, lymphatics), 120 µA; H6 (large intestine) 90 µA; F1 (spleen), 70 µA; F2 (liver), 100 µA; F5 (gallbladder), 20 µA; F6 (stomach), 20 µA.

Treatment and outcome: The reactive points were each stimulated for 5 seconds using a 0.2-mm needle with electrical stimulation (120 V, 100 µA). This was followed by multiple non-scarring moxa on a major acupoint on the leg below the knees.

During the week after treatment, the patient felt better. When a hospital examination indicated some improvement, she was very encouraged. She returned for treatment almost daily for an extended period, with hospital tests every 4 weeks. During this time her symptoms essentially disappeared; only a little pressure in the epigastric region remained. Blood tests also revealed a continued improvement in her condition. On her discharge from treatment, *Ryodoraku* measurement revealed only the liver (F2) showing slight abnormality. The patient was instructed to continue applying moxibustion at home, with monthly hospital follow-ups. Ten years after treatment, all improvement has been maintained.

Clinical adaptation

The following case is from Marc Coseo, a former world-ranked tennis player whose acupuncture clientele consists of professional and amateur

---

> **Box 7.7** Brief case: male, 50 years, USA
>
> The patient, an architect, chose to see a particular internist in Los Angeles because he heard that he was more open than most and practiced acupuncture as well as regular medicine. The patient was frustrated by doctors; several had failed to relieve the chronic head, neck, shoulder, and back pain that began after a skiing accident more than 8 years previously. He had tried various pain, anti-inflammatory, and muscle-relaxant medications, as well as two courses of powerful injections, all with little effect. He could work without too much difficulty, but often had trouble sleeping and could exercise only rarely.
>
> The internist, a man in his late forties, performed a thorough examination, taking particular interest in how the patient felt, what he ate, and how he responded to weather and food. He then performed a very unusual physical examination, mostly palpating for sore points in many areas. After he had finished, he informed the patient that he had a problem with his *tai yang* system, and that he should respond well to acupuncture.
>
> With the patient lying on the treatment bed, the internist inserted needles at points in his hands, arms, feet, and legs, heating a few of the needles with a cigar-shaped stick of burning moxa. Besides feeling sensations at all the needles, some of which were a little tight but nonetheless strangely comfortable, the patient found the heat very relaxing. After re-palpating certain points, the internist needled points on the patient's abdomen and lower chest. After a few more minutes he removed these, and needled points on his back, neck, and shoulders, adding heat to a few of these needles as well.
>
> When he got up to dress, the patient found that more time had elapsed than he imagined, and thus became aware of how relaxed he felt. He also felt much less pain and experienced more mobility than he had for some time. He was very pleased to leave his insurance information with the receptionist and to schedule an appointment for 5 days later.
>
> Explanatory model of sources: 3–4
> Main pattern identification method: 3–4
> Medical acupuncture root treatment logic: 3–4
> Symptom-control treatment logic: 3–4
> Source of tools used: 3
> Stimulus level: 3–5
> Relative cost to patient: none, or insurance co-payment (*c* US $2–10)

athletes. From this specialization, Coseo has not only adapted influences from ion-pumping and *keiraku chiryo*, but has also incorporated electro-acupuncture and standard biomedical diagnostic tests that allow him to work cooperatively with physicians. One of the interesting aspects of

Coseo's practice — self-acupressure use for injury prevention and rehabilitation — has been published as the *Acupressure Warmup*.[28] Keep in mind the Chinese doctor's shoulder treatment (Case 4, p. 272) while you read this case. Although the trauma to Coseo's patient was of greater severity and the two cases are separated by time, distance, and culture, the essential clinical logic, the biomedical integration, and the treatment strategy are essentially the same. You can also see cultural differences in the approach to treatment, in particular the Western emphasis on self-responsible care.

Case 17

Patient: Female, 55 years.

Main complaint: Reaching for a parking ticket while driving, the patient's foot slipped from the clutch, causing the car to lurch forward, wrenching her arm backward. Under the care of an osteopathic surgeon, her arm was immobilized in a sling for 6 weeks, during which time she completed a course of anti-inflammatory medication. Following the immobilization she was unable to lift her arm to the front or side. During the next 6 weeks she went for physical therapy daily, but the pain was unrelenting. She was unable to sleep, and the range of motion in her shoulder was extremely limited. For an additional 8 weeks she continued three sessions of physical therapy per week, along with a course of three cortisone injections.

Symptoms: During the initial evaluation, the patient described herself as 'at wits end.' A throbbing pain kept her awake at night, she was unable to lift her child, comb her hair, brush her teeth, or attend to her daily activities. The pain was so severe and the injury so physically limiting that her job performance had been affected (the patient was an investment executive).

Examination: (Biomedical) The range of motion measurements were: shoulder abduction was 30° (180° is considered full range); medial rotation was 10° (55° is a full range); and lateral rotation was 15° (45° is a full range). (Palpation) Pressure sensitivity was noted on

acupoints on the shoulder. (Inspection) No swelling or redness was noted.

Diagnosis: The biomedical diagnosis was adhesive capsulitis (frozen shoulder), a condition that results when the sleeve-like structure that holds the ball and socket of the shoulder joint together adheres to itself. In traditional thought this is a *qi* and blood obstruction.

Treatment and outcome: The main point of the treatment plan was to avoid the next step in the biomedical treatment program, physical manipulation of the joint through its full range of motion while under general anesthesia. This typically follows failed cortisone treatment. Thus electroacupuncture, in conjunction with home therapy, was undertaken. Acupoints were selected to stimulate *qi* and blood circulation. Both local and distal points were chosen. The patient was taught to stimulate three treatment points by bringing her body weight to bear on tennis balls positioned to stimulate the acupoints.

After six treatments, given over 3 weeks, shoulder abduction had increased from 30° to 68°, medial rotation from 10° to 20°, and lateral rotation from 15° to 28°. The primary throbbing pain was reduced sufficiently for nightly sleep, but the patient's self-assessed improvement rating was only 25%. When asked if she had kept up with the tennis-ball exercise, she replied 'Yes, once a day.' Coseo stressed the importance of the regular acupressure.

After six more treatments the patient's self-assessment was 80% improvement. Shoulder abduction was now 145°, medial rotation was 45°, and lateral rotation was 38°. She experienced no further pain while sleeping, was fully functional at home and work, and had self-prescribed an increase of the acupressure to four times daily. After four more treatments the patient was discharged with full range of motion by all measures, no further pain, and full functionality. In a follow-up phone interview, she reported that all the treatment benefits remained.

Coseo's incorporation of biomedical measurement standards reflects his need to interact with the physician sports medicine specialists, trainers, and insurers who are so often involved with his patients. Just as acupuncturists in China have adapted to work within a biomedically dominated system, Coseo's practice shows how acupuncture is able to adapt clinically through integration. Not only has he adapted measures derived from biomedicine, but he has also selected techniques from different stimulus levels to meet the needs of his patients. The lighter-stimulus techniques are appropriate for Coseo's patients whose lifestyle, awareness of their bodies, and training habits make a readily available self-responsible approach ideal. The electro acupuncture, on the other hand, is TCM-derived, and Coseo uses it because he finds a stronger (level 4–5) physiotherapeutic stimulation useful for traumatic damage. This case, coupled with that of the Chinese school teacher (Case 4, p. 272), are excellent examples of the practical clinical adaptability that has shaped acupuncture's diversity, while essential observations and approaches are consistent across cultures and clinical settings.

SUMMARY

We cannot select cases to illustrate a range of treatment styles and then suggest that acupuncture is typified by those selections. Conclusions about the techniques of acupuncture used worldwide will have to wait until there are agencies and funds to collect and collate the necessary records. However, some of the trends exemplified in our selections may be worth looking for in larger and more representative samples. For example, acupuncturists draw from a broad but coherent set of treatment strategies. Although there are many such strategies, it is the ideas of channels and acupoints that are most critical to the clear majority of treatment styles. Thus, rather than discussing acupuncture treatment as it is usually discussed (i.e. as an expression of one theory or another) it may be more productive to discuss the various styles of acupuncture in a more holistic way. The theories applied to pattern identification and point selection are only part of the story. Without considering the types and strength of acupoint stimuli in relation to acupoint selection, it is probably impossible

adequately to describe or test any practice style. Some point-selection strategies might be better with stronger stimuli; some acupoints or combinations may work better with a lighter touch.

Seeing stimulation as tied to technique and labeling it as a continuum, like the one we have described, may better represent actual practice. In these cases, the Chinese TCM practitioners placed a greater emphasis on stimulation, its course and direction, strength, and duration. In fact, these cases are reminiscent of the clinical instructions given by pre-TCM acupuncturists such as Tin Yau So. But, even within these cases, there is also variability. Some Chinese practitioners use stronger stimulus than others, and most probably vary their technique in accord with at least their patient's age and state of health. This is true among Japanese acupuncturists as well. Relatively strong techniques are not infrequently used in conjunction with those that are light and refined.

Once, when Yoshio Manaka was teaching in the USA, he was in the midst of a clinical demonstration when a student asked a question about stimulus. While he answered, his clinician's instincts drew him to a area of vascular spiders and string-like moles on the demonstration patient's arm. (These are signs of advanced stagnation.) Seeing his attention shift, his colleague Kazuko Itaya immediately handed him a case of sterile bloodletting instruments. The entire audience was then presented with the ironic image of a gentle and articulate grey-haired Japanese physician speaking animatedly of light stimulation as he bled his patient. In other words, it is probably better to think of acupuncture techniques as technical wholes related to particular principles, rather than as expressions of a theoretical perspective or an ethnic approach.

Other trends that may hold true on a wider scale in the cases discussed are listed in Table 7.1. Perhaps the most obvious trend is the home-therapy component of the Western approaches. Although this may be in large part due to the less socialized medical delivery systems in the USA and Japan, it may also be a product of Western populations' demands for greater control over their own health care. This may also

Table 7.1 Summary of the qualities of cases 1–0

Case No.	Western medical correspondence	Pattern	Practice system	Stimulus Level	Treatments sequence
1	Constipation	Phlegm–rheum panting	TCM	0.5–2	7
2	Loss of night vision	Lack of nutrition	TCM	5–4	6
3	Stroke	Channel stroke	TCM	5	8
4	Pericarditis of the shoulder	*Qi* and blood obstruction by cold evil	TCM	3–5	12
5	Gastroptosis	Spleen and stomach vacuity	TCM	3–5	12
6	Loss of visual acuity	Liver *qi* depression	TCM	3	12
7	Interstitial cystitis	Damp heat in the small intestine; liver *yin* vacuity	TCM	3	28
8	Acute dizziness	Liver vacuity	*Keiraku chiryo*	1	3
9	Asthma	Liver vacuity	*Toyohari* and *shonishin*	1–3	30
10	Chronic migraine	Earth, with wood imbalance	Traditional acupuncture	2–3	*c* 30
11	Alcohol and cocaine addiction	*Yin* vacuity	NADA and TCM	2–3	*c* 164
12	Lower back pain	Cross-syndrome	Japanese *yin-yang* balancing	2	6
13	Atrial fibrillation	*Yin wei-chong mai*	Japanese *yin-yang* balancing	2	10
14	Recurrent infection	Whole body	*Shonishin*	2	1 + home therapy
15	Cerebral palsy	Whole body	*Shonishin*	2	1 + home therapy
16	Chronic hepatitis	Measured channel imbalance	*Ryodoraku*	2–3	30 + home therapy
17	Adhesive capsulitis	*Qi* and blood obstruction	TCM and *keiraku chiryo*	3–5	12 + home therapy

be true of the greater psychological attentiveness seen in the US cases. This observation, however, should not be overly elaborated. Chinese patients' greater control of their own clinical record and the consequent ability to scrutinze the information they have reported must certainly encourage a sense of participation and control that can fairly be labeled 'holistic.' Although it is known that Chinese patients tend to report symptoms rather than feelings,[29] this may, to some extent, be an artifact of the more public clinical settings in which acupuncture is practiced in China. Note for example, that both the American executive (Case 17, p. 286) and the Chinese school teacher (Case 4, p. 272) reported their debility in exactly the same terms (i.e. not being able to comb their hair).

There is a similar technical congruence. For example, although TCM is often said to have no palpation component, Jiang You Guang's case (Case 3, p. 271) included the palpatory investigations typically associated with Japanese practice. This further suggests that ethnic labels such as 'Japanese' or 'Chinese acupuncture' are inherently inadequate, and would be better replaced by labels that reflect the theoretical and clinical perspectives employed.

Another clear trend is that acupuncture is practiced as courses of treatment, typically 6–12 treatments. Although this seems obvious, as we saw in regard to research, this difference from biomedicine has not been well understood in the West, and is generally poorly reported in Western literature. At a typical cost of US $50 per treatment, most of the cases presented here cost $300 to $600. This is more expensive than a single visit to a physician followed by a prescription, but can be considerably less than the total cost of many of the biomedical tests and procedures undertaken for these conditions. However, it is also clear that, in these cases, at least, integration with biomedicine is inescapable. Even those practitioners who do not use biomedical information must understand biomedical data because it has become the standard language of patients worldwide.

We also feel that it is fair to suggest that acupuncture works on many levels. Channels and points are transducers that seem to be able to initiate regulatory effects. Acupuncture can alter the body's functional status, including, for example, measurable changes in physical structure. How does this happen? Can we be satisfied with simple mechanistic answers? We think not. And, as with all else we have investigated in this book, is it probably wise not to try to lock acupuncture in too small a box.

NOTES

1 Ellis A, Wiseman N, Boss K 1991 Fundamentals of Chinese acupuncture, rev edn. Paradigm Publications, Brookline, MA, p 249
2 See note 1, p 201
3 See note 1, p 131
4 See note 1, p 154
5 Shudo D 1990 Japanese classical acupuncture: introduction to meridian therapy. Eastland Press, Seattle, WA, pp 160–168
6 Soulie de Morant G 1994 Chinese acupuncture. Paradigm Publications, Brookline, MA, pp 86–87
7 See, for example: note 6, pp 151–171
8 See note 1
9 Auteroche, Gervais, Auteroche, Navailh, Tovi–Kan 1992 Acupuncture and moxibustion
10 Jayasuriya A 1980 Acupuncture science. The Acupuncture Foundation, Sri Lanka
11 Fukushima K 1991 Meridian therapy. Toyo Hari Medical Association, Tokyo
12 See note 5
13 So JTY 1982 Lecture at the New England School of Acupuncture, Spring
14 There is no source of definitive information about the tools and techniques applied by working acupuncturists. Thus we cannot reference the information in this section to authoritative sources. The information presented is founded on a review of the clinical manuals listed in the Bibliography, interviews with suppliers, and replies to a practitioner questionnaire by which we cross-checked our conclusions
15 Zhang FR, Geng JY 1991 Zhong Guo Jiu Liao Xue: Chinese moxibustion treatments. Zhi Yin Publishing Company, Taipei, p 10
16 Epler DC 1980 Bloodletting in early Chinese medicine and its relation to the origin of acupuncture. Bulletin of the History of Medicine 54: 337–367
17 See, for example: Lu G-D, Needham J 1980 Celestial lancets: a history and rationale of acupuncture and moxa. Cambridge University Press, Cambridge, p 295
18 (a) For elaborations on this method see: Matsumoto K, Birch S 1988 Hara diagnosis: reflections on the sea. Paradigm Publications, Brookline, MA, ch 16
(b) Manaka Y, Itaya K, Birch S 1995 Chasing the dragon's tail. Paradigm Publications, Brookline, MA
19 Kenner D 1994 A taxonomy of acupuncture. In: Proceedings of the first symposium of the Society for Acupuncture Research. Society for Acupuncture Research, Bethesda, Maryland
20 There is no source of definitive information about the disease treated, the systems and approaches applied, or the choice of acupoints relative to diseases or patterns. Assembling such information is far beyond our resources and the needs of this discussion. However, without such data there is naturally a bias to our case selections. Because standard translation methods ask translators to translate many pages and conduct many interviews with

clinicians as a foundation for any translation of medical Chinese, Nigel Wiseman and his colleagues were a convenient source of Chinese-language cases. Because Bill Prensky, Stephen Birch, Pat Culliton, and Zoe Brenner are involved in projects where formal case documentation is required, their cases offered similar advantages. In other words, the cases presented here are biased by our editorial needs and designs. The aim was to assemble 'real-life' cases, actual therapeutic events, from the range of theoretical, stimulus, and research models discussed in this chapter. Instead of listing the acupoints chosen, we have listed the indications to which they were applied, in order to make comparison with information presented in earlier chapters easier. As limited as this approach may be, isolating these cases from the didactic cases (cases fictionalized to demonstrate theory or procedure) provides a better view of the clinical reality of an acupuncturist. A recently published book contains many cases from practitioners of multiple traditions and models of practice, and thus a more complete example of how clinical practice manifests; see: MacPherson H, Kaptchuk T 1997 Acupuncture in practice: case histories from the West. Churchill Livingstone, Edinburgh

21 Kenner D. Personal communication.
22(a) Shudo D 1989 *Shinkyu Chiryo Shitsu*, 2nd edn. Ido no Nippon Sha, Yokosuka, p 215
(b) For an English presentation of Shudo's work, see note 5
23 Wen HL, Cheung SYC 1973 Treatment of drug addiction by acupuncture and electrical stimulation. Asian Journal of Medicine 9:138–141
24 Bullock ML, Culliton PD, Olander RL 1989 Controlled trial of acupuncture for severe recidivist alcoholism. *Lancet* 24: June 1435–1439
25 Helms JM 1995 Acupuncture energetics: a clinical approach for physicians. Medical Acupuncture Publishers, Berkeley, CA
26 See, for example: Mussat M 1972 Physique de l'acupuncture: hypotheses et approaches experimentales. Librairie le Francois, Paris
27 Suzuki H 1989 *Shinkyu Chiryo Shitsu*, 2nd edn. Ido no Nippon Sha, Yokosuka, pp 168–169
28 Coseo M 1992 The acupressure warmup. Paradigm Publications, Brookline, MA
29 Wiseman N, Ellis A, Zmiewski P 1985 Fundamentals of Chinese medicine, 1st edn. Paradigm Publications, Brookline, MA, p xxii

Conclusion and strategies for the future

During the interviews and research from which this book was composed, it was obvious that the single most important question about acupuncture's future was whether it is to be an alternative or a complement to biomedicine. The strategy that has brought acupuncture to the end of the 20th century is that of an alternative — a practice seen by both supporters and detractors as separate from the principles, standards, and delivery systems of biomedicine. As we have seen, a common expression of this assumption has been for systems of acupuncture that have found their way West, or have developed in the West, to seek legitimacy through association with the long history of the practice of acupuncture in East Asia. This, as Kevin Ergil[1] has noted, is obvious in the use of 'traditional' or 'classical' in the titles by which proponents attempt to associate their practices with an extensive history of presumably reproducible clinical success. It is also seen more subtly, as Wiseman[2] notes, in a preference for translations that emphasize contrast with biomedicine, or that deemphasize the militaristic metaphors of medical Chinese.

With exceptions, acupuncture's proponents have sought Western acceptance for the 'test of time,' instead of adopting the truth-testing mechanisms of the West. This not only contrasts with Asian opinion and powerful cultural trends, but is also poorly founded in history. For example, Chen Keji, President of the Chinese Association of Integrated Medicine, People's Republic of China, has told the *Wall Street*

Journal: 'We believe fundamentally that the outside world will only take us seriously if we modernize.'[3]

The broad consistency in pattern recognition, and in acupoint and stimulus selection, was not based on a 'one and only,' biomedical-style labeling of reality, but on the practical utility of the intellectual tools of acupuncture. Acupuncture is like computer programming, in that there is a variety of styles and languages. Each is capable of accomplishing a task, but no two programmers will produce exactly the same code, even from the same design. Regardless, the common body of theory, experience, and training regularly results in equally reliable solutions to problems, just as we saw with different approaches in the practice of acupuncture (see Ch. 7). Thus, regarding acupuncture, what has survived the test of time are the observational, logical, and technical skills of acupuncture, and the traditional-language algorhythms for solving health problems.

It is not that what any particular clinician may do is justified by history; rather, it is that the tool set developed through the centuries has proven adaptable to a vast variety of medical, social, political, and economic conditions. In its most generic sense, acupuncture is a set of physical and sensory skills for assessing the human body and its relation to the environment. It uses those assessments to describe an image of condition in a language that corresponds to therapeutic stimulations. This set of skills and patterns is larger than that used by any individual practitioner, during any particular era, in any school of practice, or in any single cultural environment. Elements are amended, added, and subtracted over time. What has survived is not the procedures of any particular school, but the skills, language, and patterns of systematic correspondence.

History denies acupuncture's proponents longevity as a blanket claim of efficacy. Just as the entrepreneurial masters of the Asian past justified their clinical visions by training apprentices whose skills were sufficient for economic survival, today's schools and leaders will succeed or fail as measured by the ability of their graduates to earn a place in the medical marketplaces of the next century. Although undoubtedly much remains to be learned in the literature of traditional Chinese medicine, and the authenticity of ideas needs to be known, it will be the opinion of today's established sciences, not the minds of ancient sages, that will determine what can be part of health care in the 21st century.

Skeptics face an equally demanding test. The root of most skeptical argument against acupuncture is that lack of scrutiny, not clinical efficacy, explains its survival. Skeptics assert that Asian peoples acquired faith in acupuncture through the biasing predispositions of their culture. They argue that acupuncture seemed to work because of a faith-strengthened placebo effect, because many diseases resolve untreated, and because failure was selectively perceived. Pointing to religious faith or the vague promises of oracular systems as parallels, skeptics dismiss acupuncture's survival.

Yet, what history shows is that acupuncture was not the work of wizard-robed religionists offering vague promises of subjective betterment. It was the daily work of marketplace practitioners who sold specific promises of cure for ills understood through the naked senses. Although it is unbelievable that there were no charlatans among them, it is equally unbelievable that acupuncturists survived in closed societies without a set of skills capable of satisfying the immediate, self-assessed complaints of their neighbors. Acupuncture's skeptics are asking us to believe that generation upon generation of Chinese were more gullible than we ever think of ourselves.

Could every Chinese mother have been so culturally blind as to not know what could, and what could not, relieve her children's fevers? Did people who labored to live not know how far they could bend before their back pain began? Do skeptics propose that Mao's patronage preserved acupuncture without any objective evidence of benefit in the penurious and powerfully antitraditional climate of post-Liberation China? Is it credible that acupuncture's Western and Eastern rise against legal prohibition, the advice of established medical authorities, cultural bias, and economic disincentive were solely the result of mystical presentations that heighten the placebo effect? Is that opinion inherently more credible than the assertion that generations of intelligent humans discovered useful ways to stimulate the body to produce predictable and desirable results?

The value of knowing the history of acupuncture is not that it offers easy answers, but that it destroys them. Although history is significantly suggestive that the observational and therapeutic skills of acupuncture have objectifiable value, it neither justifies nor dismisses acupuncture. Instead, it offers an opportunity to contextualize its practice fairly.

The alternative assumption has also influenced how acupuncture is evaluated and taught. This is easily seen by comparing Western academic ideas to those common among acupuncturists. In contrast to the as yet unachieved ideal of interdisciplinary integration, and the powerful demands for integration in East Asian nations, the opinion of Western experts in fields that impact on the evaluation of traditional ideas — philology, anthropology, linguistics, and history, among others — are rarely considered and have yet to be addressed in the education of either Western-trained physicians practicing acupuncture or specifically trained acupuncturists. Because these experts are not practitioners, their contributions are dismissed with diminutive labels such as 'nonclinically practicing sinologist,' as if either medicine or sinology were occupations best performed part-time. As we saw with the extraordinary vessels in Chapter 2, this dismissal of non-alternative evidence and opinion has spawned Western ideas that disregard not only academic or historical information but also the Asian clinical record.

If there is no doubt that acupuncture has been presented as an alternative, neither is there any doubt that the strategy has been successful. Considering the traditional disinterest of academic sinology in Chinese medicine, and biomedical disinterest in nontechnological therapies, it is hard to imagine that acupuncture could have been transmitted in any other way. Given the Gordian knot of interlocking social, political, scientific, and financial interests that is modern medicine, the current extent of acupuncture's Western adoption was everything but an obvious outcome. Many Westerners, even those who have never been treated by an acupuncturist, believe that acupuncture works. Acupuncture has not only touched upon needs broadly perceived by Western populations, it has also earned patient loyalty. That it has achieved this without any organized support from medical or social authorities — and at times against their opposition — is a testament to the dedication of acupuncture's pioneers, and an insight into the functionality of acupuncture.

However, as Paul Unschuld has noted, this advancement is not itself evidence of clinical efficacy; instead, it demonstrates that the rationale of acupuncture makes sense to people.[4] Although there is no doubt that the idea of an alternative is welcome and that the perceived dangers of biotechnology provide acupuncture an opening into Western societies, there is reasonable doubt that this alone will be sufficient. It will take more than a warm welcome for acupuncture to be deeply absorbed by Western societies. This too is a lesson of history, particularly when the extent of the use of acupuncture — not simply its survival — is considered.

In Europe, acupuncture has been welcomed in the past. However, only where practitioners were empowered by the biomedical system has lasting adoption resulted. The successful strategy that George Soulie de Morant pioneered in France promoted acupuncture as a physician-based clinical exploration, not as an alternative. Even in Asian societies where acupuncture is an indigenous practice, it is the relation and integration of acupuncture with biomedicine that determines the extent of its use. In the USA, licensing, educational authority, and the development of a professional degree were accomplished only when alternative degrees and labels were sufficiently suppressed to permit accommodation to local, state, and national standards.

Neither did acupuncture survive in its generative cultures as an alternative. In fact, it has a long history of complementary use. So-called 'herbal medicine' which, other than its name implies, is a sophisticated pharmacotherapy, has more often than not been the big brother of acupuncture, as is true today. In fact, it would be hard to justify describing acupuncture in isolation at any time or place in its long history. Thus the fairest question might be: Can the alternative strategy continue to succeed? In practical terms, can any alternative approach firmly establish the efficacy of acupuncture, make it available at the highest and best utility, or to the largest populations? There is already some evidence that it cannot.

After reviewing all the studies evaluating clinical trials of acupuncture, and after participating in both the 1994 US Food and Drug Administration (FDA) Workshop on Acupuncture, and the 1997 National Institute of Health (NIH) Consensus Development Conference on Acupuncture, it is clear that much of the scientific literature on acupuncture has been rejected as methodologically flawed. However, there seems to be an increasingly positive response, with a growing benefit of doubt. Only 2 years ago not one indication for acupuncture could be approved. There were only four conditions approved at the 1997 NIH conference, and 12 listed as promising. Clearly, the need for rigorous studies has not gone away. Many questions about the efficacy of acupuncture remain unanswered, and the manner in which those questions must be answered has not changed. The only building consensus among researchers is that, whatever the result of the outcomes study debate, a considerable body of needle-controlled, randomized controlled clinical trials will be required before treatment by acupuncture can be broadly accepted as effective. This brings the moment of the decision between alternative and complementary strategies closer to hand. It is reasonable to suggest that the strategy of alternative acculturation has brought acupuncture as far as it can, at least with regard to access to mainstream medical delivery and finance.

Although many familiar with the research literature have long warned that the proofs of the efficacy of acupuncture were on tenuous ground, some in the acupuncture community feel that Western medical authorities have taken a purposefully combative position, a confrontational exercise of authority. Therefore, suggestions of complementary acculturation are often greeted with distrust — the sense that cooperation will lead to co-option and the loss of the traditional essence of acupuncture. Our correspondence and interviews give us instead the sense of a clean slate — a decision to retain a standard that is clearly and unequivocally trusted. It should not be forgotten that implicit in this ruling is the public, simultaneous, and equal rejection of the flawed work that has been deeply harmful to acupuncture. The US FDA decision to grandfather the acupuncture needle eliminates the most obvious and easily exercised method of wresting control of acupuncture from acupuncturists. Thus, as a matter of opinion, at least the official US position seems deliberately neutral.

It seems that the most conservative estimate has always been that, if acculturated at a professional level, acupuncture would reflect the contemporaneous trends of the culture into which it is arriving, just as it has in the past. No matter what acupuncture is or was in Asia, what it will be in the West must be determined by Western social, economic, and intellectual trends. Given the power of scientific and technological thought in the world, and the dependence on statistical information that accompanies every version of public-health strategy in both capitalist and socialist economies, it is hard to imagine that acupuncture will not need to accommodate to these methods.

Whether our judgement is right or wrong, whether or not acupuncture is being held to a standard forced by inimical powers or derived from the biases and standards of science and economics, acupuncture probably needs to do very little to remain an alternative system of health care. The question is not its survival, but the extent of its application. Public faith remains, and will bring acupuncture attention, patients, and a new generation of practitioners worldwide. It is hard to imagine that acupuncture will do anything but grow. On the other hand, it is equally hard to imagine that an alternative acupuncture would not remain isolated from mainstream education, medical delivery, and health-care finance. As commercial or governmental medical reimbursement systems are the norm of the world, the strategy of alternative acculturation has characteristics of the proverbial two-edged sword.

We see no direct challenges to the status quo of the teaching, licensing, and legality of acupuncture, because the operative criteria for these matters are public responsibility and safety, neither of which has been seriously challenged. However, efforts to access reimbursement systems, public funding, and biomedical facilities are more likely to be sensitive to scientific evidence. With currently less than 1–5% of most industrialized populations using acupuncture, substantive growth of public funding for acupuncture research, acupuncture schools, training residencies, or public health programs seems unlikely without scientific support. Furthermore, the status that attaches to acupuncturists, and particularly the extent of their diagnostic authority, will be largely determined by scientific evidence, if only when tested by malpractice law.

Historically, the status of traditional physicians was hierarchical and there was always variety in clinicians' attachment to the qi paradigm. Today, in the People's Republic of China acupuncturists are secondary in pay and position to traditional physicians. Pharmacotherapy leads acupuncture in both public and professional perceptions, as it has for some time. This, as Marnae Ergil's research has shown, impacts on the career choices of China's best graduates.[5] Traditional physicians enjoy lower pay and prestige than biomedical physicians, and must obtain access to biomedical budgets to pursue their research interests. Since the 1980s, China has directed funding for clinical research toward the integration of traditional medicine and biomedicine. This is in no small

way because the Chinese interest in Traditional Chinese Medicine (TCM) lies in its economic application in a huge public-health system, a concern not unlike those of governments in the West.

In the West, the standing TCM infrastructure is not well prepared to raise the level of acupuncture or to counter pressures for scientific approbation. Worldwide, the infrastructure arose to meet not a demand from the health-care system, but the need to prepare student clinicians for private practice. Its center of gravity today is proprietary acupuncture and Oriental medical schools. The few nonprofit state and private academic institutions, whether for specialists or Western-trained physicians practicing acupuncture, are also tuition funded, and have similar budgetary constraints.

These schools support a service economy of teachers and writers. There is also commercial continuing education. There is a product-centered economy of suppliers to practitioners. Judging by the advertising in clinician's journals, the largest of these are prepared herbal formula suppliers. Virtually everyone in the field reports an upward trend. These supplier organizations are proprietary and, apart from the Asian-based producers, are cash-flow driven. However, they have recently been joined by larger established concerns that now see the field as financially viable. These organizations, particularly the schools, are already supporting the field's various governing bodies, some of which remain in active competition.

In short, beyond the efforts of individual schools, it is difficult to see how funding for acupuncture's development can be generated from within the field. It is equally difficult to see how commercial investment can provide development funds. Acupuncture is the labor-intensive occupation of individuals, and thus offers few opportunities for capital investment. After that for tools and devices, the most obvious influx of venture capital has been directed toward larger scale TCM treatment centers, particularly in Europe, but now also in the USA. In these centers acupuncturists are typically employees. This is in contrast to traditional pharmacotherapy where research funding can provide access to large established markets. For example, the company that brought a Chinese medicinal with cholesterol-lowering abilities to market raised over US $21 million.

Thus the current economic infrastructure is delicately balanced on the capital and cash-flow available to entrepreneurial organizations. Yet, the customer base is expanding from a largely one-on-one retail trade (clients for private practices) to a highly leveraged, massively capitalized whole-sale market, access to which is controlled by HMOs, Preferred Provider Organizations (PPOs), the state, and private medical insurance providers. The field is subject to new forces and economic consequences. However, these trends are not essentially a challenge to acupuncture but to the structures created by those who have introduced it to the West. In the established medical-delivery system, acupuncture will belong to whoever arrives at the doorway of academic medicine with a package of methodologically sound research that shows practitioners making statistically reliable diagnoses leading to statistically justified treatments. If those acupuncture treatments are cost effective for diseases, symptoms, or patterns for which the medical insurance and managed-care industries can establish cost-justified payment programs, those treatments will become practically indistinguishable from biomedicine in terms of legitimacy and availability. The extent to which these treatments utilize the powers of acupuncture, and the extent to which holism and quality of life are recognized, will be limited only by the extent to which these qualities have been studied as scientific and economic issues. The role of traditional patterns and their underlying theories will be determined by the extent to which the study designers recognize their importance.

Whoever designs these trials will design the future of acupuncture. Acupuncture will become what it can be statistically proven to do. If these trials are accomplished by biomedicine, any of its subspecialties, or midlevel professions, parts of acupuncture will almost certainly be subsumed and attached as techniques to bio-medicine. If the procedures thus established

prove to be cost effective, the pressure brought to bear by insurers could be intense — remember the figures for chronic pain, which is already a common target of insurance and HMO-sponsored clinical trials. Although there is no present attack on the status quo of acupuncture, and it seems very unlikely that there will be any successful challenge to acupuncturists' right to practice, neither is there any obvious guarantee that the present practitioner population will continue to be the exclusive providers of acupuncture.

An observation common to many who have witnessed the 30-year acculturation of foreign concepts from *aikido* to *zen* is that social, intellectual, and commercial entrepreneurs often survive start-up adversity only to be overwhelmed by established and better capitalized organizations when the idea reaches commercial viability. In other words, in very practical ways, until acupuncture achieves control of its body of knowledge and firmly roots its diagnostic authority in the standards of the recipient culture, increasing recognition and popularity are good for acupuncture, but not necessarily good for acupuncturists.

Considering these possibilities, the inescapable need for scientific proof should not be taken as 'bad news.' It is in the realm of science that acupuncture is most equal. It is there that the rules are most standard for all. It is there that the unfairness of judging one practice by the methods of another can be addressed. It is there that it will be easiest for acupuncture to join to the mainstream, and it is there that a single scientific paper can change the minds of many. Compared with the brute force of politics and the vast power of economic interest, the intellectual realm is easily moved. Compared with moving the interests entrenched in the economics of medical treatment, the cost of controlled clinical trials is small. Of all the places in Western culture where acupuncture could be required to compete, medical science is the one where two millenia of marketplace survival make it best prepared.

Acupuncture thus has the possibility of determining its own future, and to us this alone is sufficient to suggest reassessment of the alternative strategy. It is perhaps a decision that is imminent and unavoidable. At the very least, the moment calls for a new assessment. This is not to say that providing scientifically sound evidence of the value of acupuncture will be a trivial undertaking; it will require the full cooperation of all the proponents of acupuncture, and it will put a strain on the available resources. Those who wish to remain in an alternative mode — as will many of our colleagues in the most traditional schools — must be shown that complementarianism is not designed as a threat to their practices. However, compared to moving the mountains of entrenched financial interests, compared to maintaining the faith of a media-saturated population that can abandon any trend at breathless speed, and compared to the quagmire of health-care politics, scientific proofs are tasks that realistically can be accomplished.

Thus, the questions become: Just what would it take for acupuncture to become a complement to biomedicine, justified to the satisfaction of science? What would it mean to provide traditional patterns with measurable reliability, to bring issues of well-being to scientific acceptability? How can a traditional medicine be justified by the standards that Western biomedical institutions have set? Again, we offer no sure answer, but repeat the observation that it would be difficult for acupuncture to progress in isolation from traditional Western science and academics. Without persons educated in traditional Western academic disciplines, acupuncture has no representation in the peer system where research is funded and matters of sufficient proof decided. The price of isolation has already been years of negative bias. Consider, for example, Melzack's trigger point research. If there had been experts knowledgeable in acupuncture to critique his work when it first appeared in the journal *Pain*, would so many have believed that acupuncture had been explained?[6]

Without journals that adopt the standards of academic publications, acupuncture is effectively refusing the information scholars could provide. Because academics interested in traditional medicine must nonetheless publish to further their careers, the existence of recognized peer publications is critical. Already, the bulk of primary materials actually translated from Chinese or Japanese are the work of academic writers funded by conventional university sources. Futhermore, without respectability for their academic foundations, acupuncturists' opinions will be ignored. This is true of clinical literature as well. Claims to have interpreted patterns, and even entire practice traditions, from personal clinical experience are so rarely accompanied by even the roughest quantifications of that experience that it is impossible to know whether the writer speaks from the basis of two or 2000 cases.

Finally, because the educational and practitioner organizations that Western acupuncturists control do not have the funds to finance research, the only realistic source will be public funds. Relatively few studies of acupuncture are funded in the West (less than 4 million dollars per year). Without a base of successful studies, funds will become harder and harder to find. It is already easy to see the beginnings of a vicious cycle, where underfunding incapacitates research, which in turn retards funding and the interest of scientists, which reduces funding still further. It is thus necessary that acupuncturists agree upon and promote studies that benefit the whole profession and reverse this trend. This means cooperation in order to meet effectively common, clear, and present needs. That is a political process, a unity within diversity that Asian practitioners have sometimes achieved. In both Japan and China, for example, the first steps taken to counter the collapse of traditional medicine were to control political infighting.

The immediate need, and the interest all hold in common, is to demonstrate unequivocally that acupuncture is able to treat the conditions for which it is most commonly used. These include, for example, back pain, headaches, arthritis, and drug addiction. Medical centers and insurance companies understand these to be the central issues, and have begun large-scale trials. Presently planned or on-going trials are: a large multicenter trial of acupuncture for tension headache in the UK; a large multicenter trial of acupuncture for cocaine addiction in the USA; a large HMO trial of acupuncture and massage for chronic back pain in the USA, and a large academic center–HMO study of acupuncture, massage, and chiropractic for acute back pain in the USA. There was a call recently for studies from the National Institutes of Health to test acupuncture for osteoarthritis. In the UK, large-scale projects concerning acupuncture for back pain and headache have been submitted. Large-scale trials of acupuncture for obstetric and gynecological problems have been completed as has a large back pain study. The focus on economically significant conditions is clear. If these studies are successful, research and private donations and capital investment will be encouraged. If these trials fail, continuing research investment will be difficult to find.

Those, including ourselves, who believe that acupuncture should be available to Western populations have typically been most interested in confirming traditional ideas. However, it is symptom–control treatments with powerful economic consequences that are most commonly shared. The lack of a track record, or a negative record, in these economically sensitive venues will benefit none. On the other hand, a dozen successful trials of formulas such as those developed in China's state system, or like those for emesis using a single acupuncture point, or Bullock and Culliton's work, would completely change scientific thinking about acupuncture.[7] A few compelling trials could bring the funds needed for more complex and traditionally oriented research.

These empirical approaches are the least complex and least expensive to accomplish as double-blinded trials. Although we believe that the full complement of the arts of acupuncture will produce the best results, a concentration on proving the efficacy of a particular traditional approach is not only more complex, but will almost certainly stimulate further competitive discord. As sociologist Arthur O'Neil proposed in his study of alternative medical education in Australia, separation from culturally established institutions contributes to internal rivalries.[8] This has been no less the case in Europe, the USA, and UK than in Australia. These debates have absorbed time and human and financial resources that would have been better applied elsewhere. It is not control of today's infrastructure or the loyalties of acupuncture students that will decide the future of acupuncture. Rather, it will be a proven economic contribution to the pressing health-care demands of modern societies.

We do not, however, suggest that the exploration of the cultural foundations of acupuncture should be forgotten in exclusive concentration on clinical research. Anthropology, philology, linguistics, and history, all the liberal arts, may teach no one how to use a needle, but they are the principal guardians of the profession's culture. Authenticity is also a powerful clinical resource. Before any trial begins, the authenticity of the treatment tested, as well as the irrelevance of the treatment used as a control, must be known, confirmed, and have achieved some degree of general agreement, even before pilot studies can begin. There must be some clear evidence for the number of treatments tested. There must be some reliable expectation of the outcome, and a demonstrable foundation in the clinical practice from which the treatment is derived. There is no bias by which misinterpretation or idiosyncratic protocols are to anyone's advantage.[9] The protocols tested must be as authentic as possible if the results are to mean anything at all.

This requires a new and additional literary effort, one based not on the creation of prose for student education, but on the practical ability to investigate the massive Asian clinical record. One demand the future makes of translators is for investigations of clinical reports and case histories. This is what will be required to establish any clinical notion as part of a common thread in Asian history. The results of these translations must be rigorously consistent databases of information prepared from dictionaries that are freely available to acupuncturists, scientists, and scholars alike. The links to Chinese, Japanese, and other Asian languages must be sufficient for intercultural communication.

Again, this will provide purely clinical benefits. All of modern medicine depends upon large-scale, multitext, multiauthor compilations prepared as computer databases. It is via systems such as MEDLINE, perhaps the best known example, that information is distributed, patient problems studied, and treatment probabilities assessed. Unless acupuncture is represented in these databases, it is practically hidden. The technical nature of these systems demands precisely the same rigorous preparation required for clinical trials.

Once a base of compelling evidence of the clinical utility of acupuncture has been achieved, the same structures — and the same funding sources — can be attached to confirmations of traditional clinical procedures. Once acupuncture's reputation among scientists has been supported by solid evidence, resistance to such studies will no longer be fueled by scientists' suspicion of 'mystical energies.' Take, for example, pulse palpation. If a statistically significant group of similarly trained practitioners can demonstrate that their pulse diagnoses are as reliable as the diagnoses of, for example, psychiatrists who must also depend on inter-rater reliability, then pulse diagnoses can be a legitimate element of a clinical trial. Once a foundation has been established, traditional concepts can be confirmed. Layered on earlier evidence, these trials become less complex.

Adjusting the selection of treatment points and techniques according to the pattern each patient presents offers a chance to increase effectiveness. Were research confirming this opinion to be accomplished, the scope of acupuncturists' diagnostic authority would be enhanced considerably. If properly founded studies confirm this opinion, not only will there be greater utilization of traditional approaches, but also researchers and clinicians will begin to conceive of how biomedicine might profit from these techniques. Perhaps whole-person approaches, rooted in systems and information theory, will find greater acceptance and utilization.

There are many such advantages to a complementary approach and, although there is no doubt that the development of acupuncture independent of the medical establishment was necessary to make acupuncture available, there is reasonable doubt that independent development remains viable. Left entirely to the biomedical establishment, acupuncture would probably never have begun its westward progress. But left only to today's acupuncture establishment, it may never become fully used. This is the double-edged nature of the current acculturation of acupuncture — the very qualities that produced its accomplishments have set its limits.

As a complementary system of health care, these limits can be vastly transcended. The potential that acupuncture offers medicine is nearly unimaginable from today's perspective. Not only will it be offered to more people, but its impact on medicine will also increase. As better research supports what current findings suggest, acupuncture will be practiced routinely in pain centers, substance-abuse treatment programs, oncology units, stroke rehabilitation programs, pulmonary units, and many, many more venues. Acupuncturists will no longer be an unusual sight in any clinical setting. There is already an acupuncturist on the staff of each of Harvard's teaching hospitals in Boston. Patients will no longer feel they must conceal visits to an acupuncturist from their physician, and the numbers of patients seeking or being referred to acupuncturists will increase as acupuncture more frequently features in clinical databases and the personal experience of primary-care physicians. The potential clinical vista is vast.

Throughout this book we have tried to make our biases clear. That the greatest contribution of acupuncture will arise if it becomes a complementary system of health care, fully joining the academic, medical, and financial systems of the nations in which it has acculturated, seems an inescapable conclusion. If acupuncture is to achieve its highest and best use in the West, if it is to become available to the most people at the lowest possible cost, it must integrate.[10] Although it will be challenged to retain its unique character, its alternative institutions lack the resources to fund an advance. A new approach is required. Acupuncturists and their colleagues in Western disciplines have already accomplished much. Research has begun; there are on-going experiments in education, and new approaches to clinical trails. The oldest and most important documents of Chinese medicine are being rigorously examined. Tools for accessing the diverse clinical experience available in East Asian societies are now realities. Every day, practitioners worldwide add to the base of public support every person whose problems they have successfully treated.

In essence, we end where we began: with no quick and easy description of acupuncture; with no one-and-only explanation we ask you to believe. We offer only the on-going pursuit of authenticity and validity as the sources of clinical success. There is only the on-going exercise of human genius applied to the universal human quest for a long, happy, and healthy life.

NOTES

1 Ergil KV 1992 Strategic representations. 'Oriental' Medicine at large. Paper presented at American Anthropological Association Annual Meeting.
2 Wiseman M 1998 Rationale for the terminology of the fundamentals of Chinese medicine, Paradigm Publications, Brookline, MA, p 11
3 Keji C Wall Street Journal 1997 Interactive Edition. A fight over rice yeast pit, Dec 3
4 Unschuld PU 1992 Epistemological issues and changing legitimation: traditional Chinese Medicine in the 20th century. In Leslie C, Young A (Eds) Paths to Asian medical knowledge, University of California Press, Berkeley, CA
5 Ergil MC 1994 Chinese Medicine in China: education and learning strategies. Paper presented at the Association for Asian Studies Annual Meetings, Boston
6 Melzack R Stillwell DM, Fox EJ 1997 Trigger points and acupoints for pain: correlations and implications. Pain 3:3–23
7 Bullock ML, Culliton PD, Olander RL 1989 Controlled trial of acupuncture for sevese recidivist alcoholism. Lancet, June 24, 1435–1439

8 O'Neill A 1994 Enemies within and without. Latrobe University Press, Bundoora, Victoria
9 As this is about to go to press the Journal of the American Medical Association just published a trial of acupuncture for the pain of HIV-related peripheral neuropathy (Shlay JC, Chalones K, Max MB, Flaws B, Reichelderfer P, Wentworth D, Hillman S, Brizz B, Cohn DL 1988 Acupuncture and amitriptyline for pain due to HIV-related peripheral neuropathy: A randomized controlled trial. JAMA, 280(18):1590–1595). This study was the first multicenter study of acupuncture in the US. It tested what can only be considered as a strange idiosyncratic treatment that had virtually no background and no reputation. It is a surprise to few acupuncturists that this flawed study found no therapeutic benefit whatsoever.
10. (a) Cooper RA, Henderson T, Dietrich CL 1988 Roles of nonphysician clinicians as autonomous providers of health care. JAMA 280(9):795–802
(b) Grumbach K, Coffman J 1988 Editorial. JAMA 280(9):825–826

Appendices

Appendix 1

Resources and questions

As a patient or referring professional, what can you expect from an acupuncturist and how should you decide whom to see?

Clinical setting. Both physician acupuncturists and licensed practitioners can be found in medical buildings and other mainstream clinical settings. However, although there is no definitive information available, it is likely that most acupuncturists work in private offices located in urban and suburban areas. In the typical office there will probably be more than one practitioner, or a practitioner in a group practice with other therapists, such as masseurs and herbalists. Some practitioners practice therapies in addition to acupuncture, typically herbal medicine, massage, homeopathy, or counseling. There is often an office manager who schedules appointments and manages payments. In some offices you may find clinical interns, students from a local acupuncture school, or graduate acupuncturists working as apprentices. Some clinics employ assistants who perform moxibustion, monitor electro acupuncture devices, and remove needles.

Patients are not typically asked to disrobe. However, loose clothing is well advised, because important treatment and diagnostic points are located on both the front and back of the torso, legs, and arms. Tight pants and metal adornments can be very inconvenient during treatment; for example, reaching an acupoint on the leg is often most easily achieved by simply rolling-up the pant leg. Make-up and excessive eating or drinking immediately before acupuncture can interfere with some aspects of the examination. For example, coffee stains the tongue and can alter the pulse.

If someone is uncomfortable with any aspect of the examination or treatment, they should inform the acupuncturist immediately. In the beginning, any sensation can be reported. The feedback a practitioner requires is quickly learned.

Treatment plans. Different practitioners approach treatment differently, but a few basic approaches are commonly found. Many practitioners will suggest a specified minimum number of treatments. This allows both patient and practitioner to make a realistic assessment of benefit and future course. It is unrealistic to expect immediate results for many conditions. Chronic conditions will probably require at least 10 treatments. Again, there is considerable variability. Some conditions will be remedied, others will be managed. Some conditions will be addressed quickly (e.g. in Denmai

Shudo's dizziness patient (case 8, p.276), the effects were immediate and the patient was quickly discharged). Others, typically those with advanced organic problems (e.g. Steve Birch's patient suffering from a damaged heart (case 13, p. 282)) will require repeated acupuncture treatment over a period of time.

However, regardless of the approach, or the severity or age of a condition, there should be observable change. An improvement may be signaled by changes that do not seem to be directly related to the primary symptoms, and the effects of acupuncture are typically cumulative; that is, there is a continuing and developing improvement. For example, a general digestive improvement may precede the diminishment of the presenting symptom. The more information the practitioner is provided with the better. Patient notes can help track improvement, and attention to even slight changes may provide an acupuncturist with useful clues. It is better to report too much than too little.

Most practitioners will suggest a regular interval for treatment. This will be something like once or twice a week for a certain number of weeks, although in some cases an acupuncturist may suggest more frequent treatments. The frequency of treatment depends on the severity of the condition, ability to pay, and the patient's work schedule. If a condition is severe or chronic, there will often be follow-up treatments once the initial course of treatments is complete. Generally, if there has been little or no improvement, people decide not to continue treatment. However, when someone experiences improvement of a severe or chronic condition and is satisfied with the progress, acupuncture can be a viable means of maintaining improvement and preventing relapses. This may require treatment every few weeks or every few months. However, in any case, the best possible strategy is for the patient to recognize quickly the premonitory signs of an acute incidence. Caught early, it is easier to prevent a relapse. Acupuncturists, like most medical personnel, leave room in their schedule for patients who need immediate attention. For 'incurable' diseases and quality-of-life improvements, some experimentation may be required to find the best schedule.

Lifestyle changes. Acupuncturists also vary in the extent to which they suggest adopting positive habits and abandoning negative ones. Because of the concentration of acupuncture on the human, climatic, and social environment, most acupuncturists will note environmental conditions or personal habits directly related to a patient's presenting problem (e.g. deleterious dietary habits). Some acupuncturists will routinely encourage specific lifestyle changes, some will not.

Length of treatment. As above, the length of treatment can vary. The critical factors are the severity of the problem, the patient's overall health (and thus ability to heal), and the skill and experience of the practitioner. It is very difficult to make precise predictions, but an experienced practitioner will be able to provide a 'rule of thumb' assessment. It is not unreasonable to set a reassessment point, after a certain number of treatments, at which to evaluate progress. For some conditions there are biomedical measures that can be monitored via concomitant biomedical assessment (e.g. range-of-motion tests). Acupuncturists vary in their familiarity with laboratory and other biomedical tests; however, many will be able to discuss and follow a patient's progress via appropriate biomedical measures.

Length of treatment sessions. Depending on the practitioner and the patient's problem, treatment may last anywhere from 20 minutes to over an hour. Most treatments last 40–60 minutes. A practitioner may not be with a patient for the entire time. In some treatments, patients are asked to relax for 5–20 minutes after the treatment has begun (e.g. after the first needles have been inserted).

Treatment techniques. Anyone who sees or refers to more than one acupuncturist will probably notice differences in how each approaches and applies treatment. Knowing that different schools of thought adopt different approaches, expect this variation. Besides differences in how the acupuncture is practiced (e.g. the depth and quality of insertion), there will also be variations because of the other modalities introduced (e.g. massage or herbal medicines). Acupuncturists, like most professionals, are often enthusiastic about the technical variations, tools, and techniques they use, and will very likely be happy to discuss these.

Costs. As with all medical care, the cost of acupuncture varies according to locale, specialization, and experience, and the setting in which care is provided. Average treatment costs in the USA are $40–50 per visit, average costs in other countries are similar. The fee schedules of Western-trained physicians practicing acupuncture tend to follow their fees for biomedical services. Some practitioners charge less and some charge more. Some practitioners work in public-health settings, such as substance-abuse centers and AIDS clinics, where treatment is given for free or at a nominal cost. Student clinics attached to acupuncture schools are usually inexpensive, and can be a very pleasant experience because of the students' enthusiasm and attentiveness.

Insurance cover. Most people pay for acupuncture out-of-pocket. The insurance industry is under both social and political pressure to reduce expenses. This creates two often contradictory tactics: one is to include fewer and fewer treatment methods, and the other is to include cheaper and cheaper treatment methods. This is a complicated issue that each insurance company decides in its own way. Some companies do not want to cover acupuncture, as its inclusion is perceived as an extra cost. Other insurance companies include acupuncture because they believe it to be less expensive than other services they already cover. However, insurance is a competitively marketed product. If there is a significant demand for acupuncture in a given population, and it is perceived that its inclusion will make a company's plans more competitive, acupuncture will be covered.

National insurance plans, state-sponsored programs, and workman's compensation programs are even more burdened by the crisis of cost in health care. There are enormous pressures brought to bear by politicians and lobbyists. Many Western countries are facing sharply spiraling increases in health-care budgets, and are looking at any measures to slow down that increase. These forces, coupled with discord about the utility of medical practices that are still perceived as alternatives, make it very difficult to predict the future of acupuncture in government insurance programs. At present, it is difficult to suggest that there will be any increase in the use of acupuncture until some definitive clinical trial evidence becomes available.

Selecting an acupuncturist. Everyone wants to see the best practitioner of any healing art. Deciding who is best is the problem. In an area where several acupuncturists are available, the best selection criterion is prior success. Seeking a practitioner reccomended by someone whose opinion is trustworthy is probably the single best strategy. Also, people who have the same or a similar problem, patient-support groups, and appropriate interest groups, are good sources of experience with local practitioners. For example, if you suffer from tennis elbow, talk to tennis players. You will quickly learn of their experiences with local practitioners. However, as people tend to speak highly but generally of their health-care providers, ask specific questions: How long? How much? Are you still bothered by the problem? Also, it is possible that biomedical personnel such as physicians, nurses, and physiotherapists will be familiar with local acupuncturists. It is our experience that some physicians are more open to acupuncture than their patients believe them to be.

In circumstances where reputation cannot be assessed, or once a general assessment has been made, call the clinic or practitioner and speak to the acupuncturist directly. Consider some or all of the questions listed in Box A 1.1. It is impossible to make an absolutely sure decision based on this or any list of questions. There are no right or wrong answers to any of these questions. But, you will very likely get honest answers that will inform you and give you a sense of the person and their skills.

As a medical provider how do you decide to whom to refer?

Medical doctors and their qualifications: In the US, only a few states have specific educational requirements for Western-trained physicians who practice acupuncture. The current standard was developed by the World Federation of Acupuncture and Moxibustion Societies under the auspices of the World Health Organization (WHO). This standard recommends a minimum of 200 hours of training in acupuncture. Various physician acupuncture groups, such as the American Academy of Medical Acupuncture and the Australian and New Zealand Medical Acupuncture Societies, have designed programs to meet this requirement. However, some physician-training programs are ongoing programs that can be more extensive. In the USA, UK and Australia, it is possible for physicians to practice with no required training. It is generally recommended that patients are referred to someone who has the above or greater training.

Specifically trained acupuncturists. Acupuncturists typically graduate from acupuncture programs of 2–4 years duration. Upon graduation, they must satisfy the licensing requirements of the state or country in which they intend to practice. Thus it is important to verify that the practitioner has graduated from at least a 2-year program (preferably a recognized school, see below), and has licensure or registration in that state or has passed a national examination such as that prepared by the National Commission for the Certification of Acupuncturists (NCCA) in the USA. In the UK, since there is as yet no licensure, verify that the practitioner belongs to one of the registers, and has graduated from one of the major schools.

Titles, the initials after an acupuncturist's name, are more difficult to assess than are academic degrees. There are variances between countries, between states, between the same states at different times, and between programs. For example, you will find some acupuncturists using the title 'Doctor' who have an MD, some who have an academic PhD, some who are chiropractors, and some who have professional (nonacademic) doctorates in a variety of unrelated fields. There are also titles that are rough translations of foreign credentials, and titles given for what are essentially programs in continuing education. Overseas certificate programs and commercial certification programs are extremely difficult to assess. In both the West and East Asia the titles awarded are sometimes grander than the courses themselves.

The assessment of Asian degrees acquired in the 1950s to 1980 is difficult. To assess these Asian titles fairly one must know the school, the date of graduation, and the curriculum accomplished. However, in China there are now two standardized ways to become a registered doctor of TCM: students study as apprentices alongside established practitioners; or students pass the national entrance examination and become students at an institute of TCM. Apprentices are registered when they pass a national examination, and institute students are automatically registered when they pass their final examinations. No matter which of these paths is taken, the same basic subjects are studied, although in the institutes modern biomedicine is also studied. There are about 20 subjects common to both paths, the number varying from year to year.

The structure of a 5- or 6-year full-time course in China is quite different from the structure of a Bachelor course in the West. In China the first 4 years are spent studying at an

---

Box A1.1 Questions to ask when selecting an acupuncturist	
Western-trained physician practicing acupuncture	**Specifically-trained practitioners**
• Have you completed a WHO recommended acupuncture program? • How many years have you been practicing? • What are your results treating this condition? • What treatment approach would you recommend for my problem? • Can I have disposable needles if I ask for them? • What is the cost of each treatment session and the initial visit? • How often will I need to see you, and for how many visits?	• Are you licensed? • How many years have you been practicing? • Which acupuncture school did you graduate from? • What are your results treating this condition? • What treatment approach would you recommend for my problem? • Can I have disposable needles if I ask for them? • What is the cost of the initial visit and each treatment session? • How often will I need to see you, and for how many visits?

institute, and the last year is spent in a hospital. Students study or train for 42 weeks a year, 6 days a week, 8 hours a day. After finishing an internship they become a registered Bachelor of TCM. At this time, they can choose to enter clinical practice or to continue studying. To continue studying, students must select a subject and pass an entrance examination on that subject, studying in that single area of special interest for another 3 years. After another examination, a master's degree is awarded. Those who enter clinical practice may, after 2 years, take up an additional degree, again after first passing an entrance examination. There are also practical master's degrees; these take another 3 years to complete. Once a master's degree has been obtained and another entrance examination passed, the student may study for a PhD, which takes another 2 or 3 years. Thus, learning that a practitioner has been formally registered in the People's Republic of China indicates a considerable degree of both didactic and practical training. However, very little of that training may be in acupuncture, and questions similar to those you would ask Western-trained physicians are appropriate for Chinese physicians:

- Were you registered in the People's Republic of China?
- What was your area of study (acupuncture, herbal medicine)?
- How many years have you been practicing?
- What are your results treating this condition?
- What treatment approach would you recommend for my problem?
- Can I have disposable needles if I ask for them?
- What is the cost of each treatment session and the initial visit?
- How often will I need to see you, and for how many visits?

These general guidelines can be used when specific recommendations are absent; there are experienced acupuncturists who, having trained prior to the current era, do not have formal credentials. There are excellent practitioners whose names are unadorned with titles. There are excellent practitioners whose names are followed by an entire alphabet soup. In the USA only those who have passed the NCCA examination may use the title Dip Ac, NCCA. A fellow of the National Academy of Acupuncture and Oriental Medicine (FNAAOM) has been nominated and accepted by his peers; however, this title does not specify any particular educational achievement, but rather a contribution recognized by the Academy's fellows.

How to find an acupuncturist

- *State acupuncture associations* usually have contact numbers for referral; these are usually found in phone books.
- *The board of medicine* for each authority that licenses acupuncturists maintains a list of acupuncturists licensed or registered by that authority.
- *National associations* have contact numbers where you can obtain referral information.

US acupuncture organizations

American Academy of Medical Acupuncture (AAMA), 5820 Wilshire Boulevard, Suite 500 Los Angeles, CA 90036. (Tel. 213 937 5514)

American Association of Oriental Medicine (AAOM), 433 Front St, Catasaqua, PA 18032–2506. (Tel. 610 266 1433)

National Acupuncture and Oriental Medicine Alliance (NAOMA) 14637 Starr Rd. S.E., Ollaia, WA 98359 (253-861-6896)

National Acupuncture Detox Association (NADA) Box 1927, Vancouver, WA, 98668-1927 (206-260-8620)

The National Certification Commission for Acupuncture and Oriental Medicine (NCCAOM), 11 Canal Center Plaza, Suite 300, Alexandria VA 22314

UK acupuncture associations

International Register of Oriental Medicine, Green Hedges House, Green Hedges Avenue, East Grinstead, West Sussex RH19 1DZ, UK

Register of Traditional Chinese Medicine, 19 Trinity Road, London N2 8JJ, UK

British Acupuncture Association and Register, 34 Alderney Street, London SW1V 4EU, UK

Traditional Acupuncture Society, 1 The Ridgeway, Stratford upon Avon, Warwickshire CV37 9JL, UK

Australian and New Zealand acupuncture associations

Australian Medical Acupuncture Society, c/o Dr Chin Chan, Bundall Clinic, 60 Ashmore Road, Bundall, Queensland 4217, Australia. (Tel. 075 926 770)

Acupuncture Association of Victoria, 126 Union Road, Surrey Hills, Victoria 3127, Australia.

Medical Acupuncture Society of New Zealand, PO Box 164 Lyleton, 64-3-3288132

Australian Acupuncture & Chinese Medicine Association, PO Box 5142, West End 4101, Queensland. (Tel. 1 800 025 334 or 07 3846 5866)

Australian Traditional Medicine Society, PO Box 1027, Meadowbank 2114, NSW. (Tel. 02 9809 6800)

New Zealand Register of Acupuncturists, PO Box 9950, Wellington 1, New Zealand. (Tel. 04 476 8578)

Canadian acupuncture associations

The Canadian Acupuncture Foundation, Ste. 302, 7321 Victoria Park Avenue, Markham, Ontario L3R 278, Canada.

Research organizations

As an interested researcher, you can contact the following organizations for information about acupuncture:

Society for Acupuncture Research, 6900 Wisconsin Ave., Suite 700, Bethesda, MD 28314, (301-571-0624).

American Foundation of Medical Acupuncture, 5820 Wilshire Boulevard, Suite 500, Los Angeles, CA 90036, USA. (Tel. 213 937 5514)

Research Council for Complementary Medicine, 60 Great Ormond Street, London WC1N 3JF, UK. (Tel. 0171 833 8897)

Acupuncture Research Resource Centre, Centre for Complementary Health Studies, Amory Building, Rennes Drive, Exeter EX4 4RJ, UK. (Tel. 01392 264 498)

As an interested academic researcher, you can contact the following for information:

Centre for Complementary Health Studies, Streatham Court, Rennes Drive, University of Exeter, Exeter EX4 4PU, UK (Tel. 01392 264 498)

Department of Complementary Medicine, School of Postgraduate Medicine and Health Studies, University of Exeter, 25 Victoria Park Road, Exeter EX2 4NT, UK. (Tel. 01392 424 989)

Center for Alternative Medicine Research, Beth Israel Hospital, Harvard Medical School, 330 Brookline Avenue, Boston, MA 02215, USA. (Tel. 617 667 3995)

Centre for the Study of Complementary Medicine, 51 Bedford Place, Southampton SO1 2DG, UK. (Tel. 01703 231 835)

Division of Complementary Medicine University of Maryland School of Medicine, James L. Kerman Hospital Mansion, 2200 Forest Park Avenue, Baltimore, MD. 21207-6697 (410 328-3784)

Acupuncture and Alternative Medicine Program, Hennepin Faculty Associates, 825 South Eighth Street, Suite 1106 Minneapolis, MN 55404, USA. (Tel. 612 347 6238)

Bastyr College, 14500 Juanitz Drive N.E. Kendall WA 98011 (425-823-1300)

Peer review journals

The following journals are not primarily concerned with clinical East Asian medicine. They review scholarly work in the field, and works in allied disciplines such as linguistics. Peer-reviewed clinical journals in acupuncture have yet to develop; all acupuncture journals are presently proprietary.

Journal of Asian Studies Department of History, University of Wisconsin, Milwaukee, WI 53201, USA.

Philosophy East and West University of Hawaii Press, 2840 Kolowaku Street, Honolulu, HI 96822, USA.

Oceanic Linguistics University of Hawaii Press, 2840 Kolowaku Street, Honolulu, HI 96822, USA.

China Review International University of Hawaii Press, 2840 Kolowaku Street, Honolulu, HI 96822, USA.

Asian Studies Review Asian Studies Association of Australia, La Trobe University, Bundoora, VIC 3083, Australia.

Australian Journal of Chinese Affairs RSPA5, Australian National University, Canberra, ACT 0200, Australia.

Journal of Oriental Studies Centre of Asian Studies, The University of Hong Kong, Pokfulam Road, Hong Kong.

International Association for the Study of Traditional Asian Medicine Department of Anthropology, Emory University Atlanta, GA 330322, USA.

ChinaMed Dipl. Kfm. Renate Hess, Herbert-Lewin-Strasse 5, 50931 Koln, Germany.

The Journal of Asian Studies The Association of Asian Studies, 1 Lane Hall, University of Michigan, Ann Arbor, MI 48109, USA.

Electronic resources

Databases in which literature searches on acupuncture are available are: MEDLINE, EMBASE, AMED, CATLINE, and LCMARC. JMEDICINE is recommended for those who read Japanese.

Other resources

We have not included commercial resources because it is impossible for us to gather the information necessary to author fair reviews or compile a comprehensive list. However, practitioner journals oriented to clinical topics, books, and products, as well as many schools and educational programs, are commercially available.

There are growing numbers of World Wide Web and other sites available through commercial online services and internet service providers. Internet searches under 'acupuncture, Oriental medicine, TCM' yield hundreds of references. Most are commercial. There are no USENET newsgroups specifically related to acupuncture; however, there are a number related to holism. Although there are practitioner 'listservs,' we are presently unaware of any for patients or referring physicians.

As a prospective student how do you find out about acupuncture schools? How do you choose between acupuncture schools?

Around 20 schools in the USA are accredited by the National Accreditation Commission for the Schools and Colleges of Acupuncture and Oriental Medicine, which itself is accredited by the US Department of Education. Some 10 other schools are in accreditation candidacy. It is a good idea to attend a school, that is accredited or in candidacy because this maximizes your options for practice locations (because of licensing requirements). Based on what you know about your interest in acupuncture, ask relevant questions, and select the school that is closest to your interests. Talk to students in their last year, or to students who have graduated. It is graduating students who know the most about a school, and it is recent graduates who can tell you how well their education prepared them for practice. To find out about schools in the USA contact:

The Council of Colleges of Acupuncture and Oriental Medicine, 1010 Wayne Avenue, Suite 1270, Silver Spring, MD 20910. (301-608-9175)

In the UK, you can contact:

The Council for Acupuncture, Suite 1, 19A Cavendish Square, London W1M 9AD.

In Australia and Canada, contact the associations listed above.

Contacting the authors

You may contact us at: bob@paradigm-pubs. com. Although we cannot guarantee an answer to every query, much less a timely reply, we will try to refer educators, interested researchers, and scholars to colleagues or sources of interest. Please do not submit questions concerning medical conditions; we cannot wisely, ethically, or accurately answer such queries. We are particularly interested in written materials and references concerning the modern history of acupuncture in the West and would appreciate any personal sources readers may offer.

Appendix 2

Major acupuncture/ moxibustion treatises

(C) Chinese; (J) Japanese; (K) Korean

−200 (C) *Zu Bi Shi Yi Mai Jiu Jing* and *Yin Yang Shi Yi Mai Jiu* from the Ma Wang-dui grave site are the oldest extant medical treatises describing the precursors of the channel system used in acupuncture and moxibustion. These two treatises did not describe the systems of acupoints, and described only the use of moxibustion along the channel pathways. At the time of this publication an authoritative English translation by Donald Harper was near publication by the Welcome Institute, Kegan Paul International.

−200 to −100 (C) *Huang Di Nei Jing Su Wen Ling Shu*, the *Nei Jing*, regarded by many as the 'bibles' of acupuncture. These two books are compilations of various authors and theories about health and disease. The *Su Wen* contains significant theory, with treatment primarily by bloodletting; the *Ling Shu* has more information on the practice of acupuncture and moxibustion. There are thought to be over 250 Chinese commentaries and more than 20 Japanese commentaries on the *Nei Jing*, many of which have been influential. The *Nei Jing* is thought by many to be the basis for the practice of traditional medicines such as acupuncture, moxibustion, and herbal medicine. There have been a few English translations of the *Nei Jing*. These are either translations of the modern editions produced in the People's Republic of China during the 1950s or of an edition individually selected from one or another period. The *Nei Jing* is only now being collated into an edition, the contents of which have been justified by the best-available scholarly investigation. Professor Unschuld's group will publish that edition, including commentaries, in approximately 2005.

c **100** (C) *Nan Jing*, attributed to Bian Que, is an extremely important text in the historical development of acupuncture. It was the first acupuncture-only text book. It is *the* text that first systematically developed and described the theory of systematic correspondence, which has been influential in acupuncture ever since. It systematized the idea of *qi* circulation, the practice of radial pulse diagnosis, abdominal diagnosis, subtle needle techniques, the five-phase classification of the acupuncture points, and the extraordinary vessels, all of which are essential in the practice of acupuncture, surviving in various traditions into modern practice in most countries where acupuncture is practiced. There are over 70 Chinese and over 50 Japanese commentaries on the *Nan Jing*, many of which have been influential. It is the one classical text with a firmly founded English translation, including commentaries. Professor Unschuld's *Nan Jing* has been available in English since 1986.

c 280 (C) *Mai Jing*, by Wang Shu-he, was the first classic on pulse diagnosis. Wang Shu-he systematized even further what the author(s) of the *Nan Jing* had begun, and described the use of acupuncture, moxibustion, and herbal medicine. Passages from the *Mai Jing* have been translated, but there is no entire English version available.

282 (C) *Zhen Jiu Jia Yi Jing*, by Huang Fu-mi, is an important text because it systematically described ideas from the *Nei Jing* and *Nan Jing*, but more importantly, it was the first text to describe systematically the locations, techniques, and uses of the acupuncture points. This trend, started by Huang Fu-mi, has continued into modern times, where description of the location, techniques of stimulation, and clinical uses (diseases and functions) of the points is routinely found in textbooks of acupuncture. There is a direct translation of the systematic classic translated by Yang Shou-zhang and Charles Chace, published by Blue Poppy Press.

610 (C) *Huang Di Nei Jing Tai Su*, by Yang Shang-shan (but probably compiled over several centuries by several authors), is an important text because it describes, explains, and expands on earlier *Nei Jing* and *Nan Jing* discussions of the practice of acupuncture and moxibustion. No translation is currently available.

652 (C) *Qian Jin Yao Fang*, by Sun Si-miao, is important because Sun Si-miao described many 'extra' points (non-channel points that have powerful symptomatic effects, especially when treated by moxibustion), and first described the '*a-shi*' point, the 'pressure–pain point.' No English translation is currently available.

762 (C) *Chong Guang Bu Zhu Huang Di Nei Jing Su Wen*, by Wang Bing, is the oldest surviving edition of the *Nei Jing*, and is important also for its new additions, in particular the biorhythm *yun qi* system. No English translation is currently available.

982 (J) *Ishin Po*, by Tamba Yasuyori, is an important historical text, not only because it is one of the oldest surviving historical texts, but also because it describes and compiles an enormous amount of medical information that was current at that time in Japan and China, including one section devoted to the practice of acupuncture and moxibustion. Parts of the *Ishin Po* have been translated into English, but no entire translation is available.

1027 (C) *Tong Ren Shu Xue Zhen Jiu Tu Jing*, by Wang Wei-yi, is important because it helped establish the standard for acupuncture-point locations and descriptions, being a systematization and authoritative statement of previous literature. It was called the 'bronze statue' textbook, because it was after this text that the bronze statue used for the point-location examination was based. No English translation is currently available.

1125 (C) *Tai Yi Shen Zhen*, by Yuan Ti, is the first book in the *shen zhen* tradition, where moxa was mixed with herbs, rolled into a pole, and used in place of moxa to heat the points. No English translation is currently available.

1126 (C) *Huang Di Ming Tang Jiu Jing*, by Dou Zhe, is an early important and influential moxibustion-only treatise. This text had a particularly strong influence on Isaburo Fukaya, an important figure in the moxibustion tradition of modern Japan. While the tradition of moxibustion specialization survived into the 20th century in China, right up to the installation of the Communist government, the tradition seems to be less important in China today, but remains very important in Japan, where moxibustion is licensed separately from acupuncture. No English translation is currently available.

1153 (C) *Zi Wu Liu Zhu Zhen Jing*, by He Ruo-yu, is the first clear and systematic description of the primary 'biorhythm' methods of acupuncture. The *Zi Wu Liu Zhu* system describes points that can be selected based on time of day, and the day in a cycle of days, that are said to be 'open' and capable of treating all diseases. Not only is this a fascinating system, but it has survived into modern practice, and has shown interesting results in modern scientific experiments. No English translation is currently available.

1220 (C) *Zhen Jiu Zi Sheng Jing*, by Wang Shu-chuan, is an important Song dynasty contribution to the acupuncture literature. No English translation is currently available.

1226 (C) *Bei Ji Jiu Fa*, by Wen Ren Qi-nian, is another significant moxibustion-only treatise. No English translation is currently available.

1241 (C) *Zhen Jing Zhi Nan*, by Dou Han-qing, is significant for a number of reasons, among them, Dou's development of four pairs of points with broad effects. These four pairs of points were later identified as the primary treatment points for the 'extraordinary vessels,' frequently used by some in modern practice. No English translation is currently available.

1289 (C) *Bian Que Xin Shu*, by Dou Cai, is an important early moxibustion-only treatise that helped establish further the tradition of moxibustion practice separately from the practice of acupuncture. No English translation is currently available.

1289 (C) *Gao Huang Shu Xue Jiu Fa*, by Zhang Zhuo, is a small moxibustion-only treatise describing the wonderful effects of applying moxibustion to the acupuncture point, *Gao Huang Shu*. No English translation is currently available.

1311 (C) *Zhen Jiu Si Shu*, by Dou Gui-fang, is important because Dou compiled four small but influential treatises into this book. No English translation is currently available.

1341 (C) *Shi Si Jing Fa Hui*, by Hua Shou, is important as Hua developed what is one of the most complete descriptions of the channel system, which has held influence into the modern literature on acupuncture. No English translation is currently available.

1361 (C) *Nan Jing Ben Yi*, by Hua Shou, is considered to be an important and influential commentary on the *Nan Jing*. No English translation is currently available.

1399 (C) *Ma Niu Yi Fang*, the *Veterinary Prescriptions for Horses and Oxen*, is a reasonably well-known veterinary acupuncture and moxibustion manual, indicating that such practices on domesticated animals had become commonplace. While veterinary treatments can be found dating from the Tang dynasty, they saw a significant increase from the Yuan dynasty onwards. No English translation is currently available.

1437 (C) *Zhen Jiu Da Quan*, by Xu Feng, is one of the most important and influential Ming dynasty compilations. This text began the tradition found throughout the Ming dynasty of compiling the best ideas of clinical practice, and interpretations of traditional ideas. This text is noted in particular for its compilation of the literature on the biorhythm treatment methods, the first description of the pairings and primary treatment points of the 'extraordinary vessels,' both of which influenced later Ming compilations and both of which survive into modern practice as influential and clinically invaluable methods. No English translation is currently available.

(?) 1500s (K) *Ui Pang Yu Ch'wi*, by many Korean physicians, compiled under the supervision of Sejong the Great, is an early influential Korean text consisting of 365 volumes. No English translation is currently available.

1505 (C) *Nan Jing Ji Zhu*, by Wang Jiu-si, is an important *Nan Jing* commentary, mostly written as a compilation of important earlier commentaries. No English translation is currently available.

1510 (C) *Tu Zhu Ba Shi Yi Nan Jing*, by Zheng Shi-xien, is an important *Nan Jing* commentary. No English translation is currently available.

1529 (C) *Zhen Jiu Ju Ying*, by Gao Wu, is another important text in the tradition of the *Zhen Jiu Da Quan*. It is important for its compilation and explication of many traditional ideas and methods. It is noted especially for its development of ideas about the five-phase points, in particular its innovation of the 'supplementation' (or 'tonification') and 'draining' (or 'dispersion') points. This classification of certain five-phase points is very important in virtually every traditional system that has survived into the modern period. No English translation is currently available.

1575 (C) *Yi Xue Ru Men*, by Li Ting, is an influential and important introductory text on acupuncture, moxibustion, and herbal medicine. This text was frequently quoted by Soulie de Morant in his influential *L'Acupuncture Chinoise*. No entire English translation is available.

1578 (C) *Qi Jing Ba Mai Kao*, by Li Shi-zhen, was the only historical treatise devoted to the extraordinary vessel channel system. While theoretically very influential, treatments were described almost totally in terms of herbal medicine, so its import in acupuncture is primarily to do with Li's excellent scholarship of the earlier theoretical literature on the extraordinary vessels. No English translation is currently available.

late 1500s (K) *Chimku Yokyol*, by Sa-Am or Do-In, is important as it was here that Sa-Am expounded his five-phase 'four point' 'supplementation' and 'draining' treatments, which have been influential in Korea ever since, being taught in the curriculum of the modern schools of Oriental medicine in Korea. Sa-Am's treatment patterns have also been influential in many other countries. They have been adopted in modern textbooks in Japan, the UK, Europe, and the USA. No English translation is currently available.

1601 (C) *Zhen Jiu Da Cheng*, by Yang Ji-zhou, is perhaps the most influential text of the Ming dynasty. It follows in the tradition of the *Zhen Jiu Da Quan*, but gained much greater recognition. It is an explanatory text of the traditional literatures dating from the *Nei Jing*, and a compilation of the most useful clinical treatment protocols known to the author at the time. This text has influenced untold numbers of practitioners in many countries into the modern era. There have been at least 30 editions through 1900, and about 50 since 1900. *L'Acupuncture Chinoise*, an important and influential French modern text on acupuncture, was heavily influenced by this book. The work of the famous clinician James Tin Yau So seems to be heavily influenced by this text; the development of the modern system of 'traditional Chinese medical acupuncture' seems also to have been strongly influenced by this text. Although the significance of this text for the modern practice of acupuncture cannot be overstated, it has not been translated into English.

1613 (K) *Tong Ui Po Kam*, by Ho Chun, was a well-known and influential dictionary of medicine, including acupuncture. No English translation is available.

1624 (C) *Lei Jing*, by Zhang Jie-bin, is an important text as it is an explanation by categorization of the *Nei Jing*. No English translation is available.

1624 (C) *Jing Yue Quan Shu*, by Zhang Jie-bin, is important because Zhang describes systematically both historical and recent medical ideas and methods. His text has been quite influential, as it pertained to concepts and methods that would prevail into the modern era, focusing primarily on acupuncture and moxibustion. No English translation is available.

1642 (C) *Nei Jing Zhi Yao*, by Li Zhong-zi, is an important systematic explanation of the *Nei Jing*. No English translation is available.

1644 (K) *Ch'im Ku Kyong Hom Pang*, by Ho Rim, was an influential Korean text on the theories and practice of acupuncture and moxibustion. No English translation is available.

1677 (C) *Su Wen Jing Zhu Jie Jie*, by Yao Zhi-an, is an important and influential commentary on the *Nei Jing*. No English translation is available.

c **1700** (J) *Sugiyama Ryu Sanbusho*, by Waichi Sugiyama, is important because Sugiyama is considered to be the 'father' of acupuncture in Japan. He invented the *shinkan*, or insertion tube, which is used by virtually every acupuncturist in Japan today, and by many others around the world. Sugiyama was also the first blind acupuncturist in Japan, and started the first school for blind acupuncturists in the late 17th century. His text is a straightforward explanation of basic principles stemming from the *Nei Jing* and *Nan Jing*, with treatment approaches that continue to influence modern practitioners today. No English translation is available.

early 1700s (J) *Mokyu Susetsu*, by Konzan Goto, is an influential Japanese moxibustion-only book. No English translation is available.

1703 (J) *Shinkyu Azeyoketsu*, by Ippo Okamoto, is a significant and influential Japanese acupuncture point text, summarizing both traditional Chinese and Japanese ideas about the uses of the points. No English translation is available.

1712 (J) *Wakan Sansai Zue*, by Ryoan Terashima, is an important text, where Terashima compiled the dominant ideas of the time (including many historical ideas) about the broad practice of medicine, including acupuncture, moxibustion, and herbal medicine. In some respects, this is similar to, but not as influential as, the *Ishin Po* of eight centuries earlier. No English translation is available.

1718 (J) *Shinkyu Chu Ho Ki*, by Masaytoyo Hongo, is an influential Japanese acupuncture and moxibustion text, describing treatment techniques, point locations, and point uses quite systematically. No English translation is available.

1727 (C) *Tai Yi Shen Zhen*, by Fan Yu-qi, is an influential text in the '*shen zhen*' moxibustion tradition. No English translation is available.

1742 (C) *Yi Zong Jin Jian*, by Wu Qian, is a major compilation of all aspects of Chinese traditional medicines, including acupuncture, moxibustion, and herbal medicine. No English translation is available.

mid-1700s (J) *Ipon Do Kyusen* and *Kagawa Kyuten*, both by Shutoku Kagawa, are influential Japanese moxibustion-only texts. No English translation is available.

1750 (J) *Nangyo Tekkan*, by Sosen Hirōka, is an influential Japanese commentary on the *Nan Jing*. No English translation is available.

1757 (C) *Yi Xue Yuan Liu Lun*, by Xu Da-chun, is important for several reasons. Xu was one of the more influential scholar-physicians of Chinese traditional medicine from this era, and was quite critical of his peers and predecessors. He bridged all the major theories and treatment systems that survived to his time with critical precision, casting a shadow that looks very modern. He wrote essays on acupuncture and moxibustion, as well as many on diagnosis and herbal medicine. Paul Unschuld's English translation (*Forgotten Traditions of Ancient Chinese Medicine*) is available.

1767 (J) *Shinkyu Soku*, by Shukei Suganuma, is a small but influential acupuncture and moxibustion text that focuses on the classical tradition of practice in Japan. No English translation is available.

1798 (C) *Zhen Jiu Yi Xue*, by Li Shou-xian, is an important and influential text describing the practice of acupuncture in relation to ideas from the famous book the *Yi Jing* (*Book of Changes*). No English translation is available.

1805 (J) *Meika Kyusen*, by Waki and Hirai, is a very famous and influential moxibustion-only text that continues to influence modern practice through the work of Isaburo Fukaya. The text is a compilation of moxa recipes and empirical famous treatment points. No English translation is available.

1811 (J) *Shinkyu Setsuyaku*, by Sōtetsu Ishizaka, is important because it marked the beginning of the Western scientific influence (Dutch medicine) in the practice of acupuncture and moxibustion in Japan. Ishizaka tried to reconcile traditional methods and ideas with modern anatomically based descriptions, and thus began a trend that continues into modern practice in all countries, being especially obvious in modern Japanese and Chinese systems of acupuncture and moxibustion practice. No English translation is available.

1813 (J) *Kaitai Hatsumou*, by K. Misutane, also attempted to reconcile the traditional with the undeniable observations of Western anatomy. Misutane tried to reconcile traditional anatomical/functional ideas with these modern anatomical ideas. No English translation is available.

1851 (C) *Shen Jiu Jing Lun*, by Wu Yan-cheng, an important Qing dynasty moxibustion-only text, shows that the tradition of moxibustion specialization had survived into the 19th century in China.

1893 (K) *Tong Ui Su Se Po Won*, by Lee Che-ma. In this text, Lee devised his theory and practice of 'four constitution' traditional medicine, which has been influential in Korean acupuncture and moxibustion practice since that time, being taught in the Korean Oriental medical schools as part of the modern curriculum. No English translation is available.

1895 (C) *Nan Jing Zheng Yi*, by Ye Lin, is an important late Qing dynasty commentary on the *Nan Jing*. No English translation is available.

Bibliography

A complete list of sources
consulted during the writing
of this book

Bibliography

Aakster CW 1986 Concepts in alternative medicine. Social Science and Medicine 22(2): 265–273

AAMA Review 1(1), 1989

Abbot NC, White AR, Ernst E 1996 Letter to the editor (complementary medicine). Nature 381:361

Agren H 1975 A new approach to Chinese traditional medicine. American Journal of Chinese Medicine 3(3):207–212

Alavi A, LaRiccia P, Sadek AH et al 1997 Neuroimaging of acupuncture in patients with chronic pain. Journal of Alternative and Complementary Medicine 3(suppl 1):S47–S53

Aldridge D 1989 Europe looks at complementary medicine. British Medical Journal 299:1121–1122

Aldridge D 1990 Pluralism of medical practice in West Germany. Complementary Medicine Research 4(2):14–15

Anon 1947 The status of the blind (acupuncturists). Ido no Nippon Magazine 6(8):45

Anon 1947 Serious news. Ido no Nippon Magazine 6(7):44

Anon 1947 Compensation for our efforts: status law is passed. Ido no Nippon Magazine 6(9):46

Anon 1947 Demonstration by the blind. Asahi Shinbun October

Anon 1948 Symposium on the business and education of acupuncture and moxibustion. Ido no Nippon Sha, Yokosuka

Anon 1975 Acupuncture anesthesia. Geographic Health Studies Program NIH, Washington, DC

Anon 1979 National symposia of acupuncture and moxibustion and acupuncture anesthesia, Beijing

Anon 1980 Essentials of Chinese acupuncture. Foreign Language Press, Beijing

Anon 1986 Bunshun library. Shukan Bunshun 128

Anon 1987 Selection from article abstracts on acupuncture and moxibustion. China Association of Acupuncture and Moxibustion, Beijing

Anon 1988 Interview with Ji Sheng Han. *Omni* February: 81 ff

Anon 1989 Abstracts of the all-union symposium with international participation on the fundamental aspects of the application of µ-range electromagnetic radiation in medicine, Kiev, May 10–13

Anon 1991 One in five Canadians is using alternative therapies, survey finds. Canadian Medical Association Journal 144(4):469

Anon 1994 Acupuncture. Consumer Reports January: 54–59

Anon 1998 Acupuncture: NIH consensus development panel on acupuncture. JAMA 280(17):1518–1524

Baldry PE 1989 Acupuncture, trigger points and musculoskeletal pain. Churchill Livingstone, Edinburgh

Becker RO 1984 Electromagnetic controls over biological growth processes. Journal of Bioelectronics 3(1&2):105–118

Becker RO, Marino AA 1982 Electromagnetism and life. State University of New York Press, Albany, NY

Becker RO, Selden G 1985 The body electric. William Morrow, New York

Beijing Foreign Languages Institute 1980 The Sino Chinese English dictionary. Sino Publishing Company, New York

Benson H, McCallie DP 1979 Angina pectoris and the placebo effect. New England Journal of Medicine 300(25): 1424–1429

Bensoussan A, Myers SP 1996 Towards a safer choice. Department of Human Services, Victoria, Australia

Birch S Preliminary investigations of inter-rater reliability of traditionally based acupuncture diagnostic assessments. (in submission)

Birch S 1989–1991 Acupuncture in Japan; an introductory survey. Parts 1–4. Review 6:12–13, 7:16–20, 8:21–26, 9:28–31, 39–42

Birch S 1992 Naming the un-nameable: a historical study of radial pulse six position diagnosis; Traditional Acupuncture Society 12:2–13

Birch S 1993 Prelude to a trial: preparatory studies for clinical research of acupuncture and east Asian medicine. Proceedings of the first symposium of the Society for Acupuncture Research. Society for Acupuncture Research, Washington DC

Birch S 1989 Plumbing the depths; a comparative study of needle depths for a number of classical and modern acupuncture texts. Unpublished manuscript

Birch S 1989 Acupuncture point contraindications; an historical survey. Unpublished manuscript

Birch S 1993 Some thoughts on the nature and timing of currently proposed changes in the acupuncture field. The Journal of the Acupuncture Society of New York 1(1):20–25; The Journal of Traditional Acupuncture XV: 11–17

Birch S 1993 So what is the *sanjiao*? The Journal of the Acupuncture Society of New York 1(1): 6–8

Birch S 1995 On the development of Japanese style acupuncture in the US. Ido no Nippon Magazine, 7, 11:84–90

Birch S 1997 Testing the claims of traditionally based acupuncture. Complementary Therapies in Medicine 5(3):147–151

Birch S 1997 An exploration with proposed solutions of the problems and issues in conducting clinical research in acupuncture. PhD thesis, Centre for Complementary Health Studies, University of Exeter, UK

Birch S 1995 (Ida J, trans) Gendai Amerika ni Okeru Nihon Igaku no Ukeirei ni Kansuru Mondaiten (Problems in the translation of Japanese medicine in to contemporary America). Ido no Nippon Magazine 7(11):84–90

Birch S 1989 Diversity and acupuncture: acupuncture is not a coherent or historically stable tradition. In: Vickers AJ (ed) Examining complementary medicine: the sceptical holist. Stanley Thomas, Cheltenham

Birch S 1997 Through the point of the needle. Reflections on the influence of acupuncture and traditional East Asian medicine on consciousness. In: Rubik B (ed) Frontiers of consciousness

Birch S 1992 A taxonomy of acupuncture. Unpublished manuscript

Birch S 1995 Testing the clinical specificity of needle sites in controlled clinical trials of acupuncture. Part 1: the importance of validating the 'relevance' of 'true' or 'active' points and 'irrelevance' of 'control' or 'less active' points proposal for a justification method. Part 2: The problem of 'diffuse noxious inhibitory control' and how to control for it. Proceedings of the second symposium of the society for Acupuncture Research. Society for Acupuncture Research, Washington DC, pp 274–294

Birch S 1997 Issues to consider in dermining an adequate treatment in a clinical trial of acupuncture. Complementary Therapies in Medicine 5:8–12

Birch S, Friedman M 1989 On the development of a mathematical model for the 'laws' of the five phases. American Journal of Acupuncture 17(4):361–366

Birch S, Hammerschlag R 1996 Acupuncture efficacy: a compendium of controlled clinical trials. National Academy of Acupuncture and Oriental Medicine, New York

Birch S, Ida J 1997 Forming a prognosis; perspectives from the works of Japanese acupuncturists: a preliminary compilation of ideas. North American Journal of Oriental Medicine 4(10):4–8

Birch S, Ida J 1998 Japanese acupuncture: a clinical guide. Paradigm Publications, Brookline, MA, in press

Birch S, Jamison RN 1998 The importance of assessing the reliability of diagnosis in traditional acupuncture. Abstracts of the third world conference on acupuncture. World Federation of Acupuncture and Moxibustion Societies, Kyoto

Birch S, Jamison RN 1998 A controlled clinical trial of Japanese acupuncture: assessment of specific and non specific effects of treatment. 14:248–255

Birch S, Tsutani K 1995 A bibliometrical study of English language materials on acupuncture. Complementary Therapies in Medicine 4:172–177

Birch S, Hammerschlag R, Berman B 1996 Acupuncture in the treatment of pain. Journal of Alternative and Complementary Medicine 2:101–124

Birch S et al 1998 Trigger point acupoint correlations revisited. Unpublished manuscript

Bischko J 1985 An introduction to acupuncture, 2nd edn. Karl F Haug, Heidelberg

Bischko J 1986 Intermediate acupuncture. Karl F Haug, Heidelberg vol 2

Blackburn BA, Smith H, Chalmers TC 1982 The inadequate evidence for short hospital stay after hernia or varicose vein stripping surgery. The Mount Sinai Journal of Medicine 49(5):383–390

Bossut D 1990 Development of veterinary acupuncture in China. Paper presented at the 16th International Veterinary Acupuncture Society Congress on Veterinary Acupuncture, Holland

Bossut D 1996 Veterinary clinical applications of acupuncture. Journal of Alternative and Complementary Medicine 2(1):65–69

Bossut DF, Mayer DJ 1991 Electroacupuncture analgesia in rats: naltrexone antagonism is dependent on previous exposure. Brain Research 549:47–51

Bossut DF, Mayer DJ 1991 Electroacupuncture analgesia in naive rats: effects of brainstem and spinal cord lesions, and role of pituitary–adrenal axis. Brain Research 549:52–58

Bossut DF et al 1991 Electroacupuncture in rats: evidence for naloxone and naltrexone potentiation of analgesia Brain Research 549:36–46

Bossy J 1993 History and present status of acupuncture in France. World Federation of Acupuncture and Moxibustion

Societies. Abstracts of the Third World Conference on Acupuncture, Kyoto

Boston Globe 246(103), 13 April 1994

Bouchayer F 1990 Alternative medicines: a general approach to the French situation. Complementary Medicine Research 4(2):4–8

Bourdiol RJ 1983 Auriculo-somatology. Maisonneuve, Moulins-les-Metz, France

Bradford H 1994 Cost effectiveness of acupuncture. Proceedings of the first symposium of the Society for Acupuncture Research. Society for Acupuncture Research, Washington DC

Bragin E 1993 Present and future of traditional medicine in Russia. In: Abstracts of the Third World Conference on Acupuncture. World Federation of Acupuncture and Moxibustion Societies, Kyoto

British Medical Association 1993 Complementary medicine; new approaches to good practice. Oxford University Press, Oxford

Broffman M, McCulloch M 1986 Instrument assisted pulse evaluation in the acupuncture practice. American Journal of Acupuncture 14(3):255–259

Brumbaugh AG 1993 Acupuncture: new perspectives in chemical dependency treatment. Journal of Substance Abuse Treatment 10:35–43

Bullock ML, Culliton PD, Olander RL 1989 Controlled trial of acupuncture for severe recidivist alcoholism. Lancet 24 June: 1435–1439

Califano JA, Kleber HD 1992 Annual report. Center on Addiction and Substance Abuse, Columbia University, Columbia, OH

Campbell J 1962 The masks of god: oriental mythology. Penguin, New York

Campbell NA 1987 Biology. Benjamin Cummings, Menlo Park, CA

Cao XD 1977 Protective effect of acupuncture on immunosuppression. In: NIH Consensus Development Conference on Acupuncture. Program & Abstracts. National Institutes of Health, Bethesda, MD, pp 129–133

Capra F 1982 The turning point. Bantam, New York

Carneiro NM, Li SM 1995 Letter to the editor (acupuncture technique). Lancet 345:1577

Carr DJ, Blalock JE 1991 Neuropeptide hormones and receptors common to the immune and neuroendocrine systems: bidirectional pathway of intersystem communication. Psychoneuroimmunology: 573–588

Chalmers TC, Block JB, Lee S 1972 Controlled studies in clinical cancer research. New England Journal of Medicine 287(2):75–78

Chang J 1992 Wild Swans. Flamingo, London

Chang PL 1988 Urodynamic studies in acupuncture for women with frequency, urgency and dysuria. Journal of Urology 140:563–566

Chapman CR, Chen AC, Bonica JJ 1977 Effects of intrasegmental electrical acupuncture on dental pain; evaluation by threshold estimation and sensory decision theory. *Pain* 3:213–227

Chen WC et al 1979 The determination of the depth of puncture for the development of needling sensation. In: National Symposia of Acupuncture and Moxibustion and Acupuncture Anesthesia, Bejing, China, pp 113–114

Chen Ze-lin 1988 Development of research on tongue diagnosis. Chinese Journal of Integrated Medicine 8(special issue 2):104–108

Chen Zhi 1979 Ci Liao Fa, methods of magnet treatment. Science and Technology Publishing, Hunan

Cheng R, Pomeranz B 1987 Electrotherapy of chronic musculoskeletal pain: comparison of electroacupuncture acupuncture-like TENS. Clinical Journal of Pain 2:143–149

Cheng R.S.S. 1989 Neurophysiology of electroacupuncture analgesia. In: Pomeranz B, Stux G (eds) Scientific bases of acupuncture. Springer-Verlag, Berlin, pp 119–136

Cheng Xinnong (ed) 1987 Chinese acupuncture and moxibustion. Foreign Languages Press, Beijing

Chiu ML 1986 Mind, body, and illness in a Chinese medical tradition. PhD thesis, Harvard University, Cambridge, MA

Coan RM et al 1980 The acupuncture treatment of low back pain: a randomized controlled study. American Journal of Chinese Medicine 1:39–42

Cohen AP (ed) 1979 Selected works of Peter A. Bodenberg. University of California Press, Berkeley, CA

Cooper RA, Henderson T, Dietrich CL 1998 Roles of nonphysician clinicians as autonomous providers of healthcare. JAMA 280(9):795–802

Cooper RA, Laud P, Dietrich CL 1998. Current and projected workforce of nonphysician clinicians JAMA 280, 9: 788–794

Coseo M 1992 The acupressure warmup. Paradigm Publications, Brookline, MA

Council of Oriental Medical Publishers 1993 Report of the publishers and translators conference. Journal of the Acupuncture Society of New York 1(2):5–7

Cui Jing, Zhang Guangqi 1989 A survey for thirty years clinical application of cupping. Journal of Traditional Chinese Medicine 9(2):151–154

Culliton P 1994 The Hennepin County experience with acupuncture research. In: Proceedings of the First Symposium of the Society for Acupuncture Research. Society for Acupuncture Research, Washington DC

Culliton PD, Resuk TJ 1996 Overview of substance abuse acupuncture treatment research. Journal of Alternative and Complementary Medicine 2(1):149–159

Cunningham A 1986 Information and health in the many levels of man: toward a more comprehensive theory of health and disease. Advances 3(1):32–45

Darras JC 1989 Isotopic and cytologic assays in acupuncture. In: Energy Fields in Medicine; A Study of Device Technology Based on Acupuncture Meridians and Chi Energy. John E Fetzer Foundation, Kalamazoo, pp 44–65

Debata A 1968 Experimental study on pulse diagnosis of rokubujoi. Japanese Acupuncture and Moxibustion Journal 17(3):9–12

de la Torre CS 1993 The choice of control groups in invasive clinical trials such as acupuncture. Frontier Perspectives 3(2):33–37

Delis K, Morris M 1994 Clinical trials in acupuncture. In: Proceedings of the First Symposium of the Society for Acupuncture Research. Society for Acupuncture Research, Washington DC

Dold C 1998 Needles and Nerves. Discover, September, pp 59–62

Dorland's illustrated medical dictionary, 26th edn, 1981. WB Saunders, Philadelphia

Dundee J., McMillan C 1992 Some problems encountered in the scientific evaluation of acupuncture antiemesis. Acupuncture in Medicine 10(1):2–8

Dung HC 1984 Anatomical features contributing to the formation of acupuncture points. American Journal of Acupuncture 12(2):139–142

Eckman P 1990 Korean acupuncture. Traditional Acupuncture Society Journal 7:1–6

Eckman P 1996 In the footsteps of the yellow emperor. Cypress Book Company, San Francisco, CA

Eckman P 1997 Tracing the historical transmission of traditional acupuncture to the West: in search of the five element transfer lineage and a higher vision. American Journal of Acupuncture 25(1):59–69

Eisenberg D 1989 Energy medicine in China; defining a research strategy which embraces the criticisms of skeptical colleagues. In: Energy fields and medicine: a study of device technology based on acupuncture meridians and chi energy. John E Fetzer Foundation, Kalamazoo, pp 78–92

Eisenberg D, Wright TL 1987 Encounters with qi. Penguin, New York

Eisenberg DM, Kessler RC, Foster C, Norlock FE, Calkins DR, Delbanco TL 1993 Unconventional medicine in the United States; prevalence, costs, and patterns of use. The New England Journal of Medicine 328(4):246–252

Eisenberg DM et al 1993 Cognitive techniques for hypertension: are they effective? Annals of Internal Medicine 118(12):964–972

Eisenberg DM, Davis RB, Ettner SL, Appel S, Wilkey S, Van Rompay M, Kessler RC 1998 Trends in alternative medicine use in the United States 1990–1997. Results of a follow-up national survey. JAMA 280(18):1569–1575

Ellis A, Wiseman N, Boss K 1988 Fundamentals of Chinese acupuncture. Paradigm Publications, Brookline, MA

Ellis A, Wiseman N, Boss K 1989 Grasping the wind. Paradigm Publications, Brookline, MA

Epler DC 1980 Bloodletting in early Chinese medicine and its relation to the origin of acupuncture. Bulletin of the History of Medicine 54:337–367

Ergil KV 1990 A challenge to medical hegemony? Epistemological issues informing the practice of TCM in the United States. Paper presented at the Third International Congress on Traditional Asian Medicine, Bombay

Ergil KV 1992 Strategic representations: 'Oriental' medicine at large. Paper presented at the American Anthropological Association Annual Meeting

Ergil MC 1993 Letter to the editor. Journal of the Acupuncture Society of New York 1–3:23–26

Ergil MC 1994 Chinese medicine in China: education and learning strategies. Paper presented at the Association for Asian Studies Annual Meeting, Boston

Erickson RJ 1992 Acupuncture for chronic pain treatment: its effects on office visits and the use of analgesics in a prepaid health plan: a feasibility study. The AAMA Review 4(2):2–6

Evans JR 1988 Medical Education in China. In: Bowers JZ, Hess JW, Sivin N (eds) *Science and medicine in twentieth century China: research and education.* Center for Chinese Studies, University of Michigan, Ann Arbor, MI, pp 239–259

Falk CX, Birch S, Margolin A, Avants SK 1900 Measurement of electrical resistance of the skin: mapping resistance at auricular acupuncture points. Submitted

Finn P, Newlyn AK 1993 Miami's 'drug court', a different approach. National Institute of Justice, US Department of Justice, Washington DC, NCJ 142412

Fisher S, Greenberg RP 1989 A second opinion: rethinking the claims of biological psychiatry. In Fisher S, Greenberg RP (eds) The limits of biological treatments for psychological distress. Lawrence Erlbaum, Hillsdale, NJ

Flaws B 1991 American acupuncture education: has a wrong turn been taken? American Journal of Acupuncture 19(1):63–70

Flaws B 1993 On the historical relationship or acupuncture and herbal medicine in China and what this means politically in the United States. American Journal of Acupuncture 21(3):267–278

Fletcher RH, Fletcher SW 1977 Clinical research in general medical journals: a 30 year perspective; New England Journal of Medicine 301(4):180–183

Foss L, Rothenberg K 1987 The second medical revolution. Shambhala, Boston, MA

Friedman M, Birch S Towards the development of a mathematical model describing the interactions of the twelve meridians. Unpublished manuscript

Friedman M, Birch S, Tiller WA 1989 Towards the development of a mathematical model for acupuncture meridians. Acupuncture and Electrotherapeutic Research International Journal 14:217–226

Friedman M, Birch S, Tiller WA 1989 A dynamical systems approach to modelling meridians and ki. In: Energy fields and medicine: a study of device technology based on acupuncture meridians and chi energy. John E Fetzer Foundation, Kalamazoo, pp 218–229

Friedman MJ, Birch S, Tiller WA 1997 Mathematical modelling as a tool in basic research in acupuncture. Journal of Alternative and Complementary Medicine 3(suppl 1):S89–S99

Fu Cong-yuan 1988 Achievements of research on pulse-taking with integrated traditional Chinese and Western medicine. Chinese Journal of Integrated Medicine 8(special issue 2):108–112

Fugh-Berman A 1996 Alternative medicine: what works? Odonion, Tucson, AZ

Fukushima K 1991 Meridian therapy. Toyo Hari Medical Association, Tokyo

Fulder S 1989 The handbook of complementary medicine. Coronet, London

Fulder SJ, Munro RE 1985 Complementary medicine in the United Kingdom: patients, practitioners, and consultations. Lancet:542–545

Fung Yu-lan 1952 A history of Chinese philosophy. Princeton University Press, Princeton, NJ

Gale H 1993 Developing national competency standards. Australian Journal of Acupuncture 20:59–62

Gao Wu 1983 Zhen Jiu Ju Ying [1529]. Hong Ye Book Shop, Taipei

Gaw AC et al 1975 Efficacy of acupuncture on osteoarthritis pain: a double blind controlled study. New England Journal of Medicine 293:375–378

Gibbs N 1993 Up in arms. Time 20 December:18–26

Gibbs N 1993 Angels among us. Time 27 December:56–65

Goldkamp JS, Weiland D 1993 Assessing the impact of Dade County's Felony Drug Court. National Institute of Justice, US Department of Justice, Washington, DC, NCJ 145302

Gorman C 1992 Is health care too specialized? Time 14 September

Greenberg RP, Fisher S 1989 Examining antidepressant effectiveness: findings, ambiguities, and some vexing puzzles. In: Fisher S, Greenberg RP (eds) Limits of biological treatments for psychological disorders. Lawrence Erlbaum, Hillsdale NJ

Greenberg RP, Bernstein RF 1992 A meta-analysis of antidepressant outcome under 'blinder' conditions. Journal of Consulting and Clinical Psychology 60(5):664–669

Greenleaf MC 1993 Acupuncture in New Zealand. In: Abstracts of the Third World Conference on Acupuncture. World Federation of Acupuncture and Moxibustion Societies, Kyoto

Grumbach K, Coffman J 1998 Editorial JAMA 280(9): 825–826

Guelrud M, Rossiter A, Souney PF, Sulbaran M 1991 Transcutaneous electrical nerve stimulation decreases lower esophageal sphincter pressure in patients with achalasia. Digestive Diseases and Sciences 36(8):1029–1033

Gunn CC 1976 Transcutaneous nerve stimulation, needle acupuncture and 'Teh Chi' phenomenon. American Journal of Acupuncture 4(4):317–322

Gunn CC 1996 The Gunn approach to the treatment of chronic pain. Churchill Livingstone, Edinburgh

Gunn CC 1988 Reprints on pain, acupuncture and related subjects. Self-published. Vancouver

Guo Qin tang et al 1991 Clinical and experimental observation on treating cholelithiasis by ear-point pressing. International Journal of Clinical Acupuncture 2(1)

Halvorsen TB, Anda SS, Naess AB, Levang OW 1995 Letter to the editor (fatal cardiac tamponade after acupuncture through congenital sternal foramen). Lancet 345:1175

Hammerschlag R 1995 Randomized controlled trials comparing acupuncture and biomedical treatment. In: Proceedings of the Second Symposium of the Society for Acupuncture Research, pp 230–240

Hammerschlag R 1997 Acupuncture efficacy: presenting the evidence. Journal of the National Academy of Acupuncture and Oriental Medicine 4(1–2):9–10

Han Jisheng 1987 The neurochemical basis of pain relief by acupuncture. Beijing Medical University, Beijing

Han Jisheng 1989 Central neurotransmitters and acupuncture analgesia. In: Pomeranz B, Stux G (eds) Scientific bases of acupuncture. Springer-Verlag, Berlin, pp 7–33

Han Jisheng 1997 Physiology of acupuncture: review of thirty years of research. Journal of Alternative and Complementary Medicine 3(suppl 1):S101–S108

Hanson RW, Gerber KE 1990 Coping with chronic pain. Guildford Press, New York

Harper D 1982 The *Wu Sh Erh Ping Fang*: translation and prolegomena. PhD thesis, University of California, Berkeley, CA

Heise TE 1986 Historical development of traditional Chinese medicine in West Germany. Journal of Traditional Chinese Medicine 6(3):227–230

Helms JM 1989 A hierarchy of acupuncture energy lines. In: Energy fields and medicine; a study of device technology based on acupuncture meridians and chi energy. John E Fetzer Foundation, Kalamazoo, pp 2–9

Helms JM 1993 Physicians and acupuncture in the 1990s, a report. The AAMA Review 5(1):1–6

Helms JM 1993 Review of medical and clinical literature paper presented at the workshop on acupuncture. Office of Alternative Medicine Food and Drug Administration, Washington DC

Helms JM 1995 Acupuncture energetics: a clinical approach for physicians. Medical Acupuncture Publishers, Berkeley, CA

Hemken A 1995 The Anglo-Dutch Institute for Oriental Medicine and the situation on alternative medicine in the Netherlands. European Journal of Oriental Medicine 1, 6:30–31

Hillier SM, Jewell JA 1983 Health care and traditional Chinese medicine in China 1800–1982. Routledge & Kegan Paul, London

Huang Fu-mi 1982 *Zhen Jiu Jia Yi Jing*, from *Zhen Jiu Jia Yi Jing Shu Xue Zhong Ji*. Science and Technology Publishing Company, Shandong

Huynh, Hoc Ku (trans) 1985 Pulse diagnosis, *Li Shi Zhen*. Paradigm Publications, Brookline, MA

Hyodo M 1975 *Ryodoraku* treatment. Japan *Ryodoraku*, Autonomic Nerve System Society, Osaka

Ionescu-Trigoviste C 1991 Acupuncture in Romania. Complementary Medicine Research 5(2):89–92

Ishihara T 1983 A compilation of pre-Meiji-era acupuncture related classical literature. *Keiraku Chiryo* 72:8–45

Itaya K, Manaka Y, Ohkubo C, Asano M 1987 Effects of acupuncture needle application upon cutaneous microcirculation of rabbit ear lobe. Acupuncture and Electrotherapeutics Research International Journal 12:45–51

Jobst KA 1995 A critical analysis of acupuncture in pulmonary disease: efficacy and safety of the acupuncture needle. The Journal of Alternative and Complementary Medicine 1(1):57–85

Johansson K et al 1993 Can sensory stimulation improve the functional outcome in stroke patients? Neurology 43:2189–2192

Kaptchuk TJ 1983 The web that has no weaver. Congdon and Weed, New York

Karlgren B 1946 Legends and cults in ancient China. Bulletin of the Museum of Far Eastern Antiquities 18

Keiraku Chiryo Journal. 50th anniversary special issue # 100, January 1990

Keji C Wall Street Journal Interactive Edition 1997 A fight over rice yeast pit, Dec 3

Kennedy DL, Burke LB, McGinnis T 1995 National postmarketing drug surveillance and reporting to the MedWatch program. Pharmacy Times August

Kenner D 1994 A taxonomy of acupuncture. In: Proceedings of the First Symposium of the Society for Acupuncture Research. Society for Acupuncture Research, Washington DC

Kenyon JN 1983 Modern techniques of acupuncture. Thorsons, Wellingborough, vols 1 and 2

Kenyon JN 1985 Modern techniques of acupuncture. Thorsons, Wellingborough, vol 3

Kim DH 1987 Oriental medicine series. Volume 2: Acupuncture and moxibustion. Research Institute of Oriental Medicine, Seoul

Kitasato kenkyujo huzoku toyoigaku sogokenkyujo rinsho koten kenkyuhan 1979 *Somon Rinsho Sakuinshu*, the *Suwen* clinical index. Kokusho Kankokai, Tokyo

Kitasato kenkyujo huzoku toyoigaku sogokenkyujo rinsho koten kenkyuhan 1982 *Reisu Rinsho Sakuinshu*, the *Lingshu* clinical index. Kokusho Kankokai, Tokyo

Kleijnen J et al 1991 Acupuncture and asthma; a review of controlled trials. Thorax 46(11):799–802

Kleinman A 1980 Patients and healers in the context of culture. University of California Press, Berkeley, CA

Kohn L (ed) 1989 Taoist meditation and longevity techniques. University of Michigan Center for Chinese Studies, Ann Arbor, MI

Krieger D 1979 Therapeutic touch: how to use your hands to help or heal. Prentice Hall, Englewood Cliffs, NJ

Kuhn TS 1970 The structure of scientific revolution. University of Chicago Press, Chicago, IL

Kuriyama S 1992 Between mind and eye; Japanese anatomy

in the eighteenth century. In: Leslie C, Young A (eds) Paths to Asian medical knowledge. University of California Press, Berkeley, CA, pp 21–43

Kurosu Y 1969 Experimental study on the pulse diagnosis of *rokujuboi* II. Japanese Acupuncture and Moxibustion Journal 18(3):26–30

Lacayo R 1993 Beyond the Brady Bill. *Time* 20 December:28–32

Lazarou J, Pomeranz BM, Corey PN 1998 Incidence of adverse drug reactions in hospitalized patients. JAMA 279:(15) 1200–1205

Le Bars D, Dickenson AH, Besson JM 1979 Diffuse noxious inhibitory controls (DNIC). I: Effects on dorsal horn convergent neurones in the rat. Pain 6:283–304

Le Bars D, Dickenson AH, Besson JM 1979 Diffuse noxious inhibitory controls (DNIC). II: Lack of effect on non convergent neurones, supraspinal involvement and theoretical implications. Pain 6:305–327

Le Bars D, Willer JC, Broucker T. de, Villanueva L 1989 Neurophysiological mechanisms involved in the pain-relieving effects of counterirritation and related techniques including acupuncture. In: Pomeranz B, Stux G (eds) Scientific bases of acupuncture. Springer Verlag, Berlin,

Lee JK, Bae SK 1978 Acupuncture. Sam Wha, Seoul

Lee MHM, Ernst M 1989 Clinical and research observations on acupuncture analgesia and thermography; In: Pomeranz B, Stux G (eds) Scientific bases of acupuncture. Springer-Verlag, Berlin, pp 157–175

Levine JD, Gordon NC, Fields HL 1978 The mechanism of placebo anesthesia. Lancet ii:654–657

Levinson JM 1974 Traditional medicine in the Democratic Republic of North Vietnam. American Journal of Chinese Medicine 2(2):159–162

Lewith GT 1984 How effective is acupuncture in the management of pain? Journal of the Royal College of General Practitioners 34:275–278

Lewith GT 1993 Every doctor a walking placebo. In: Lewith GT, Aldridge D (eds) Clinical research methodology for complementary therapies. Hodder & Stoughton, London

Lewith GT, Machin D 1983 On the evaluation of the clinical effects of acupuncture. Pain 16:111–127

Lewith G, Vincent C 1996 On the evaluation of the clinical effects of acupuncture: a problem reassessed and a framework for future research. Journal of Alternative and Complementary Medicine 2(1):79–90

Li Y, Tougas G, Chiverton SG, Hunt RH 1992 The effect of acupuncture on gastrointestinal function and disorders. American Journal of Gastroenterology 87(10):1372–1381

Li Ding Zhong 1984 *Jing Luo* phenomena 1. Yukonsha, Tokyo

Li Ding Zhong 1985 *Jing Luo* phenomena 2. Yukonsha, Tokyo

Liao SJ 1992 Acupuncture for low back pain in *Huang Di Nei Jing Su Wen*. Acupuncture and Electro-therapeutics Research International Journal 17:249–258

Liao SJ, Liao MK 1985 Acupuncture and tele-electronic infra red thermography. *Acupuncture and Electro-therapeutics Research International Journal* 10:41–66

Linde K, Worku F, Stor W et al 1996 Randomized clinical trials of acupuncture for asthma: a systematic review. Forschung for Komplementarmed izinische 3:148–155

Lipman RS 1989 Pharmacotherapy of anxiety disorders. In: Fisher S, Greenberg RP (eds) The limits of biological treatments for psychological disorders. Lawrence Erlbaum, Hillsdale, NJ

Liu Bing-quan 1988 Optimum time for acupuncture. Shandong Science and Technology Press, Jinan

Lock MM 1978 Scars of experience; the art of moxibustion in Japanese medicine and society. Culture, Medicine and Psychiatry 2:151–175

Lock MM 1980 East Asian medicine in urban Japan. University of California Press, Berkeley, CA

Lock MM 1980 An examination of the influence of traditional therapeutic systems on the practice of cosmopolitan medicine in Japan. American Journal of Chinese Medicine 8(3):221–229

Lock MM 1980 The organization and practice of East Asian medicine in Japan: continuity and change. Social Science and Medicine 14B:245–253

Lock MM 1985 The impact of the Chinese medical model on Japan or, how the younger brother comes of age. Social Science and Medicine 21(8):945–950

Lu Gwei-Djen, Needham J 1980 Celestial lancets: a history and rationale of acupuncture and moxa. Cambridge University Press, Cambridge

Lynoe N 1990 Is the effect of alternative treatment only a placebo effect? Scandinavian Journal of Social Medicine 18:149–153

Lytle CD 1993 An overview of acupuncture. US Department of Health and Human Services, Public Health Service, Food and Drug Administration, Center for Devices and Radiological Health, Washington DC

Lytle CD 1997 Safety and regulation of acupuncture needles and other devices. Presentation at the Consensus Development on Acupuncture, National Institutes of Health, November 3–5, Bethesda, MD

MacDonald AJR, Macrae KD, Master BR, Rubin AP 1983 Superficial acupuncture in the relief of chronic low back pain. Annals of the Royal Colleges of Surgeons of England 65:44–46

Maciocia G 1989 Foundations of Chinese medicine. Churchill Livingstone, Edinburgh

Manaka Y 1948 Treatment by disease name and treatment by '*sho.*' Ido no Nippon Magazine 7(1):50

Manaka Y 1980 *Ika no Tameno Shinjutsu Nyumon Kuoza*: introductory lectures on acupuncture for medical doctors. Ido no Nippon Sha, Yokosuka

Manaka Y, Itaya K 1994 Acupuncture as intervention in the biological information system: meridian treatment and the X-signal system. Journal of the Acupuncture Society of New York 1(3 & 4): 9–18; 2(1) 15–22

Manaka Y, Itaya K, Birch S 1995 Chasing the dragon's tail. Paradigm Publications, Brookline, MA

Mann F 1972 Acupuncture; the ancient Chinese art of healing and how it works scientifically. Vintage, New York,

Mann F 1974 The treatment of disease by acupuncture. Heinemann, London

Margolin A, Chang P, Avants SK, Kosten TR 1992 Effects of sham and real auricular needling: implications for trials of acupuncture for cocaine addiction. American Journal of Chinese Medicine 21:103–111

Margolin A, Avants SK, Chang P, Kosten TR 1992 Auricular acupuncture for the treatment of cocaine dependence in methadone-maintained patients. The American Journal on Addictions 2(3):194–200

Margolin A, Avants SK, Chang P, Birch S, Kosten TR 1995 A single-blind investigation of four auricular needle puncture configurations. American Journal of Chinese Medicine 23(2):105–114

Margolin A, Avants SK, Birch S 1997 Letter to the editor. Complementary Therapies in Medicine 5:53–54

Margolin A, Avants SK, Birch S, Falk CX, Kleber HD 1997 Methodological investigations for a multisite trial of auricular acupuncture for cocaine addiction. A study of active and control auricular zones. Journal of Substance Abuse Treatment 13(6):471–481

Maruyama M Kudo K 1982 *Shinpan Shiraku Ryoho*: blood-letting therapy. Sekibundo, Tokyo

Matsumoto T 1968 Experimental study on *fukushin* (abdominal palpation). Japanese Acupuncture and Moxibustion Journal 17(3):13–16

Matsumoto H 1994 Acupuncture and moxibustion in Japan. North American Journal of Oriental Medicine 1(2):11–17

Matsumoto K, Birch S 1986 Extraordinary vessels. Paradigm Publications, Brookline, MA

Matsumoto K, Birch S 1988 Hara diagnosis: reflections on the sea. Paradigm Publications, Brookline, MA

Matsunaga T 1983 Socio-cultural transformation of Japanese medical systems. PhD thesis, Western Michigan University, Michigan

McLellan AT, Grossman DS, Blain JD, Haverkos HW 1993 Acupuncture treatment for drug abuse: a technical review. Journal of Substance Abuse Treatment 10:569–576

McQueen DV 1985 China's impact on American medicine in the seventies: a limited and preliminary inquiry. Social Science and Medicine 21(8):931–936

Melzack R, Stillwell DM, Fox EJ 1977 Trigger points and acupoints for pain: correlations and implications. Pain 3:3–23

Mendelson G, Selwood TS, Krantz HK, Loh TS, Kidson MA, Scott DS 1983 Acupuncture treatment of chronic pain: a double blind placebo controlled study. American Journal of Medicine 74:49–55

Mori H, Yoneyama H 1983 *Shonishin ho:* acupuncture for children. Ido no Nippon Sha, Yokokusa

Morohashi T (ed) 1976 *Daikanwa jiten:* Morohashi encyclopedic dictionary of Chinese, 5th edn. Daishukan Sha, Tokyo

Moskowitz G et al 1983 Deficiencies of clinical trials of alcohol withdrawal. Alcoholism: Clinical and Experimental Research 7(1):42–46

Motoyama H 1981 Biophysical elucidation of the meridians and ki energy. What is ki energy and how does it flow? International Association for Religion and Parapsychology 7(1):1–78

Motoyama H 1986 Meridians and ki: measurements, diagnoses and treatment principles with the AMI. International Association for Religion and Parapsychology 16

Mussat M 1972 Physique de l'acupuncture: hypotheses et approches experimentales. Libraire le Francois, Paris

Naeser M 1996 Acupuncture in the treatment of paralysis and stroke. Journal of Alternative and Complementary Medicine 2(1):211–248

Nagatomo T, Nagatomo MP 1976 Shinkyu kuowa hachiju hachisyu: Nagatomo's 88 Lectures on the Minus-Plus Needle Therapy. Shinkyu Shinkuokai Sha, Kyoto

Nakatani Y, Yamashita K 1977 *Ryodoraku* acupuncture. Ryodoraku Research Institute, Tokyo

National Accreditation Commission for Schools and Colleges of Acupuncture and Oriental Medicine 1989 American acupuncture: a historical perspective. Journal of Traditional Acupuncture Spring:12–19

National Commission for the Certification of Acupuncturists 1989 Clean needle technique manual, 3rd edn. National Commission for the Certification of Acupuncturists, Washington DC

National Commission for the Certification of Acupuncturists 1993 State acupuncture laws. National Commission for the Certification of Acupuncturists, Washington, DC

National Council Against Health Fraud 1991 Acupuncture: the position paper of the National Council Against Health Fraud. The Clinical Journal of Pain 7(2):162–166

Needham J 1954 Science and civilisation in China, vol I. Cambridge University Press, Cambridge

Needham J 1956 Science and civilisation in China, vol II. Cambridge University Press, Cambridge

Needham J, Lu G-D 1974 Science and civilisation in China, vol V, part 2. Cambridge University Press, Cambridge

Needham J, Lu G-D 1975 Problems of translation and modernisation of ancient Chinese technical terms. Annals of Science 32:491–502

Ng LKY 1996 Effect of auricular acupuncture in animals. Journal of Alternative and Complementary Medicine 2(1):61–63

Nogier PFM 1983 From auriculotherapy to auriculomedicine. Maisonneuve, Saint-Ruffine

Norbeck E, Lock M (eds) 1987 Health, illness and medical care in Japan. University of Hawaii Press, Honolulu

Norheim AJ, Fonnebo V 1995 Letter to the editor (adverse effects of acupuncture). Lancet 345:1575

Norheim AJ, Fonnebo V 1996 Acupuncture adverse effects are more than occasional case reports: results from questionnaires among 1135 randomly selected doctors, and 197 acupuncturists. Complementary Therapies in Medicine 4:8–13

O'Connor J, Bensky D 1981 Acupuncture: a comprehensive text. Eastland Press, Seattle, WA

Oda H 1989 *Ryodoraku* textbook. Naniwasha, Osaka

Ohnuki-Tierney E 1984 Illness and culture in contemporary Japan. Cambridge University Press, Cambridge

Omura Y 1974 Effects of acupuncture on blood pressure, leukocytes and serum lipids and lipoproteins in essential hypertension. Federal Proceedings [Physiology 1242] 33:430

Omura Y 1975 Some historical aspects of acupuncture and important problems to be considered in acupuncture and electro-therapeutic research. Acupuncture and Electrotherapeutics Research International Journal 1:3–44

Omura Y 1979 The effects of acupuncture on the cardiovascular and nervous systems, including the release of ACTH and endorphins. British Journal of Acupuncture 2(1):17–19

Omura Y 1986 Practice of "bi-digital O-ring test". Ido no Nippon Sha, Yokosuka

O'Neill A 1994 Enemies within and without. La Trobe University Press, Bundoora, Victoria

Oschman JL 1994 A biophysical basis for acupuncture. In: Proceedings of the First Symposium of the Society for Acupuncture Research. Society for Acupuncture Research, Bethesda, MD

Paldan D (trans), M. Lee M (rev) 1991 Tung's acupuncture by Dr Ching-Chang Tung. Blue Poppy Press, Boulder, CO

Parfitt A 1994 Placebo treatments. In: *Proceedings of the First Symposium of the Society for Acupuncture Research.* Society for Acupuncture Research, Bethesda, MD

Parfitt A 1996 Acupuncture as an antiemetic treatment. Journal of Alternative and Complementary Medicine 2(1):167–174

Patel MS 1987 Problems in the evaluation of alternative medicine. Social Science and Medicine 25(6):669–678

Patel M, Gutzwiller F, Paccaud F, Marazzi A 1989 A meta-analysis of acupuncture for chronic pain. International Journal of Epidemiology 18(4):900–906

Pomeranz B 1989 Research into acupuncture and homeopathy. In: Energy fields and medicine: a study of device technology based on acupuncture meridians and chi energy. John E Fetzer Foundation, Kalamazoo, pp 66–77

Pomeranz B 1991 Scientific basis of acupuncture. In: Stux G, Pomeranz B (eds) Basics of acupuncture. Springer-Verlag, Berlin pp 4–55

Pomeranz B 1993 Change in the medical science of acupuncture. In: Abstracts of the Third World Conference on Acupuncture. World Federation of Acupuncture and Moxibustion Societies, Kyoto

Pomeranz B 1996 Scientific research into acupuncture for the relief of pain. Journal of Alternative and Complementary Medicine 2(1):53–60

Pomeranz B, Stux G (eds) 1989 Scientific bases of acupuncture. Springer-Verlag, Berlin

Porkert M 1974 The theoretical foundations of Chinese medicine. MIT Press, Cambridge

Prance SE, Dresser A, Wood C, Fleming J, Aldridge D, Pietroni PC 1988 Research on traditional Chinese acupuncture science or myth: a review. Journal of the Royal Society of Medicine 81:588–590

Praznikov VP 1993 The role of acupuncture in modern medicine. In: Abstracts of the Third World Conference on Acupuncture. World Federation of Acupuncture and Moxibustion Societies, Kyoto

Qian Cun-ze 1981 Simulated human body information in bio-medical therapy: experimental investigation in human body field (II). Shanghai Jiao Tong University, Shanghai

Raccah D, Petti F, Liguori A 1993 A survey on the diffusion of acupuncture in Italy. In: Abstracts of the Third World Conference on Acupuncture. World Federation of Acupuncture and Moxibustion Societies, Kyoto

Rasmussen NK, Morgall JM 1990 The use of alternative treatment in the Danish adult population. Complementary Medicine Research 4(2):16–22

Ratcliffe JW 1983 Notions of validity in qualitative research methodology. Knowledge, Creation, Diffusion, Utilization 5(2):147–167

Reed JC 1996 Review of acute and chronic pain published studies. Journal of Alternative and Complementary Medicine 2(1):129–144

Requena Y 1986 Terrains and pathology in acupuncture. Paradigm Publications, Brookline, MA

Richardson PH, Vincent CA 1986 Acupuncture for the treatment of pain: a review of evaluative research. Pain 24:15–40

Rosenthal MM 1987 Health care in the People's Republic of China: moving toward modernization. Westview Press, Boulder, CO

Rosted P 1996 Literature survey of reported adverse effects associated with acupuncture treatment. American Journal of Acupuncture 24(1):27–34

Rozman P 1993: Integration of acupuncture into Western health system: the role of national acupuncture association's strategy. In: Abstracts of the Third World Conference on Acupuncture. World Federation of Acupuncture and Moxibustion Societies, Kyoto

Rudenko M, Kabaruchin B 1993 The system of education in traditional Chinese medicine in Russia. In: Abstracts of the Third World Conference on Acupuncture. World Federation of Acupuncture and Moxibustion Societies, Kyoto

Rughini S, Marino F, Bangrazi A 1993 The demand for acupuncture in the treatment of painful syndromes: a survey carried out in Italy. In: Abstracts of the Third World Conference on Acupuncture. World Federation of Acupuncture and Moxibustion Societies, Kyoto

Sacks HS, Berrier J, Reitman D, Pagano D, Chalmers TC 1992 Meta-analyses of randomized controlled trials. In: Bailar JC, Mosteller F (eds) Medical uses of statistics. NEJM Books, Boston, MA

Schimmel HW The segment electrogram. Vega, Grieshaber KG, Postfach 10, D-7622, Schiltock, Schwarzwald

Schwartz SA, DeMattei RJ, Brame EG, Spottiswoode SJP 1990 Infrared spectra alteration in water proximate to the palms of therapeutic practitioners. Subtle Energies 1(1):43–72

Sermeus G 1990 Alternative health care in Belgium: an explanation of various social aspects. Complementary Medicine Research 4(2):9–13

Seto A, Kusaka C, Nakazato W, Huang T, Seto T, Hisamitsu T, Takeshige C 1992 Detection of extraordinary large biomagnetic field strength from human body during external qi emission. Acupuncture and Electro-Therapeutics Research International Journal 17:75–94

Shanghai College of Traditional Chinese Medicine n.d. *Zhen Jiu Zhi Liao Xue*. Shao Hua Cultural Service, Hong Kong

Shcheglov VS, Teppone MV n.d. Method of determining therapeutic frequency when carrying out microwave therapy with the use of temperature sensors

Sheldrake R 1981 A new science of life: the hypothesis of causative formation. JP Tarcher, Los Angeles, CA

Shi Dian-bang 1991 Development and prospect of traditional Chinese medicine at the contemporary era. In: International Congress on Traditional Medicine. State Administration of Traditional Chinese Medicine, Beijing

Shichido T 1996 Clinical evaluation of acupuncture and moxibustion (32). Clinical tests of acupuncture in Japan. Ido no Nippon Magazine 623(8,7):94–102

Shifrin K 1993 Setting standards for acupuncture training: a model for complementary medicine. Complementary Therapies in Medicine 1(2):91–95

Shiroda Bunshi 1986 *Shinkyu Chiryo Kisogaku*, 6th edn. Ido no Nippon Sha, Yokokusa

Shlay JC, Chalmers K, Max MB, Flaws B, Reichelderfer P, Wentworth D, Hillman S, Brizz B, Cohn DL 1998 Acupuncture and amitriptyline for pain due to HIV-related peripheral neuropathy. A randomized controlled trial. JAMA 280(18):1590–1595.

Shudo D 1989 *Shinkyu Chiryo Shitsu*, 2nd edn. Ido no Nippon Sha, Yokosuka, p 215

Shudo D 1990 Japanese classical acupuncture: introduction to meridian therapy. Eastland Press, Seattle, WA

Sivin N 1987 Traditional medicine in contemporary China. Center for Chinese Studies, University of Michigan, Ann Arbor, MI

Skrabanek P 1989 Acupuncture: past, present, and future. In: Stalker, Glymour (eds) Examining holistic medicine. Promethers Books, NY, pp 181–196

Smith MO 1988 Acupuncture treatment for crack: clinical survey of 1500 patients treated. American Journal of Acupuncture 16(3):241–247

So JTY 1985 Book of acupuncture points. Paradigm Publications, Brookline, MA

So JTY 1987 *Treatment of disease with acupuncture*. Paradigm Publications, Brookline, MA

Sodipo JA 1979 Acupuncture and gastric acid studies. American Journal of Chinese Medicine 7(4):356–361

Song Jang-Heon 1985 The role of Korean oriental medicine. Korean Oriental Medical Association, Seoul

Sonoda K 1988 Health and illness in changing Japanese society. University of Tokyo Press, Tokyo

Soulie de Morant G 1994 Chinese acupuncture. Paradigm Publications, Brookline, MA

Stedman TL 1982 Stedman's medical dictionary, 24th edn. Williams & Wilkins, Baltimore, OH

Stephenson D 1990 Acupuncture in Australia: past, present, future. Complementary Medical Research 4(1):18–20

Stux G, Pomeranz B 1991 Basics of acupuncture. Springer-Verlag, Berlin

Sun KL, Li YL, Liu H, Yan QL, Sun PS 1987 The experimental study on the conduction of quantitative acoustic frequency signals along the large intestine channel of hand *yangming*. In: Selection from article abstracts on acupuncture and moxibustion. China Association of Acupuncture and Moxibustion, Beijing, pp 341–343

Sun PS, Zhao YZ, Li YL, Yan QL, Liu H 1987 The study of acoustic information along channels. In: Selections from article abstracts on acupuncture and moxibustion. China Association of Acupuncture and Moxibustion, Beijing, pp 334–336

Sun PS, Li YL, Yan QL 1987 Analysis on the forming factors and the changing regulations of the background sound in measuring the sound information along the meridian. In: Selections from article abstracts on acupuncture and moxibustion. China Association of Acupuncture and Moxibustion, Beijing, pp 336–337

Sun PS, Zhao YZ, Li YL, Yan QL, Liu H 1987 The spectrum analysis of the propagation of sound information along meridians. In: Selections from article abstracts on acupuncture and moxibustion. China Association of Acupuncture and Moxibustion, Beijing, pp 337–338

Sun PS, Zhao YZ, Tian QN, Zhu FS, Wang DS 1987 Contrast observation between sound information along meridians and muscular electricity. In: Selections from article abstracts on acupuncture and moxibustion. China Association of Acupuncture and Moxibustion, Beijing, pp 340–341

Suzuki H 1989 *Shinkyu Chiryo Shitsu*, 2nd edn. Ido no Nippon Sha, Yokosuka, pp 168–169

Takeshige C 1989 Mechanism of acupuncture analgesia based on animal experiments. In: Pomeranz B, Stux G (eds) Scientific bases of acupuncture. Springer-Verlag, Berlin, pp 53–78

Temple R (eds) 1989 Government viewpoint of clinical trials of cardiovascular drugs. Medical Clinics of North America 73(2):495–509

Ter Reit G, Kleijnen J, Knipschild P 1990 A meta-analysis of studies into the effect of acupuncture on addiction. British Journal of General Practice 40:379–382

Ter Reit G, Kleijnen J, Knipschild P 1990 Acupuncture and chronic pain: a criteria-based meta-analysis. Journal of Clinical Epidemiology 43(11):1191–1199

Thomas KJ Carr J, Westlake L et al 1991 Use of non-orthodox and conventional health care in Great Britain. British Medical Journal 302:207–210

Tian Conghuo, Wang Yin 1987 Clinical and experimental research on the antipyretic effects of moxibustion. In: Selections from article abstracts on acupuncture and moxibustion. China Association of Acupuncture and Moxibustion, Beijing, pp 221–222

Tiller WA 1987 What do electrodermal diagnostic acupuncture instruments really measure? American Journal of Acupuncture 15(1):15–23

Tiller WA 1989 On the evolution and future development of electrodermal diagnostic instruments. In: Energy fields in medicine: a study of device technology based on acupuncture meridians and chi energy. John E Fetzer Foundation, Kalamazoo, pp 257–328

Toda K, Iriki A, Tanaka H 1980 Electroacupuncture supresses the cortical evoked responses in somatosensory I and II areas after tooth pulp stimulation in rat. Japanese Journal of Physiology 30:487–490

Toda K, Suda H, Ichioka M, Iriki A 1980 Local electrical stimulation: effective needling points for suppressing jaw opening reflex in rat. Pain 9:199–207

Todd SA 1994 Acupuncture: individual differences and response factors. In: Proceedings of the First Symposium of the Society for Acupuncture Research. Society for Acupuncture Research. Bethesda, MD

Toyohari Association 1998 *Kaiin Meibo*, Association membership, 1990. Toyohari Association, Tokyo

Tsutani K 1993 The evaluation of herbal medicines: an East Asian perspective. In: Lewith GT, Aldridge D (eds) Clinical research methodology for complementary therapies. Hodder & Stoughton, London

Tsutani K, Namiki T, Muramatsu S 1993 List of serials in the field of 'Toyo-Igaku' indexed in JMEDICINE. Nihon ToyoIgaku Zashi 43(4):63–67

Tsutani K, Shichido T, Sakuma K 1990 When acupuncture met biostatistics. Paper presented at the Second World Conference of Acupuncture and Moxibustion, Paris

Turk DC, Melzack R 1992 The measurement of pain and the assessment of people experiencing pain. In: Turk DC, Melzack R (eds) Handbook of pain assessment. Guilford Press, New York

Uddin J 1993 Acupuncture: Europe and the law. European Journal of Oriental Medicine 1(1):53–55

Ulett GA 1982 Principles and practice of physiologic acupuncture. WH Green, St Louis, MI

Ulett GA 1992 Beyond yin and yang. WH Green, St Louis, MI

Unschuld PU 1979 *Medical ethics in imperial China*. University of California Press, Berkeley. CA

Unschuld PU 1985 Medicine in China: a history of ideas. University of California Press, Berkeley, CA

Unschuld PU 1986 Medicine in China: a history of pharmaceutics. University of California Press, Berkeley, CA

Unschuld PU 1986 Medicine in China: *Nan Ching*: the classic of difficult issues. University of California Press, Berkeley, CA

Unschuld PU 1987 Traditional Chinese medicine; some historical and epistemological reflections. Social Science and Medicine 24(12):1023–1029

Unschuld PU (ed) 1989 Approaches to traditional Chinese medical literature. Kluwer, Dordrecht

Unschuld PU 1990 Forgotten traditions of ancient Chinese medicine. Paradigm Publications, Brookline, MA

Unschuld PU 1992 Epistemological issues and changing legitimation: traditional Chinese medicine in the twentieth century. In: Leslie C, Young A (eds) Paths to Asian medical knowledge. University of California Press, Berkeley, CA

Unschuld PU 1995 The reception of Oriental medicine in the West. Lecture given in Kobe, Japan, May

Unschuld PU Plausibility or truth. Unpublished manuscript

Vernejoul P, Albatede P, Darras JC 1992 Nuclear medicine and acupuncture message transmission. Journal of Nuclear Medicine 33(3):409–412

Vickers AJ 1996 Can acupuncture have specific effects on health? A systematic review of acupuncture antiemesis trials. Journal of the Royal Society of Medicine 89:303–311

Vickers AJ 1996 Research paradigms in mainstream and complementary medicine. In: Ernst E (ed) Complementary medicine: an objective appraisal. Butterworth, Oxford, pp 3–17

Vincent CA 1990 Credibility assessment in trials of acupuncture. Complementary Medical Research 4(1):8–11

Vincent CA 1993 Acupuncture as a treatment for chronic pain. In: Lewith GT, Aldridge D (eds) Clinical research methodology for complementary therapies. Hodder & Stoughton, London, pp 289–308

Vincent CA, Richardson PH 1986 The evaluation of therapeutic acupuncture: concepts and methods. Pain 24:1–13

Vincent CA, Richardson PH 1987 Acupuncture for some common disorders: a review of evaluative research. Journal of the Royal College of Practitioners 37:77–81

Vincent C, Tsutani K 1993 Can acupuncture survive into the 21st century? Report of the WFAS Third World Conference on Acupuncture, Kyoto. In press

Vincent CA, Richardson PH, Black JJ, Pither CE 1989 The significance of needle placement site in acupuncture. Journal of Psychosomatic Research 33(4):489–496

Volkov MV, Oganesyan OV 1987 External fixation: joint deformities and bone fractures. International Universities Press, Madison, CT

Voll R 1975 Twenty years of electroacupuncture diagnosis in Germany: a progress report. American Journal of Acupuncture 3:7–17

Wang Fengyi, Ren Huan Zhao (Kaname Asakawa, trans) 1985 *Kyugyoku Ryoho*, cupping therapy. Toyo Gakujutsu, Ichikawa City

Wang KM, Yao S, Xian Y, Hou Z 1985 A study on the receptive field of acupoint and the relationship between characteristics of needling sensation and groups of afferent fibres. Scientica Sinica *(Series B)* 28(9):963–971

Wang PS, Ma YR, Zhao Y 1987 The experimental observation on sound information of propagated sensations along channels (PSC). Selection from article abstracts on acupuncture and moxibustion. China Association of Acupuncture and Moxibustion, Beijing, pp 344–345

Wang Wei-yi 1976 *Tong Ren Shu Xue Zhen Jiu Tu Jing* [1027]. Wu Zhou, Taipei

Wang Yin, Tian Conghuo, Li Zhiming 1987 Preliminary observation on the treatment of fever due to the invasion of exogenous pathogenic wind cold with warm moxibustion. In: Selections from article abstracts on acupuncture and moxibustion. China Association of Acupuncture and Moxibustion, Beijing, pp 220–221

Wang Shu-Chuan 1980 *Zhen Jiu Ji Sheng Jing* [1220] In: *Zhen Jiu Ji Sheng Jing; Shi Si Jing Fa Hui.* Xuan Feng, Taipei

Wen HL 1979 Acupuncture and electrical stimulation (AES) outpatient detoxification. Modern Medicine in Asia 15:23–24

Wen HL, Cheung SYC 1973 Treatment of drug addiction by acupuncture and electrical stimulation. Asian Journal of Medicine 9:138–141

Wetzel MS, Eisenberg DM, Kaptchuk TJ 1998 Courses involving complementary and alternative medicine at US medical schools. JAMA 280(9):784–787

White A 1996 Economic evaluation of acupuncture. Acupuncture in Medicine 14(2):109–113

White AR, Abbot NC, Barnes J, Ernst E 1996 Self-reports of adverse effects of acupuncture included cardiac arrhythmia. Acupuncture in Medicine 14(2):121

White AR, Eddleston C, Hardie R, Resch KL, Ernst E 1996 A pilot study of acupuncture for tension headache using a novel placebo. Acupuncture in Medicine 14(1):11–15

Wickramasekera I 1985 A conditioned response model of the placebo effect. In: White, Tursky Schwartz GE (eds) Placebo theory, research and mechanism. Guilford Press, New York

Wiseman N 1995 A Chinese–English English–Chinese dictionary of Chinese medicine. Hunan Science and Technology Press, Hunan

Wiseman N 1997 A practical dictionary of traditional Chinese medicine, database edn. Paradigm Publications, Brookline, MA

Wiseman N 1998 Rationale for the terminology of the fundamentals of Chinese Medicine, Paradigm, Brookline MA, p 11

Wiseman N, Boss K 1990 Glossary of Chinese medical terms and acupuncture points. Paradigm Publications, Brookline, MA

Wiseman N, Ellis A 1985 Fundamentals of Chinese medicine Paradigm Publications, Brookline, MA

Wiseman N, Ellis A 1991 Fundamentals of Chinese medicine, rev edn. Paradigm Publications, Brookline, MA

Wolpe PR 1985 The maintenance of professional authority: acupuncture and the American physician. Social Problems 32(5):409–424

Wong KC, Wu LT 1985 History of Chinese medicine, 2nd edn. Southern Materials, Taipei

World Health Organization 1980 Use of acupuncture in modern health care. WHO Chronicle 34:294–301

World Health Organization 1985 The role of traditional medicine in primary health care. WHO, Geneva, WPR/RC36/ Technical Discussions

World Health Organization 1991 A proposed standard international acupuncture nomenclature; report of a WHO scientific group. WHO, Geneva

World Health Organization 1993 Standard acupuncture nomenclature, 2nd edn. Regional Office for the Western Pacific, WHO, Manila,

Worsley JR 1973 Is acupuncture for you? College of Traditional Chinese Acupuncture, Leamington Spa

Xie Zhu-fan 1988 Researches on 'cold' and 'heat' in traditional Chinese medicine. Chinese Journal of Integrated Medicine 8(special issue 2):93–96

Xue Xing-lu (chief ed) 1991 The international Chinese Medicine Union book catalogue. Chinese Medical Ancient Books, Beijing

Yanagiya S 1948 *Shinkyu Ijutsu no Mon:* an introduction to the medical arts of acupuncture and moxibustion. Ido no Nippon sha, Yokosuka

Yanagiya S 1948 The future of acupuncture. Ido no Nippon Magazine 7(1):50

Yanagiya S 1952 The real value of acupuncture and moxibustion. Ido no Nippon Magazine 11(2):99

Yang Ji-zhou 1982 *Zhen jiu da cheng* [1601] Da Zhong Guo Tu Shu, Taipei

Yoo TW 1988 *Koryo sooji chim: koryo* hand acupuncture, vol 1. Eum Yang Mek Jin, Seoul

Zaslawski C, Rogers C, Garvey M, Yang CX, Zhang SP 1997 Strategies to maintain the credibility of sham acupuncture as a control treatment in clinical trials. Journal of Alternative and Complementary Medicine 3(3):257–266

Zen nippon shinkyu gakkai 1982 *Hari, kyu ni kansuru gakkai, kenkyukai ichiran.* List of acupuncture and moxibustion associations and study groups. Zen Nippon Shinkyu Gakkai, Tokyo

Zhang Xin Shu 1979 *Wan ke zhen:* wrist, ankle acupuncture (trans Matsutane Sugi). Ido no Nippon sha, Yokokusa

Zhao YZ, Sun PS, Li YL, Yan QL, Liu H 1987 Study on the relations between the production of the sound information along meridian and the exciting pressures. In: Selections from article abstracts on acupuncture and moxibustion China Association of Acupuncture and Moxibustion, Beijing, pp 339–340

Zhu Baoxia 1993 State gets tough with TCM tests. *China Daily*, 1 March

Zhu FS, Peng JS, Wang PS, Wan YG 1987 Transfer of sound signals along acupuncture meridians: an experimental study. In: Selections from article abstracts on acupuncture and moxibustion. China Association of Acupuncture and Moxibustion, Beijing, p 349

Zhu ZX 1981 Research advances in the electrical specificity of meridians and acupuncture points. American Journal of Acupuncture 9(3):203–216

Zhukovsky VD n.d. Microwave resonance therapy (MRT) a new principle of disturbed organism function restoration.

Zimmerman J 1990 Laying-on-of-hands and therapeutic touch: a testable theory. Newsletter of the Bio-Electro-Magnetics Institute 2(1):8–17

Zmiewski P, Feit R 1990 Acumoxa therapy; reference and study guide. Paradigm Publications, Brookline, MA

Index